PALMER CHIROPRACTIC GREEN BOOKS

The Definitive Guide

THE INSTITUTE CHIROPRACTIC

THE INSTITUTE CHIROPRACTIC is dedicated to the publication of important books and media, which shed new light on topics such as chiropractic history and philosophy, spirituality, enlightenment, philosophy, integral theory, and subtle energies. The Chiropractic Series is designed to bring forth important works from the history and philosophy of chiropractic, publish original new works, and inspire dialogue. Membership in The Institute Chiropractic is open to chiropractors and chiropractic students. Membership includes extensive on-line learning, scholarly discussion, and professional connections with the leading chiropractors around the world, those dedicated to acknowledging the profession's history, fostering a discipline of philosophy in the profession, and leading chiropractic into the future.

MORE TITLES FROM THE INSTITUTE CHIROPRACTIC

THE CHIROPRACTOR'S PROTÉGÉ
The Untold Story of Oakley G. Smith's Journey with D.D. Palmer (2017)
Timothy J. Faulkner

THE COMPLETE CHIROPRACTOR
R. J. Watkins, DC, PhC, FICC, DACBR (2017)
Stevan Walton

EARLY HISTORY OF CHIROPRACTIC
The Palmer's and Australia (2014)
Rolf Peters

THE SECRET HISTORY OF CHIROPRACTIC
D.D. Palmer's Spiritual Writings: Second Edition (2014)
Simon Senzon

THE CHIROPRACTIC CHART
Ralph W. Stephenson (2017)

PALMER CHIROPRACTIC GREEN BOOKS

The Definitive Guide

by
TIMOTHY J. FAULKNER
JOSEPH FOLEY
SIMON SENZON

THE
INSTITUTE
CHIROPRACTIC

Asheville, N.C.

Second Edition 2025

Published in the United States by The Institute Chiropractic
218 E. Chestnut St. Asheville, N.C. 28801

Timothy J. Faulkner, b. 1966.
Joseph Foley, b. 1966.
Simon Senzon, b. 1971.
Palmer Chiropractic Green Books: The Definitive Guide.
Volume 16 of The Institute Chiropractic Books.

Includes bibliographical references.
"Palmer Chiropractic Green Books: The Definitive Guide is the first book to describe every chiropractic Green Book. It includes a master list of all Green Books, information for collectors, and a historical, theoretical, and philosophical overview of the books." -Provided by publisher.

ISBN 978-8-9922397-2-0

For current information about all releases from The Institute Chiropractic, visit the web site at http://www.institutechiro.com

Dedicated to the Green Book authors,
their students, and their readers.

Acknowledgments

Thank you to all who made this book possible. We would like to especially thank our families and our wives, without whom this book could not have happened. Also, to our children, for their loving patience and inspiration.

Editorial thanks go to Barbara Homziuk, Stevan Walton, DC, and Dave Russell, DC, Eric Springer, DC, Scott Jackson, DC, and Tyler Evans, DC.

Also thanks to Roger Hynes, DC and Donald McDowall, DC.

Special thanks goes to Caroline Webb, MA, MLIS, of the Texas Chiropractic College Library for her assistance in locating the photo of D.D. Palmer and Alva Gregory.

For assistance with procuring and scanning many of the images a special thank you goes to Rosemary Riess, MLIS, Missy Wright, MA, and the Palmer College of Chiropractic Archives.

Many images were published courtesy of Special Collections and Archives, Palmer College of Chiropractic. The pages containing images from the Palmer Archives are listed in the references.

Contents

PALMER CHIROPRACTIC GREEN BOOKS

Foreword

I have known two of the authors, Faulkner and Foley, since the early days of the Internet in the 1990s. I have known Senzon for the past few years. My expertise as a collector of Green Books as well as a scholar of chiropractic's early theories gives me a unique perspective on this book. Senzon's analysis of the forty-four Green Books as described in Chapters Two through Fifteen is outstanding. As to Senzon's overview, I recommend you take the time to study it carefully, read the references, and then study it again. It is the best introduction to the Green Books ever written. I would however like to provide more context for the important the work of Faulkner and Foley.

The authors, chiropractors Dr. Joe Foley and Dr. Tim Faulkner were computer savvy, Internet addicts as well as chiropractic literature scavenging devotees who competed with me for some of the rare documents, books and memorabilia listed on the used bookstore networks and the Ebay auction website.

In those early days there were few sources for acquiring chiropractic literature and memorabilia outside of being gifted with a retiree chiropractor's collection or purchasing an estate collection from advertisements. Many retired chiropractors simply packaged their collections and sent them to their Alma Mater for the library archives. Some padded their retirement funds and sold them to the highest or quickest Internet bidder. Much rare historical literature was destroyed when chiropractors passed away.

These old books and relics of the early chiropractors became treasures for a few collectors like Foley, Faulkner and myself. However, the disadvantage I had in this competition to find chiropractic treasures, was where I lived. Canberra, Australia was a long way from where most chiropractors lived in the heartland of chiropractic, the good old USA. The other problem I had was the 14-hour time difference between Australia and the USA.

Sometimes we would bid against each other over a book listing. Dr. Foley and I met battling each other on Ebay.com for a leather-bound edition of D.D. Palmer's great 1910/11 tomes. Dr. Foley won that battle. However, I was able to win the 1904-1906 leather bound editions of *The Chiropractor* journal from the same collection. That was an interesting experience because the dealer only listed the first of the three volumes. When I won it, I telephoned the dealer and asked if she had any other items from the same collection that she had not yet listed for sale. She said there were two others and asked if I would like to purchase them as a group without them being listed on Ebay.com. Of course I said yes and was able to score the whole collection. I eventually found out they were a set of only six that B.J. Palmer ever bound and sold. As books they predated *Modernized Chiropractic* published in 1906 by Smith and Langworthy and *The Science of Chiropractic* by D.D. and B.J. Palmer, also in 1906.

Collectors are often criticized for hoarding without sharing their knowledge. This publication is a testament to both authors for giving of their knowledge of this very specialized collector's niche. I have followed their research and papers published in the *Association for the History of Chiropractic Journal* with great interest, enjoying their adventures as they uncover the most unusual history of the chiropractic profession.

This book focuses on identifying, grading and rating the Palmer Green Books published by the Palmer School and College of Chiropractic. The books were written from 1906 to 1961 and are generally identified by their green cloth covers. These books are important to chiropractors because they describe the history and challenges of the profession. Some describe the arguments and contentions that arose and were resolved or continued by the Palmers, others are texts that have gone through multiple prints and occasional additional editions.

Knowing what books to look for and how to identify these original books from modern reprints is essential to gauge a reasonable price. The authors show you how to identify the characteristics of the original books and assess their condition. Some of these books may appear new and others will be so well used they are covered in notes, handed down to many generations of students until the covers fall off and the pages fragmenting.

Over time some books became very hard to find. In fact, only 15 copies of D.D. Palmer's original 1910 book are known to exist. There may be even less copies of his 1914 book. The variations in prices of these books are well described for the beginning collector.

The book describes how to begin your collection and how to expand it. The Introduction describes Foley and Faulkner's journey as collectors. Many of the documents and books are housed at the special collections section of the Palmer University Library, the mecca for chiropractors, where they can visit and see complete sets of the various editions of these famous books. This library also contains many original publications from before the beginning of the profession that may inspire you to broaden your collection. The book also includes an extensive collection of photographs of the books to best illustrate the variety of collections possible to achieve.

Why go to this much trouble to collect the history of this unique profession? For many it will be a family heritage in the chiropractic profession, for others it will be the knowledge found in the books that may soon be lost as the profession transitions into a back pain care model. Many chiropractic schools worldwide are not teaching today's students their chiropractic history, philosophy and some of its science. Today's students may never know the unique features of their profession without having this founding education recorded by the Palmers.

Chiropractic began in a healing culture that included homeopathy (eclectics), naturopathy, medical gymnastics (pilates), pharmaceuticals, orthopedics and surgery, and still people suffered chronic conditions with no hope for further help. D.D. Palmer found that adjusting the spine rebooted the human nervous system to reset and restore tissues, organs and structures where other methods had failed. With so few copies of these early books available many chiropractors may need to refocus their current practice using the information in this book.

D.D. Palmer was a genius and defended the profession he founded in his 1910 thesis much to the dislike of those who misunderstood or misused his work. B.J. Palmer carried the flame and continued to defend his father's work until 1961. He added new methods of analysis and adjustment as described in these books. Today's chiropractors risk having a profession by name only without knowing its foundations as recorded by its founders. Drs. Faulkner, Foley, and Senzon have narrowed that gap with this work. I encourage every chiropractor to study this book and reclaim their heritage by developing their own collection of chiropractic history.

Donald McDowall
DC (PCC), DNBCE, DIBAK, MAppSc.
Canberra, Australia

Introduction

The Green Books embody the chiropractic profession's fundamental elements. The first of the books were written by D.D. Palmer, the founder of chiropractic, and his son B.J. Palmer, often referred to as the developer of chiropractic. The entire series includes more than 40 books published between 1906 and 1966. Most of the books were written by B.J. and over a dozen were written by faculty of the Palmer School of Chiropractic (PSC) as teaching texts. The books themselves cover the original chiropractic paradigm, various topics viewed from the chiropractic perspective, the development of theory and ideas from the first chiropractic school, as well as a unique historical account of chiropractic events, scientific research, and the evolution of clinical methodologies over the profession's first 60 years.

Few material items in the chiropractic profession stir up more passion and emotion than the Palmer Green Books. Some consider the books as the "alpha and omega" of the profession, with the very essence of chiropractic written within their pages. Others in the profession would like to see the Green Books burned and the Palmer ideas abandoned.

For the chiropractor who chooses to practice chiropractic as it was originally developed, the Green Books are akin to sacred texts. The Green Books are original source material containing the words of the founder and the developer. For many in the profession the Green Books define what chiropractic is and what chiropractic is not. Answers to countless questions may be found within the more than 20,000 written pages. For those looking to learn about the science, art, and philosophy of chiropractic, there is but one source, the Palmer Green Books.

The Definitive Guide was written as a comprehensive introduction to the Green Books. We hope it will appeal to anyone interested in the history, philosophy, science, or art of chiropractic. It could be read by chiropractic patients and practice members to better understand the foundations of chiropractic theory. It might also be read by historians, scholars, and health care providers interested in chiropractic. Specifically, we wrote *Palmer Chiropractic Green Books: The Definitive Guide* for practicing chiropractors, Green Book collectors, and the chiropractors of the future.

The Overview

Few chiropractors have read any Green Books. Of those few, an even smaller number have read more than two or three of the books. The most commonly read Green Books are probably D.D. Palmer's two books, B.J. Palmer's *Subluxation Specific Adjustment Specific* and his *Bigness of the Fellow Within*, and Ralph Stephenson's *Chiropractic Textbook*. Of the D.D. Palmer books it seems common for most readers to skim or selectively read passages, especially of his 1910 book, which takes a commitment to read from cover to cover. For these reasons we decided to create not only an introduction to every Green Book for beginners and collectors alike but an overview of the books. By discussing how the books developed, why they were written, and the central theories in each book, it is our hope that *The Definitive Guide* will become a resource for generations of chiropractors.

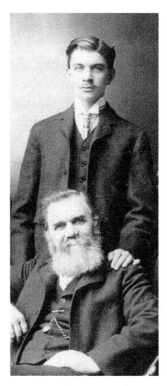

D.D. Palmer & B.J. Palmer, 1902

The first fifteen chapters are about the content of the books. Most chapters cover at least two books. Some chapters include up to eight books. Chapter One was written as a collaboration by all three authors: Faulkner, Foley, and Senzon. It provides a historical context for the books, how the chiropractic paradigm emerged, what the first teaching methods were like, and also some early conflicts in the profession, including the clash between D.D. Palmer and B.J. Palmer. The chapter also covers the legal pressures on the young profession and the emergence of the Chiropractic Book Series.

Chapters Two through Thirteen were written by Senzon, with historical and editorial insights from Faulkner and Foley. These chapters were developed to provide the modern reader with an accurate understanding of what is in Volumes 1-39 with an emphasis on the philosophical and theoretical developments. The goal was to provide an overview not a critique. So, we've glossed over things like typographical or other perceived errors. Our plan was to share what the books are about. Future works might take a more critical stance and examine the many theories against current insights from philosophy and science. However, some of the chapters do offer limited critiques, contexts, and philosophical perspectives. This was necessary in order to demonstrate the relevance of the texts for today's chiropractor.

Since the focus of the book is the Green Books themselves, we chose to highlight any mention of the Green Books in advertisements, and reference within the books to the other volumes. We also highlighted quotes about the writing process and the development of the series.

Overall, the use of quotes is designed to assist the reader to understand the writing styles and learn important concepts from the authors themselves. We included many extended quotes so that the reader might develop a feel for the writings and to make sure the quotes are viewed in context. In that regard, in Vol. 38, B.J. Palmer writes:

> It is unfair and unjust to any author for any reader to take any section or sentence out of pretext, text, or context, and misinterpret the author's overall premises of his book, in the light of what ONE SENTENCE might imply. Any book must be studied in its ENTIRETY and OVER-ALL elucidation of problems it solves.

In a few instances, we abridged quotes with "..." to jump from one statement to another. This was done purely for aesthetics. Keeping such full quotes would have required unnecessary explanations in order to add the proper context. Readers may go to the original in such instances and read the complete text.

Unfortunately, the improper use of quotes is common in the chiropractic literature, often leading to misunderstandings about the history of ideas in chiropractic. This is another reason why a thorough study of the Green Books is essential so that the development of ideas in chiropractic might be more fully understood.

Also, please note that some of the language and writing style in the Green Books is unique. For example, D.D. and B.J. Palmer used shortened words, like "thot" replacing "thought." This was a linguistic style from the early twentieth century. Additionally, both D.D. and B.J. Palmer had their own way with words. By providing extended quotes, we hope the reader might come to understand the complexity of the ideas and also develop an appreciation for the texts in a new way. Becoming acquainted with the unorthodox writing styles of the Palmers will better prepare readers for a more thorough reading of the Green Books.

In addition to the emphasis on theory and the books themselves, we highlighted writings about the history and research. This focus of *The Definitive Guide* is important because it offers a counterbalance to trends in the current chiropractic literature that is often divorced from historical fact. For example, several of the Green Books demonstrate a robust attempt to research and document the vertebral subluxation, written from first-person accounts. Some peer-reviewed literature today takes the stance that either the subluxation was never researched or that any research from earlier eras should be dismissed. We hope that by providing a more in-depth perspective on these topics the reader might judge the value of chiropractic science based on historical fact.

We have opted not to cite references throughout the text. A list of references is included at the end of the book. This was an aesthetic choice designed for the general readers and chiropractic students. We feel this way of learning about the Green Books, without being distracted by an overabundance of numbered endnotes or author's names in parenthesis, will assist the new student of the books to focus on the ideas themselves. In that regard, we have also opted to leave out page numbers alongside each quote. All quotations are associated with each volume's section or chapter. We expect that scholars and historians will study the references, especially if they have a question about any assertions made in the book.

The overall emphasis of the first part of the book is the chronological development of ideas throughout the Green Books. In this regard, an effort was made to limit repetition. This could be misleading for the reader who hopes to get a complete overview of each book. Many of the Green Books include the same basic definitions of terms like vertebral subluxation and Innate Intelligence. Some books even repeat chapters and passages from previous books. However, each book is unique in its overall focus and development of ideas. Please assume that the core ideas are congruent throughout the books unless we refer to a distinct change from one book to another, such as the shift to an upper cervical model of vertebral subluxation or years later to a full spine analysis. So, even if one of the central concepts from the chiropractic paradigm is not mentioned in regards to a particular volume, that does not mean the book skips the topic. By emphasizing the unique contribution from each book, rather than repeating identical definitions, *The Definitive Guide* explores the evolution of the ideas while offering an overview of the books. In order to acquire a complete understanding of any Green Book, it is essential to go to the source and read it.

The Writings

Chapter Two is about D.D. Palmer's first writings on chiropractic, with an emphasis on his writings between 1902 and 1906. D.D. Palmer's writings from this period laid the foundation of the chiropractic paradigm and also comprised the core chapters of Vol. 1 of the Green Book Series. Chapter Two also includes some of the historical background of his early writings, a few references to his pre-1900 writings, as well as discussions of his earliest thoughts on disease, structure and function, mixing chiropractic, vertebral subluxation, Innate Intelligence, Educated Intelligence, and Universal Intelligence. Some of these early articles were also included in D.D. Palmer's 1910 book.

Chapter Three includes an overview of 1906-1910. This includes an historical account of how Vol. 1 ultimately got published without D.D. Palmer's final approval, even though he was listed as the primary author. The chapter explores his 1906 theories about displaced articular surfaces and disease. The chapter also includes a chronological look at his Portland writings between 1908 and 1910, which were all included in his 1910 book. The examination of those writings emphasizes his critiques of other chiropractors, his theory of impingement, as well as his new thoughts on Innate. For example, in September 1909 he critiqued his own essay on Innate Intelligence originally written in 1903 and updated his theory. The chapter also includes a brief discussion of his 1910 book. This section emphasizes his theories that had not been significantly written about prior to 1910 such as tone and neuroskeleton.

Chapter Four is about D.D. Palmer's final book, *The Chiropractor*, published posthumously in 1914. Since the book was a compilation of his final lectures from 1912 and 1913, the chapter explores the lectures as one body of thought. Thus, rather than viewing the book as a cohesive text, the ideas are broken down and explained in a logical order. For example, the initial sections include his ideas about tone, biological principles, health and disease, life and death, vital force and energy, impulse, neuroskeleton as a nerve-tension frame, vertebral subluxation, pinching versus impinging, etiology, inflammation, nerve tracing, and palpation. The second part of the chapter explores his theory of neurological habit grooves, the relationship between organism and environment, consciousness, Innate, and inspiration. The final sections of the chapter examine his proposed religious legal strategy, his views on subjective and objective religion, as well as chiropractic as a moral and religious duty, his "doctrine," and also his thoughts about chiropractic's impact on society and culture, along with his view of individual greatness and what he referred to as "the great advancement."

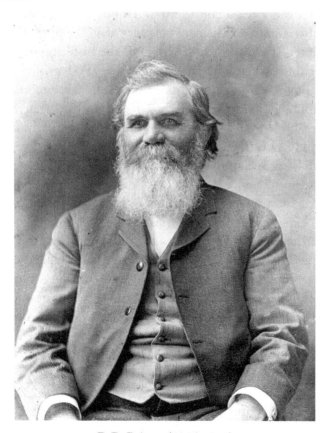

D.D. Palmer (1845-1913)

Chapters Five and Six include overviews of Vols. 2-13. These books formed the canon of the textbooks that were used to teach the first generation of chiropractic students at the PSC. Chapter Five covers B.J. Palmer's first six books. In those books, B.J. introduced new theories and practices, some of which became the foundation of the profession for decades. His new clinical applications and philosophical contributions were developed from the paradigm initiated by his father. For example, D.D. Palmer's practice of nerve tracing was developed into the meric system, and his theory of dis-ease and abnormal function were developed into B.J.'s models of momentum, retracing, and nine primary functions. B.J. Palmer's models were also developed in the context of his expanding clinical empiricism. He officially took over the school from his father in 1906 even though he had been running it since 1902. By 1909, the student clinic at PSC in Davenport was seeing more than 100 patients per day. Textbooks were needed for the growing student body, not only for philosophy and technique but for every core subject. Chapter Six explores the first textbooks written by PSC faculty between 1914-1920 on topics like Symptomatology, Physiology, Anatomy, Spinography, Chemistry, and Gynecology.

These first books in the PSC faculty series, which came to be known as the Green Books, demonstrate a pioneering philosophical approach to biology for the early twentieth century. The books shared a common viewpoint, the view from Innate. That is, not only did they consider the organism in terms of neurologically mediated self-organizing and self-healing processes but they tried to convey each physiological and clinical topic based on what Innate was attempting to do at any moment. This was in regard to normal function, interacting with the environment, and dealing with the consequences of vertebral subluxation. B.J. referred to this as "the chiropractic standpoint." The early Green Books represent the first comprehensive attempt by a school of thought to publish a series of textbooks from an Innate perspective. These chiropractic texts foreshadowed late twentieth century theoretical biology with its theories of autopoiesis, complex systems, dissipative structures, and self-organization. Future chiropractic research and theory might build upon this foundation by understanding the ways these early chiropractors integrated the chiropractic paradigm into each discipline.

Chapters Seven, Eight, and Nine include the books published in the 1920s. Chapter Seven is about what we refer to as the Humanities Green

Books: *The Spirit of the PSC*, *Chiropractic Advertising*, and *Chiropractic Malpractice*. The first book, *The Spirit of the PSC* was written as a novel by Leroy Nixon, a student, to capture the atmosphere of the school at its peak in the early 1920s. *Chiropractic Advertising* was written by Harry Vedder, a faculty member. It includes an overview of marketing practices in common use and also advice on communication and professionalism. *Chiropractic Malpractice* was written by Arthur Holmes, one of the chief lawyers who defended chiropractors in court. It includes legal advice, communication strategies, and a legalistic perspective on chiropractic from that era. Chapter Eight covers the legacy of John H. Craven, DC. He wrote two Green Books: *Chiropractic Orthopedy* and *A Textbook on Hygiene and Pediatrics from a Chiropractic Standpoint*, and, he also collaborated with B.J. Palmer on new editions of Vols. 1, 2, and 5. Those were B.J.'s main books of philosophy. As head of the Department of Philosophy, Craven was the teacher of Ralph W. Stephenson, DC.

Chapter Nine covers the life and work of R.W. Stephenson. Stephenson's *Chiropractic Textbook* has had more impact on the profession than any of the books. His 1927 book was used for decades as the main philosophy text at the PSC. It is still used today to teach the core principles of chiropractic at several colleges around the world. The chapter provides a look at Stephenson's life, his writings prior to and after 1927, and also an exploration of his second book, *The Art of Chiropractic*. Many of the main ideas published in his textbook were already described in his articles and his thesis, written in 1924. The chapter provides a context for the book and emphasizes his contributions to chiropractic theory.

Like the earlier Green Books, Stephenson's integration of the chiropractic paradigm might be viewed as a precursor to late twentieth century theoretical biology, systems views on clinical practice, and body/mind approaches to health and healing. Additionally, his text could be viewed as contemporary for the time. It was written at a time in Western culture when biology was a relatively new discipline and biologists were seeking to establish definitions of life based on the holistic organizing relations of parts rather than on the parts themselves. Here is one example of the holistic perspective inherent to

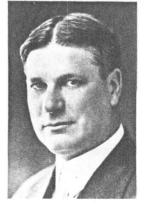

R.W. Stephenson

Stephenson's text. He writes:

> If a number of interdependent parts are to have a cooperative relation with each other, they must be grouped about a central idea, a common need or governing principle. This governing principle is Innate Intelligence.

What theoretical biologists refer to today as "self-organization," the biologist of the 1920s referred to as "organization." The Green Books used the term "organization" more than eighty times to refer to the body's innate ability to self-organize. Stephenson refers to Innate Intelligence as the scientific "law of organization." Understanding how the chiropractic paradigm and its development in the Green Books was a part of wider trends in biological thinking within the culture may help today's chiropractor to find new relevance in the texts and also provide new avenues of exploration for the chiropractic researcher.

Even though Stephenson and other chiropractic theorists of that era published ideas that were congruent with early twentieth-century theoretical biologists, chiropractic texts were not integrated with mainstream health or science literature. The Green Books were mostly self-published by the PSC. This was a common practice of chiropractic colleges, many of which published two or three texts.

Chapters Ten and Eleven are about the research pamphlets and the research textbooks from the 1920s and the 1930s. Chapter Ten includes an overview of the many pamphlets B.J. Palmer published between 1924 and 1933. These were his yearly reports delivered at Lyceum about the various research studies undertaken, starting with the first thermography research and ending with the upper cervical model of the torqued subluxation. Most of these pamphlets were integrated into future Green Books. Chapter Eleven covers the research textbooks published between 1934 and 1938. The first book, Vol. 18, introduced B.J. Palmer's approach to the upper cervical subluxation specific adjustment. In 1936, Vol. 19, B.J. gave his first report on the new B.J. Palmer Chiropractic Research Clinic. In 1938, Vol. 20, B.J. Palmer published a text on x-ray analysis using comparative graphs and Percy Remier, DC, published *Chiropractic Spinography* as Vol. 21, which included the latest advances in x-ray technology and analysis.

Chapter Twelve explores B.J. Palmer's tomes. Between 1949 and 1953, he published Vols. 22-29. Each book was more than 700 pages

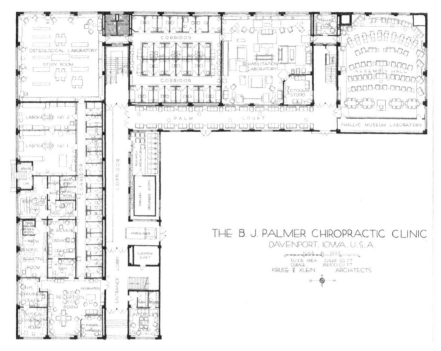

THE B. J. PALMER CHIROPRACTIC CLINIC
DAVENPORT, IOWA, U.S.A.

Architectural plans for the B.J. Palmer Chiropractic Clinic including NCM reading rooms, shielded grounded booths, ambulance parking, timpograph research lab, x-ray lab, rehab lab, osteological lab, phallic museum, and aquarium (1930s)

in length. The chapter includes the main philosophical and theoretical contributions of the books along with several important details. These texts lay the foundation for B.J. Palmer's final refinements and evolution of the Innate philosophy, including his emphasis on Innate Thot Flashes and the integration of his 14 years of clinical research using thermography, x-ray analysis, and other innovations like shielded grounded booths, and the invention of the electroencephalneuromentimpograph. The chapter also describes much of what is in the books including letters, research studies, older philosophy essays, as well as historical and autobiographical accounts. Additionally, until this chapter was written, there was no account in the literature of the way older pamphlets were used in later Green Books. One of the reasons why B.J. Palmer was able to publish so many thousands of pages in such a short time was because dozens of chapters are comprised of pamphlets, some of which were written as early as 1911. He did not include the dates for most of the original writings and so it is probable that many chiropractors have viewed these chapters as if they were written in the 1950s.

Chapters Thirteen, Fourteen, and Fifteen cover B.J. Palmer's final writings; Vols. 32-39. B.J. published these final eight books between 1955 and 1961. The books focused on philosophy, research, technique, theory, and reflect on his life in the context of the development of chiropractic. He started publishing one book per year and delivered the talks at Lyceum. His nephew, William H. Quigley wrote about B.J.'s dedication to teaching during those last years of his life. Quigley writes:

> During the summers of 1955 through 1960 B.J. wanted to keep in touch with the students and planned on addressing each of the school's 12 classes. He would lecture from eight until ten, taking time to answer questions from the student body. He would rarely have time during the year to meet this schedule, because of travel and other commitments, yet each year he would try again. He did make certain that he had at least one opportunity to talk with each class before their graduation.

In spite of B.J. Palmer's debilitating health challenges during the 1950s, he continued to write, to meet with his team running the PSC and Palmer Broadcasting, and he started planning for the inevitable. Quigley writes:

> As B.J. pondered his mortality he did what many other men did before him, he sought means of perpetuating his name and work...
>
> During the last years he clearly seemed compelled to publish what he considered proof of chiropractic in general and his philosophic beliefs in particular.

The last of the Green Books convey an evolution of B.J. himself. This evolution is most notable in his more spiritual writings as well as his attitude towards critics and detractors. He became more accepting and seemed to acquire a new type of insight about human nature. He recognized that his audience was targeted. He wrote for them.

Chapter Thirteen covers Vols. 32-34, Chapter Fourteen covers Vols. 35 and 36, and Chapter Fifteen covers Vols. 37-39. Each book represents a distinct body of knowledge. The chapter sections dedicated to each volume are categorized with topical subheadings so as to better introduce the reader to the complexity and range of ideas. The books build upon new avenues of Innate philosophy, many of which were first described in Vol. 22 published in 1949. In these, his last writings, it is possible to track new developments of ideas, an evolution of theories, and a historical perspective that brings context to chiropractic as a profession.

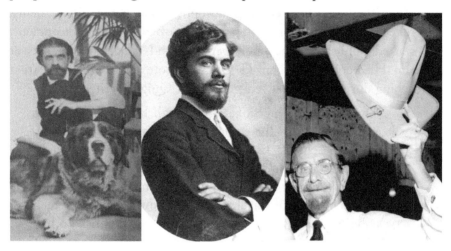

B.J. Palmer, 1921 (left), 1900 (middle), & 1957 (right)

B.J. Palmer's final eight books are an ideal place to begin any study of his life and work. The books themselves are relatively short, especially in comparison to the tomes. Any study of the Green Books could begin with Vol. 32 and, over the course of several months, systematically continue through Vol. 39. In this way, B.J. Palmer's final writings offer any student of chiropractic an excellent place to get started. These books provide a glimpse into a life of continual growth and discovery, as well as the development of theory in relation to all aspects of chiropractic.

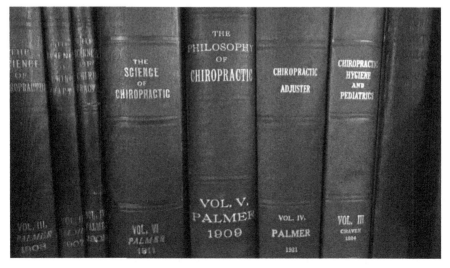

For Green Book Collectors

Chapters Sixteen, Seventeen, and Eighteen, were written by Faulkner and Foley, with editorial and historical insight from Senzon. These chapters were the inspiration for *The Definitive Guide*, which was originally intended to be a resource for Green Book collectors and gradually evolved into the current form. The detail in these chapters include the definition of a Green Book, ways to determine authenticity, rarity, and value of a book, an exploration of the history of Green Book publications, and a novel category system to distinguish between every edition of every Green Book.

Generations of chiropractors have been collecting Green Books. Many chiropractors have claimed to own a complete "set" of Green Books. Usually this means they have all the books that were issued while they or their relative was a student at Palmer. It was common for Palmer graduates to keep their Green Books even after they had retired and stopped practicing. Many kept their books until they died, their Green Books meant that much to them. Since the Green Books were produced over a nearly sixty-year span, it is doubtful that any chiropractor was ever able to purchase each book as it was initially issued. Even B.J. Palmer could not have owned a complete set of published books because the last two Green Books were published posthumously.

After B.J. Palmer died in 1961, the profession entered a "dark age" of chiropractic philosophy. The philosophy of chiropractic was not stressed as strongly in chiropractic schools. Most of the early Green Books were long out of print. New chiropractic books discussing philosophy were rare. Young chiropractors began to search for Green Books. The authors have found small want-ads from the early 1970s, when chiropractors were seeking Green Books. One chiropractor told us that in the late 1960s and early 1970s, he advertised in the classified "wanted" section of chiropractic magazines. Generally speaking, he paid $100 for a Palmer-authored Green Book and $50 for non-Palmer books. He did not know what books existed and was always excited to find a book he did not have. Oftentimes the buyer would have to purchase all the books in a lot. He would be contacted in response to his ad by a retired doctor or the family of a deceased chiropractor. They would say they have a specific number of books and a price would be negotiated. This method led to duplicates in collections, which were often traded with other chiropractors also seeking Green Books.

Some of the initial volumes from the 1920s and earlier are on their third or even fourth owners. Books from the late 1950s are just coming available because their original owners are now elderly and parting with their prized possessions.

BOOK WANTED

Anyone having for sale a Volume No. 1, By D. D. Palmer, published in 1906, kindly communicate with

J. C. HARRISON, D. C.,
16 Central Ave., Newark, N. J.

An Advertisement for Book Wanted, *The Chiropractor* (1917)

Our intent is to disseminate the most detailed knowledge available of the physical books themselves. This is the first significant update to the literature about the Green Books since Glenda Wiese and Michelle Lykens published *A Bibliography of the Palmer Green Books in Print*, in 1986. We hope that the collector may better understand the subtle nuances of the various books and make informed collecting decisions. This book provides knowledge for the Green Book collector about the individual Green Books to be sought and offers an idea of the rarity and value. Collecting Green Books is an extension of passion for the chiropractic profession.

The Wiese and Lykens bibliography introduced the profession to facts about how many Green Books were actually produced over the years. Prior to their bibliography, the only accurate lists of the books were old PSC catalogs, which listed books that were available but not books that were out of print, reissued volume numbers, or those not yet written. For example, doctors tried to collect every volume number but did not know that some numbers were used twice. Wiese and Lykens demonstrated that several volume numbers had been used on completely different books and that two volume numbers were missing from the series: Vols. 30 and 31. Their bibliography became a "shopping list" for the modern Green Book collector. It is only since their Green Book bibliography that collectors have been able to truly collect a complete set of Green Books.

Chapter Sixteen covers special considerations about the Green Books such as reissued volume numbers, missing volume numbers, unnumbered Green Books, other Palmer books, covers, leather bound special editions, private collections, author mock-ups, signed and inscribed editions, numbered editions, non-traditional sized Green Books, the difference between editions and printings, supplements to editions, and modern reprints.

Chapter Seventeen answers the question: What is a Green Book? There is some debate among collectors as to the definition. A Green Book is defined as:

> A Green Book is any one of the books written by D.D. Palmer, B.J. Palmer or other authors while they were considered faculty of the Palmer School of Chiropractic or its predecessors, with the intent of teaching chiropractic principles and methods. In addition, if a book was published with a volume number as part of the B.J. Palmer chiropractic series, all future or past editions are considered a Green Book even if the volume number was dropped.

According to the definition, there are some Palmer-authored books, such as *'Round the World with B.J.* and *Radio Salesmanship* that are not considered Green Books and there are books published without volume numbers that are considered Green Books like Stephenson's *Art of Chiropractic* and Pharaoh's *Correlative Chiropractic Hygiene*.

Chapter Seventeen introduces the new classification system called the Green Book Master List, which includes 123 books, or every edition of each book and supplement that fits within the definition of a Green Book. The entire list is included in the chapter with images of many of the books. The chapter also defines different types of sets a collector might have, which we delineate as Level 1 through 5.

Chapter Eighteen covers the rarity and value of a Green Book. Since collectors traditionally did not know what books even existed, pricing was arbitrary. We will attempt to take some of the guesswork out of collecting. The chapter includes a rarity and desirability scale (also used in the Green Book Master List); how to value Green Books; the art of trading, buying, and selling Green Books, as well as how to assess book condition and guidelines for repairing damaged books.

Before the Internet, finding Green Books was limited to advertising in chiropractic journals, from estate sales of deceased chiropractors, and contacting used bookstores in person. The Internet opened the inventory of every bookstore in the world to online buyers. In an instant, the inventory of thousands of used bookstores could be searched, and Green Books bought for the listed price. And yet, booksellers had no idea how to price these books. Some would be listed for only a dollar or two, others would be listed for exceptionally high prices.

Green Book pricing, rarity, value, and desirability became more established with online auctions such as eBay and other auctions listing Green Books for sale. This system of buying and selling began to set a true market-price for Green Books. In an online auction, as buyers bid against each other, prices began to be established. The rarer books had serious bidding wars resulting in high prices. The more common books would sell for as low as $20 and were readily available. If there were no interested buyers, the Green Book would not sell at all. Over the past fifteen years prices have fluctuated based on supply and demand. During a period of oversupply and less demand, prices dropped. The rarer Green Books continue to command a high value.

When B.J. officially took over the PSC in 1906, there were not many students. In those early years, B.J. did not need many books printed. However, he did print more books than he needed for the current students. Some books were sold to former students as well as potential students studying at home. Of course the future PSC student would need books. By 1919, the PSC had several thousand students. At that point many thousands of books were printed and sold by the PSC to its students. This simple detail is a big factor in the rarity of Green Book editions. Many of the early books were printed in such limited amounts that they are very rare today. Green Books for the 1920s were printed by the thousands, and as such, many have more supply than demand.

This Book

The Definitive Guide was also written to act as an anchor to the chiropractic paradigm. The rhetoric in the chiropractic profession today needs such an anchor. There are articles published in the peer-reviewed literature attacking the chiropractic paradigm without adequate historical references. Some of these articles suggest that philosophy and vertebral subluxation should be dropped in the trash bin of history because they are no longer needed and perhaps never were. This type of ahistorical rhetoric, usually backed up by a plethora of circular and faulty references, is taking root in the profession and influencing board decisions, institutional policies, and threatening the ability of good chiropractors to practice. On the other end of the spectrum, philosophy is sometimes used in chiropractic to support unfounded claims, historical facts are too often mistaken, and narrowly focused beliefs limit the profession's ability to develop. It is our fervent hope that this book will guide the next generation of chiropractors like a candle lit in the darkness.

Chapter 1
The Historical Context for the Green Books

The chiropractic profession traces its beginnings to a pivotal event in Davenport, Iowa, in September of 1895. Daniel David (D.D.) Palmer, at the time a practicing magnetic healer, used a spinous process of Harvey Lillard as a lever and performed what would become known as the first chiropractic adjustment.

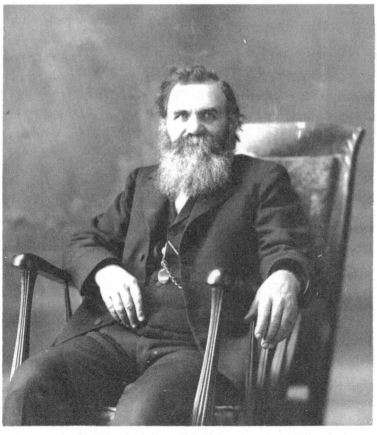

D.D. Palmer (1902) - From *The Chiropractor's Protégé*

Lillard struggled to hear and was nearly deaf. He worked as the janitor of the building where Palmer lived and conducted a large magnetic healing infirmary. Lillard reported to Dr. Palmer that his loss of hearing was related to an apparent spinal injury many years prior. Palmer examined his spine and noted a painful vertebra that seemed out of place. Palmer reasoned that if the spinal trauma caused the vertebra to be displaced and the loss of hearing coincided, returning the vertebra to its normal position should restore Lillard's hearing.

D.D. Palmer described a specific segmental contact and spinal thrust to Lillard's 4th dorsal vertebra. This resulted in a marked improvement of Lillard's hearing. D.D. Palmer was knowledgeable of the treatment of various illnesses prior to this event. However, the thrust upon Lillard's vertebra led him to better understand the fundamental spinal and neurological cause of the illnesses he had been treating as a magnetic. With the adjustment of Harvey Lillard, D.D. Palmer discovered what became known as the chiropractic vertebral subluxation. This was the birth of the chiropractic profession.

The theory and practice of chiropractic was chronicled by D.D. Palmer in dozens of essays, articles, and lectures, which were eventually published in his three books. By studying these writings in the context of his life story, it is possible to understand the development of his ideas. In fact, each book is the culmination of several years of practicing, teaching, and writing.

D.D. Palmer's Early Inspiration

D.D. Palmer's initial theories and practices can be traced to the Spiritualist movement. The movement involved practices like magnetic healing and non-materialist worldviews. This was a different perspective on reality, one that included consciousness, intelligence, and energetic phenomena as central. According to his first known published writings, D.D. Palmer began studying Spiritualism around 1866 and practiced some methods related to magnetic healing by 1872 (Appendix 1). After trying various trades such as school teacher, beekeeper, and grocer, he opened a magnetic healing practice in Burlington, Iowa, in 1886, and referred to himself as Dr. Palmer.

One of the earliest and most prominent influences on Palmer was his first wife, Abba Lord. They were married in 1871. She was active in the Spiritualist movement, serving as secretary of the local group, and advertised herself as "Dr. Abba Lord Palmer... Wonderful Psychometrist and Clairvoyant Physician,

Soul Reader and Business Medium." Diagnosis and treatment of disease were her primary services. The advertisements stated that she:

> Can diagnose disease by likeness, autograph, lock of hair, without a failure, and give prescription, which, if followed will surely cure.

After witnessing her successes, D.D. Palmer was convinced that some Spiritualist healers were honest and endowed with abilities (Appendix 1).

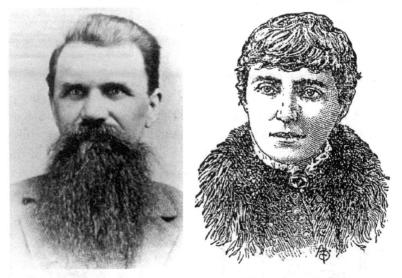

D.D. Palmer (1880s)   Abba Lord (1892)

It is possible that D.D. became acquainted with Abba Lord after reading the Religio-Philosophical Journal, which is where she ran her advertisements. The journal also advertised to beekeepers, which was Palmer's trade at the time.

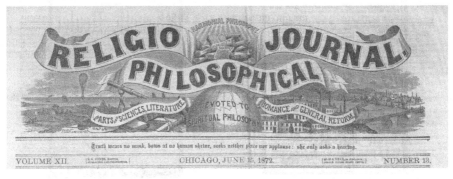

Religio-Philosophical Journal issue with D.D. Palmer's Letter (Appendix 1)

The journal may have influenced Palmer's thinking in other ways as well. Several of the books he owned were also advertised there. Books and pamphlets by Spiritualists and magnetic healers like A.B. Severance, William Denton, Warren Felt Evans, William B. Fahnestock, and Edwin Dwight Babbitt were found with D.D. Palmer's papers in a file cabinet on the Palmer campus in the 1980s. Some of these books include his signature and a date. *D.D. Palmer's Traveling Library*

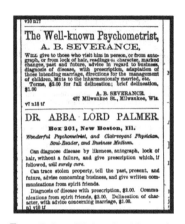

From *Religio-Philosophical Journal*

was published in 2014. The book includes selections from his personal library. It emphasizes the theories and practices that were precursors to Palmer's theory and practice of magnetic healing, and later, chiropractic. For example, Evans, Babbitt, and Caldwell promoted the use of the hands for manipulation and magnetic healing in the treatment of illness.

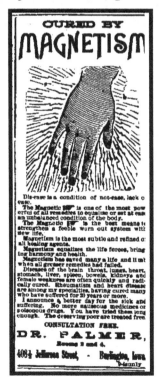

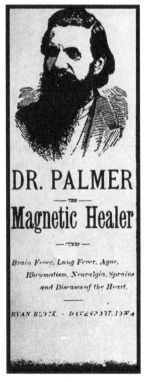

D.D. Palmer ads from Burlington and Davenport (1887 and 1891)

In his advertising as a magnetic, D.D. Palmer described some of his methods. He would locate an area of the body related to the symptom, usually associated with an organ system, then he would direct his personal energies through his hands in an effort to break up the "congestion" around the diseased organs. According to Palmer and several testimonials from other magnetic healers, his methods were an innovation.

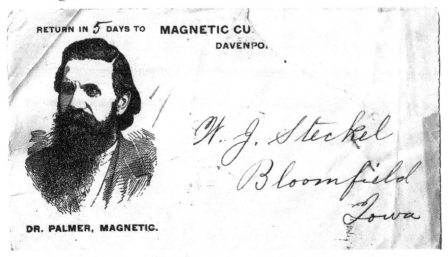

D.D. Palmer envelope (1892)

Evidence suggests D.D. Palmer saw a high volume of patients daily in his Davenport magnetic healing practice. Treating many patients allowed him to work out his chiropractic ideas and techniques.

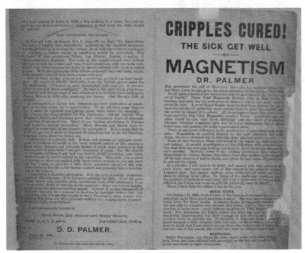

D.D. Palmer pamphlet, Davenport, IA (1889)

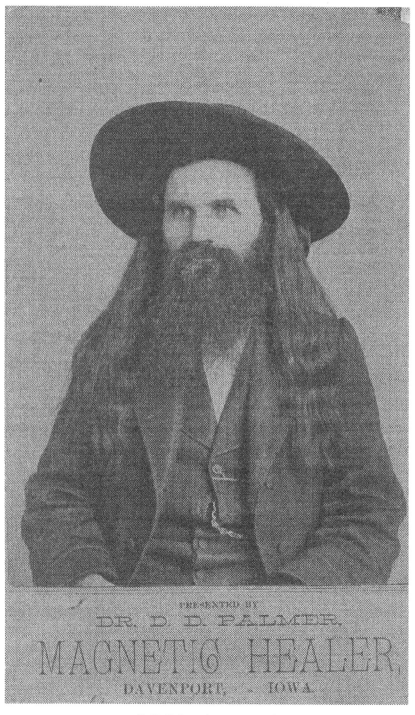

D.D. Palmer business card

The Chiropractic Paradigm

After the Lillard event, D.D. Palmer reasoned that spinal misalignment and resulting nerve irritation were the cause of the congestion. He expanded on this viewpoint after his clinical experience with another patient. He writes:

> Shortly after this relief from deafness, I had a case of heart trouble which was not improving. I examined the spine and found a displaced vertebra pressing against the nerves which innervate the heart. I adjusted the vertebra and gave immediate relief—nothing "accidental" or "crude" about this. Then I began to reason if two diseases, so dissimilar as deafness and heart trouble, came from impingement, a pressure on nerves, were not other diseases due to a similar cause? Thus the science (knowledge) and art (adjusting) of Chiropractic were formed at that time.

His books demonstrate that he continued to develop his theories over the next seventeen years but the central ideas did not change.

With suggestions provided by his patient, Reverend Samuel Weed, in January of 1896, Palmer named his new profession "chiropractic" from the Greek "hand practice" or "done by hand."

This was the emergence of D.D. Palmer's chiropractic paradigm. The paradigm viewed the body as a self-regulating and self-healing system run by intelligent life energy traveling through the nervous system. If the spine was mechanically malfunctioning, the resultant change in function to the nervous system created abnormal function in the body. Chiropractic adjustments were given to the spinal levels that were thought to be impinging nerves with the intent of decreasing the tension on the nerves, reducing the nerve irritation, and allowing the body to naturally self-regulate. Chiropractic was not a therapeutic method of treating a condition or disease. Its intent was to normalize the neurophysiology, reverse the pathophysiology, and create a state of high-level body function where the disease process was absent. This was a new and unique system of health care.

D.D. Palmer's books became the only references where doctors could go to learn his theories and practices.

Teaching Chiropractic

D.D. Palmer taught Leroy Baker, his first student, in 1896. The Palmer School and Cure was officially opened in 1897. The first graduate was William Seeley in January 1898. By the end of 1898, D.D. Palmer had taught ten students including A.P. Davis and O.G. Smith.

Palmer's initial teaching of chiropractic consisted of an apprenticeship in his practice. Students would assist Dr. Palmer in his Davenport infirmary for a period of time. There were no classroom instructions and Palmer had no books or notes of any kind. He was still developing and refining his ideas. This method of teaching allowed for an abundance of practical clinical application; however, it lacked the systematic dissemination of core fundamental ideas and thought.

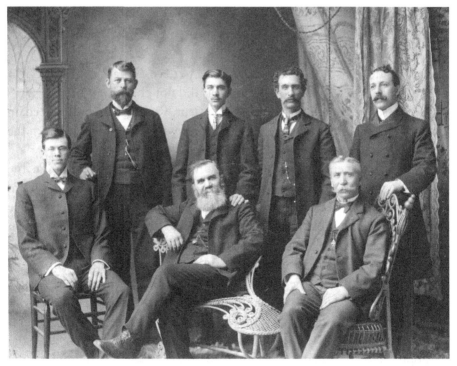

Class reunion. From left to right: (seated) O.G. Smith, D.D. Palmer, Thomas Storey, E.E. Sutton, B.J. Palmer, O.B. Jones, S.M. Langworthy (January 1902)

The very first book written to teach chiropractic can be attributed to Oakley Smith's 1899 copyrighted but unpublished vade mecum titled *Chiropractic*. It contained the original ideas that the founder of chiropractic taught at the time. Smith taught students at D.D. Palmer's Davenport school. The intent of the book was likely to instruct others at the Palmer School in the ideas and methods of chiropractic. It could arguably be considered the very first Green Book.

Early students paid $500 for their schooling. In 2018, that would be equivalent to $14,194 for tuition. Depending on the student's prior knowledge, the apprenticeship lasted from one day up to six months. His early students watched Palmer treat sick people in his infirmary with a chiropractic thrust. They were taught three things:

- A philosophy

- Nerve tracing

- How the thrust treated disease

Even though he used the word "treating," Palmer considered his approach non-therapeutic because it focused on cause not symptoms. People must have found value in his chiropractic methods because students paid the tuition and his patients paid for the care they received.

When Dr. Palmer thought the student knew enough, he issued them a diploma as a Chiropractic Practitioner or CP. The last CP diploma was granted by Palmer from his school in Santa Barbara in 1903. By that time, he did have a classroom for instruction but his California school did not last very long. After he left California and returned to his school in Davenport in 1904, the degree was changed to DC or Doctor of Chiropractic diploma.

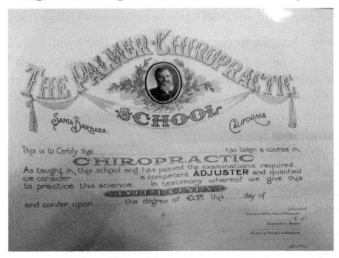

Blank Diploma, for The Palmer Chiropractic School, Santa Barbara, Competent Adjuster, degree of C.P. (1903)

Other Chiropractic Paradigms

The apprentice style of teaching was common in medicine during this time. Many of D.D. Palmer's early students were medical doctors, homeopaths, or osteopaths. Each viewed health care from the perspectives they had already studied.

D.D. Palmer thought students would abandon their previous therapeutic ideas in favor of his concepts. This did not happen as he had hoped. There were no written books or notes. There was no standard base of knowledge to impart to each student. They relied on what Dr. Palmer told them while treating patients, and supplemented their other theories and practices to fill in perceived gaps.

They applied Palmer's methods and theories from their own viewpoints. Many of them incorporated his ideas and techniques into what they were already doing when treating patients. Some took a more eclectic approach and included chiropractic along with naturopathy. Others tried to bring chiropractic into medical practice. This led to a schism in the early profession that still exists today.

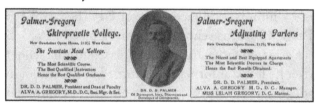

Advertisement for Palmer-Gregory Chiropractic College (1908)

Two more chiropractic paradigms emerged. Those who included natural methods as an adjunct to the chiropractic adjustment eventually became the middle chiropractic paradigm. Others sought to include chiropractic as a part of medicine. That became the biomedical chiropractic paradigm. Most students focused on D.D. Palmer's spinal thrust and less on the chiropractic ideas of health.

The result was that many early students were not practicing chiropractic as the founder had taught them. They were mixing his chiropractic ideas and techniques with other health care systems to treat illness and disease.

The profession's identity was blurred from the beginning. However, all of the earliest chiropractors advertised the same philosophy that D.D. Palmer taught. Furthermore, even two decades after he started teaching, all of the approaches developed by Palmer's students shared adjustment and correction of vertebral subluxation as the central focus.

The Conflict Between Father and Son

In order to more fully understand the Green Books, it is important to explore D.D. Palmer's relationship with his son, B.J. Palmer.

In January 1888, D.D. and his three children, May, Jessie, and B.J., who was six years old, moved to Davenport, Iowa. On November 6, 1888, D.D. married his fourth wife, Villa. The family lived in the back rooms of D.D. Palmer's magnetic healing offices. As the practice grew, more rooms were rented, until the entire floor of the Ryan block became the Palmer Infirmary. B.J. observed his

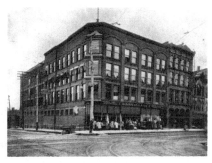

The Ryan Block, Davenport, IA

father caring for patients throughout his childhood and teen years. In Vol. 24, published in 1950, B.J. reminisced about how he was curious about his father's ideas and methods from an early age. He writes:

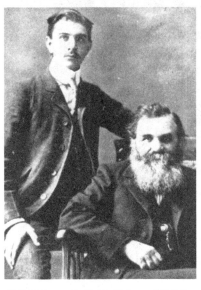

B.J. Palmer & D.D. Palmer (1902)

Father was a perfect Spencerian penman. He wrote ideas in long-hand. Would write and rewrite them, much as we do today in these articles. He would discard earlier copies by throwing them in waste basket. He never tore them up. Even as a youngster, from 1890 on—at nine years of age—we used to go each night and gather these writings. We saved them. We have them today in our scrapbook. (See The Story of S.B., in THE BIGNESS OF THE FELLOW WITHIN, Vol. XXII, Palmer, 1949.)

By 1899, at age 17, B.J. was studying chiropractic with O.G. Smith and adjusting patients. There is evidence he practiced chiropractic in the summer of 1901 in Manistique, Michigan. B.J. Palmer was given a CP diploma in January 1902 from his father's school in Davenport. Soon after, he practiced briefly in Spring Grove, Minnesota.

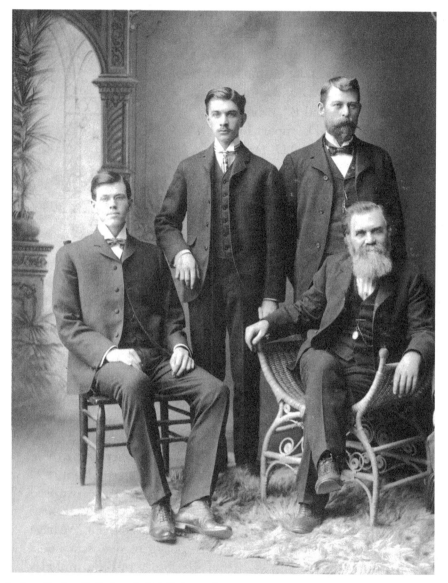

Left to Right: O.G. Smith, B.J. Palmer, E.E. Sutton, and D.D. Palmer (January 1902)
- From *The Chiropractor's Protégé*

D.D. Palmer left Davenport for about two years starting in mid 1902. He moved to Pasadena, California and taught there. He also started a school in nearby Santa Barbara in 1903 and next started a school in Chicago, Illinois, in 1904. He returned to Davenport in 1904. During those years, his son ran the Palmer School of Chiropractic (PSC) at Davenport and grew the early profession.

According to private letters from D.D. to B.J. in 1907, their time working together at the school was fraught with interpersonal difficulties between them. After all, when D.D. returned to Davenport in 1904, B.J. had been running the school for two years. The school business was booming. It was not easy for the older Palmer to adapt to those circumstances, with his son as the boss. D.D. Palmer was in his sixties and B.J. was in his twenties. The clash between the two might be viewed as dysfunctional family dynamics and as an inter-generational conflict.

The Palmers started *The Chiropractor* in December 1904 and published seventeen issues together through April 1906. Vol. 1 or *The Science of Chiropractic*, which was published in 1906, was mainly a collection of articles from the journal. A few of the articles were written by B.J. Palmer. Most were written by D.D. Palmer. *The Chiropractor* was published monthly until 1961.

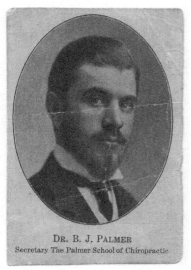

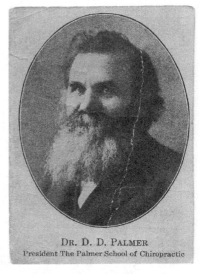

DR. B. J. PALMER
Secretary The Palmer School of Chiropractic

DR. D. D. PALMER
President The Palmer School of Chiropractic

B.J. Palmer, Secretary, PSC   D.D. Palmer, President, PSC

D.D. Palmer left Davenport in 1906 after spending 23 days in jail for practicing medicine without a license. The Palmers agreed to split the school assets. B.J. and his wife, Mabel, became the official owners of the school. The arrangement was mediated through arbitration with the help of two local friends chosen by the Palmers for their impartiality. Both father and son signed the terms of the separation agreement.

The conflicts between father and son deepened after D.D. left Davenport and moved to Medford, Oklahoma. For example, in one letter to B.J. written from Medford in 1907, D.D. writes:

> How much I would like to be a teacher in the school of which I was the founder; but I was crowded out of it. You always wanted me to get down and lose my manhood, be under you, so that you might run the whole thing.

He also complained about the conflicts between B.J. and his late wife, Villa, who died in November 1905. And, he complained about the conflicts between his new wife, Mary, with B.J., Mabel, and her mother. D.D. and Mary, an old flame from thirty-years prior, were married in winter 1906.

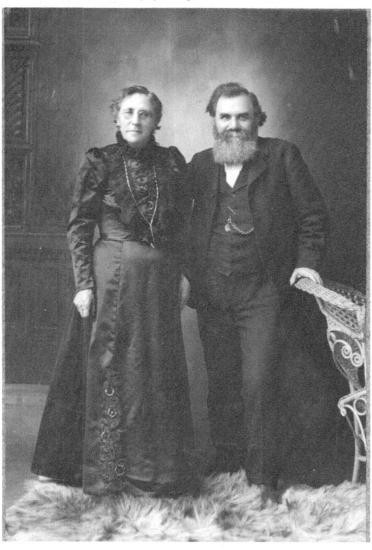

Villa Palmer and D.D. Palmer (1902) - From *The Chiropractor's Protégé*

Another source of their conflict described in the letters was about money. In the spring of 1906, while D.D. Palmer was still in jail, B.J. continued to expand operations. He built a new classroom using monies from the school's savings. D.D. Palmer had other plans for those funds but was helpless to do anything about it. He reflected on this from Oklahoma, wishing that he had more cash on hand to start the next phase of his life. He ended up borrowing money from his brother and opened a grocery store. Soon after, he got back into the school business.

In the early fall of 1906, B.J. Palmer published Vol. 1, with D.D. Palmer listed as first author and himself as second author. This would become a new source of conflict between them because D.D. had no say in the final version of the book they were planning.

Also in the fall of 1906, B.J. delivered 12 lectures on diseases at the PSC. The students asked him if he would transcribe the next lectures, which he did. The lectures from winter 1907 became Vol. 2 of his new chiropractic book series. The lectures in the fall of 1907 became Vol. 3.

D.D. Palmer grew bitter and contemptuous of his son in the years after his imprisonment. This was compounded when he moved to Portland, Oregon, in October 1908, only to meet students of B.J.'s like Leroy Gordon, who were probably reading Vols. 2 and 3. Gordon became D.D.'s partner in his new school and new journal, *The Chiropractor Adjuster*. Many of the journal articles were dedicated to criticizing or "adjusting" the new ideas put forth in B.J.'s first two books and his many articles.

Besides specific critiques of B.J.'s theories, D.D. Palmer complained that B.J. started to refer to himself as "developer of chiropractic." D.D. scoured the monthly issues of *The Chiropractor* to determine exactly when this title took hold. He determined it started in August or September of 1907. The new self-designation of "developer" rankled D.D. Palmer and he shared his thoughts about it publicly without holding back his animosity or his wit. In January 1909, he even accused B.J. of kleptomania.

The disagreements between the two impacted the profession and chiropractic theory for decades. By studying their early writings in chronological order, in the context of their disagreements, it is possible to understand how both of their theories were refined and developed as a result of the conflict. D.D. critiqued several different chiropractor's theories as a type of peer-review. Instead of just critiquing his colleagues however, he used their ideas as a way to elucidate his own theories. For example, D.D. refined and explained his impingement theory as a way to criticize B.J.'s use of the compression model as described in Vol. 3 in 1908. In response to this critique, B.J. incorporated the cord pressure model from a neurosurgical case series in his second edition of Vol 3, in 1911. B.J. and his students built on the cord pressure model for decades.

Another important impact their conflict had on the chiropractic profession is the way in which other chiropractors took sides, even decades later. After all, future students may have read D.D. Palmer's barbs against his son and assumed that every critique was correct without having any context about the bias, the bitterness, and even some of the errors found in D.D.'s criticisms. Perhaps D.D.'s bitter criticism of B.J., which was sometimes clouded by his temperament, hurt feelings, and overall frustration at his circumstances near the end of his life, was overzealous. Even though B.J.'s early theories were not without flaw, D.D.'s assessment was hardly objective. It is difficult to gauge how the conflict between father and son influenced future chiropractic educators, researchers, and theorists.

The Legal Question

The early chiropractors faced thousands of court battles, eventually securing laws in all fifty states and many countries. The chiropractic literature was used in the courtroom and was shaped, in part, by the early legal battles. As early as 1907, the courts ruled that chiropractic was a distinct and separate profession with its own art, philosophy, and science. Chiropractic books were a means to demonstrate this body of knowledge.

The most famous case from that time period was in the summer of 1907, when Shegetaro Morikubo went on trial in LaCrosse, Wisconsin, for practicing medicine, surgery, and osteopathy without a license. His lawyer, Tom Morris, got the charges reduced to practicing osteopathy without a license because his client did no surgery and prescribed no medication. Morris proved in court that chiropractic was distinct from osteopathy. Morikubo was acquitted. It was a landmark decision. Morris became the lead council for B.J. Palmer's new Universal Chiropractor's Association. Morris and his law firm went on to defend chiropractors in court for decades.

Morikubo studied chiropractic under both Palmers, taught philosophy for B.J. in the fall of 1906, and was sent to LaCrosse by B.J. in hopes of forcing the courts to rule for chiropractic. An osteopath in LaCrosse, named Jorris, brought a case against chiropractors in 1905. Jorris was their target. B.J. had already sent him a copy of Vol. 1. in 1906. Soon after

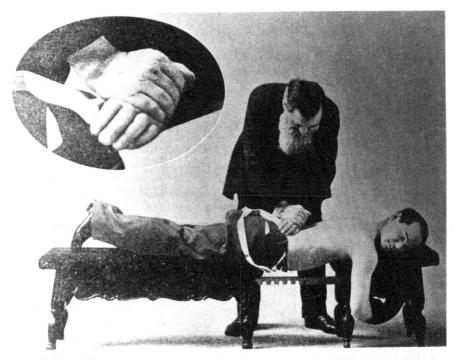

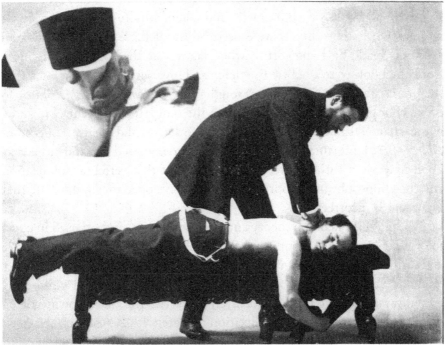

Adjusting Demonstrations from Vol. 1 with Morikubo as subject (1906)

Morikubo arrived in LaCrosse and opened a practice in the building where Jorris practiced osteopathy. Morikubo took out a full-page advertisement in January 1907, in a local newspaper. The advertisement was a four column article that described the science of chiropractic. Morikubo included many of B.J. Palmer's latest ideas about brain impulses, Innate brain, Educated mind, and the relationship between science, art, and philosophy. He even critiqued the limitations of osteopathy because "Osteopathy does not understand the nature of the mind as concerns its relations with the functions of the body." Jorris took the bait and brought charges against Morikubo.

After the trial, Morikubo wrote that he and B.J. had prepared his case for six months. It is possible that the publication of B.J. Palmer's Vol. 2 was part of their preparation. The copyright office reports that two copies were received on June 20, 1907. The trial was in August 1907. Along with Vol. 1, Vol. 2 was probably used as evidence by Tom Morris, their attorney.

This landmark case is important to understand because chiropractic historians have mistakenly thought that *Modernized Chiropractic*, written by Smith with contributions from Paxson and Langworthy, all students of D.D. Palmer, was used by the defense in the case. There is no evidence for that. There is one news article about the case, which states Morikubo furnished all books on chiropractic and osteopathy to the prosecution. It is unknown if those books were used by the defense. There was also an assertion made by Langworthy, who was not at the trial, that his ideas from the book were used by the defense. However, Morikubo states that the prosecution (not the defense) sought to use *Modernized Chiropractic* to prove chiropractic and osteopathy were the same (not different). He and a witness named Linniker, both stated that the defense did not use *Modernized Chiropractic*. Unfortunately, papers in the peer-reviewed literature as late as 2018 have cited this incorrect story to suggest that vertebral subluxation and the philosophy of chiropractic was only developed to win the case. That argument is incorrect.

Vertebral subluxation theory and philosophy were indeed used in court to prove chiropractic's distinction. However, the philosophy of chiropractic and vertebral subluxation were not developed as a mere legal maneuver. D.D. Palmer's writings dating back to the 1890s demonstrates that philosophy was always a central component of chiropractic. The first known written document with the term "sub-luxation" is dated 1902. And yet, the need to demonstrate chiropractic's separateness increased the importance of chiropractic books.

This court victory by Morikubo and B.J. Palmer set a precedent for the fledgling profession. It established chiropractic as a unique profession with a scientific rationale, a philosophy, and clinical techniques. The trial showed B.J. Palmer that if chiropractic was to be a distinct profession in the eyes of the law, it must have even more books to demonstrate its professional identity.

The Chiropractic Book Series

Under the leadership of B.J. Palmer, the PSC grew from a handful of students to the premier chiropractic school in the world of its day. As it grew, the PSC was no longer teaching the apprentice style of schooling. More formal classes and subjects were developed. The PSC became a traditional educational institution focused on teaching the ideas and methods to generations of chiropractors. Textbooks were needed to teach the ever-growing population of chiropractors. By the 1920s, the PSC had a full-time faculty, several thousand students enrolled, and eighteen distinct books, some of which were in second or third editions.

B.J. reasoned that chiropractic students could not be taught chiropractic principles using medical texts, which were written from the therapeutic viewpoint. The PSC was going to require a complete series of textbooks, booklets, and pamphlets for students to convey the chiropractic idea. In addition, basic science textbooks were needed written from the perspective of chiropractic's idea of Innate and health.

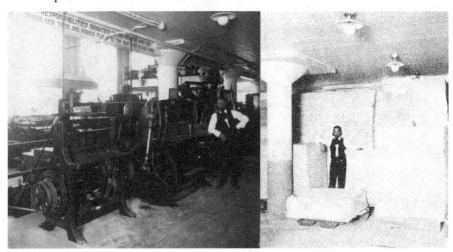

B.J. Palmer with Printing Presses and Reams of Paper at the PSC Printery

Between 1907 and 1911, B.J. Palmer published five volumes of his lectures as Vols. 2-6. In 1910, he issued a second edition of *The Science of Chiropractic*, Vol. 1, which was originally published in 1906, and listed himself as the sole author. Collectors consider the 1906 edition and the 1910 edition of Vol. 1 as separate books. Various sets of the first volumes were advertised between 1913 and 1915. In 1911, B.J. announced the titles of the next volumes in the Palmer chiropractic series. Vols. 6-13 were planned as written below but were never produced.

Vol. VI - The Science of Chiropractic
Vol. VII - The Superior and Inferior Meric System
Vol. VIII - Concussion of Forces, Cause and Adjust Subluxations
Vol. IX - 1,000 Chiropractic Questions and Answers
Vol. X - Nerve Tracing
Vol. XI - Chiropractic vs. Osteopathy
Vol. XII and XIII - Morat Criticisms and Chiropractic Orthopedy

Some of these topics were incorporated into Vol. 6 (1911) and the second edition of Vol. 2, which included the entirety of Vol. 4, and was published in 1913. Other topics were included in new books authored by PSC faculty between 1914 and 1920. By the 1920s, advertisements included 14 volumes in a set.

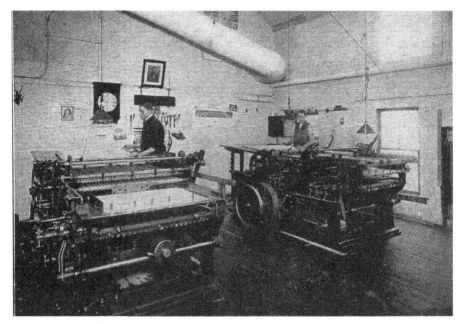

Postcard of PSC Printery (1919)

Of the 46 official Green Books, 14 were authored by faculty at the PSC, one was authored by a student, one by a lawyer, and one by a PSC alumni. These books taught a wide variety of topics such as diagnosis, anatomy, physiology, x-ray analysis, malpractice, orthopedy, pediatrics, and hygiene. All of the books were written from the perspective of the chiropractic paradigm with its emphasis on vertebral subluxation and Innate theory in relation to normal and abnormal functions. The Green Book series is the first attempt in the modern era for a school of thought to present a cohesive body of knowledge to its students on a variety of topics written from an Innate perspective.

By the early 1920s, B.J. completed the last of his revisions and updates to his six-volume, *Science of Chiropractic* series. The initial faculty-authored PSC textbooks were also completed by 1920 and only specific topic books like *Malpractice*, *Advertising*, *Orthopedy*, and *Hygiene* were added in the middle 1920s. In 1927, Ralph Stephenson produced the *Chiropractic Textbook* which was a summation of Palmer chiropractic theory. After the 1930s, the Green Books took on a new character and focus. The books embodied decades of innovation in chiropractic theory, research, and clinical application. By the 1950s, the Green Books became B.J. Palmer's distillation of a worldview that emerged from the chiropractic paradigm and from a lifetime of contemplation of the Innate philosophy. Of this last epoch, the golden age of chiropractic publications, Quigley famously writes, "He had hoped his books would become his greatest memorial."

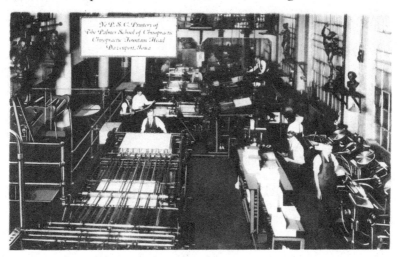

Ye PSC Printery of The Palmer School of Chiropractic,
Chiropractic Fountain Head, Davenport, Iowa (1923)

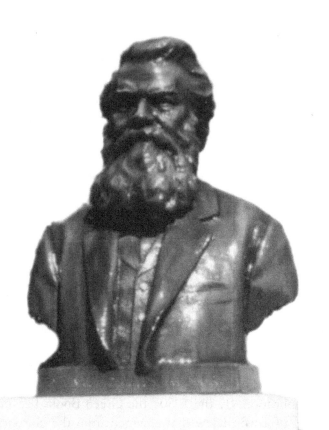

DANIEL · DAVID
PALMER

FOUNDER · OF
CHIROPRACTIC
SEPTEMBER · 18
1895

Chapter 2
D.D. Palmer's Early Chiropractic Writings

The period from 1897 to 1907 laid the foundation of the chiropractic paradigm. It included all of the early writings of D.D. Palmer as well as B.J.'s first book. Before exploring B.J.'s works and the publications of his students, it is vital to understand D.D. Palmer's core ideas, his paradigm, and how it developed through the course of his writings.

The First Writings on Chiropractic

D.D. Palmer's first writings on chiropractic were published as advertisements in 1897, where he wrote that adjustments freed nerves, arteries, and veins. His early definition statement of chiropractic can be dated to 1902 based on letters between D.D., B.J., and Langworthy. Also, in 1903, he published a two-part essay called *Innate Intelligence*. It was later published as a chapter in Vol. 1. Most of his early writings were published as broadsides, essays, and articles.

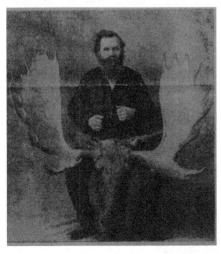 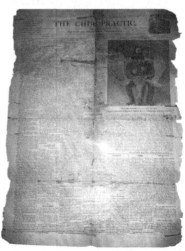

D.D. Palmer on a moose head from the cover of *The Chiropractic* (1899)

D.D. Palmer's 1902 Chiropractic Theory

In August 1902, an advertisement titled *This is the "Ultimatum of Chiro" Chiropractic,* D.D. Palmer writes about vertebral subluxation, Innate Intelligence, Educated Intelligence, the intervertebral foramina, and the chiropractic adjustment. In the advertisement he writes:

> That a disease is a condition in which Innate Intelligence is trying to carry on its work of growth and repair with the Machinery out of Gear – a human machine out of order.

He reasoned that treating effects was an incorrect approach and that all therapies treat effects. Symptoms are effects and the result of derangement, wrong action, and an "altered human mechanism." The unpleasant sensations, pains, distress, and uneasiness of the body are all related to disturbed natural functions. Disorder of the human frame leads to all illness and sickness. Thus, correcting the disorder was the only true way to allow for the functions to continue naturally.

D.D. Palmer no longer felt that the words "treat" and "treatment" effectively captured what he was doing in practice. He writes, "Chiropractors do not treat; they fix, adjust, put to right, replace, restore, do anything but treat, manipulate or operate." The reasoning was that only effects could be treated. Causes cannot be treated. They can only be made right. This is done by putting the parts into relative position. He considered the words operate, treat, and manipulate, to be allopathic, not chiropractic, and relied on the new terminology to articulate his theory. Waters observed that this advertisement is the first time D.D. used the phrase "adjust the cause." He would use this again and again in his writings through 1910.

The Chiropractor

Between December 1904 and March 1906, D.D. Palmer published monthly articles in the new journal, *The Chiropractor.* The journal was published by the PSC and copyrighted by his son, B.J. Palmer. The issues included the most comprehensive explanation of chiropractic to date including testimonials, the Lillard story, reprints of older articles, an updated definition

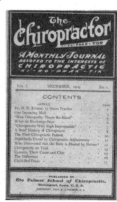

Vol. 1 No. 1

of chiropractic, and an account of his new discoveries, such as his theory of heat emanating from nerves.

D.D. Palmer writes:

> In 1886 I began healing as a business. Although I practiced under the name of magnetic, I did not slap or rub as others. I questioned many M.D.'s as to the cause of disease. I desired to know why such a person has asthma, rheumatism or other afflictions. I wished to know what difference there was in two persons that caused the one to have certain symptoms called disease that his neighbor living under the same conditions did not have. Physicians answered me by saying that they would give such and such remedies. I did not want to know what remedies they would give; I desired to learn what difference there was in the man of health, and the one who was diseased. I wanted to learn the cause of disease; why one was afflicted and the other was not.

Palmer also describes the turning point when he discovered and developed chiropractic after years of experience as a magnetic healer. He concluded that there was a cause of disease. Here is an abridged version of his statement:

> Ninety-five percent of all deranged nerves are made by sub-luxations of vertebrae which pinch nerves in some one of the 51 joint articulations of the spinal column. Therefore, to relieve the pressure upon these nerves means to restore normal action - hence, normal functions, perfect health... A large share of diseases are caused by nerves being impinged in the foramina, which is occluded by the displacement of the vertebra. These vertebrae are replaced by the hands; using the processes as handles.

The articles in *The Chiropractor* also included Palmer's theory of disease as well as his theories on cancer. Based on numerous clinical observations of tumors sloughing off after chiropractic adjustments, he conjectured that cancers were symptoms of abnormal and deranged nerves. His earliest theories on the topic were from 1893. In 1897, he proposed a dual causation theory of cancer: injury to nerves and obstruction of circulation. In 1904, D.D. Palmer states that "cancers are but the symptoms of impinged nerves." The injury to the nerves causes irritation, which leads to abnormal actions in the body. He proposed that disease is decreased or increased normal functions. He writes:

> All ailments are but the result of either repressed or exaggerated innervation, caused by irritation or paralysis of nerves. This excited or depressed condition has as its cause pressure on nerves near their origin.

This theory would comprise the core of Palmer's teaching for the rest of his life.

In these early writings, D.D. Palmer also expanded on his thoughts about the non-therapeutic approach, criticized mixing other therapies with chiropractic, and further developed his definitions of vertebral sub-luxation and the chiropractic adjustment.

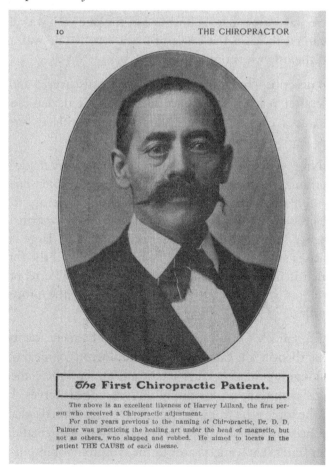

10   THE CHIROPRACTOR

The First Chiropractic Patient.

The above is an excellent likeness of Harvey Lillard, the first person who received a Chiropractic adjustment.
For nine years previous to the naming of Chiropractic, Dr. D. D. Palmer was practicing the healing art under the head of magnetic, but not as others, who slapped and rubbed. He aimed to locate in the patient THE CAUSE of each disease.

Harvey Lillard from *The Chiropractor*, Volume 1, Number 1 (1904)

D.D. Palmer's Chiropractic Theory in 1905

The twelve issues of *The Chiropractor* published in 1905 represent D.D. Palmer's most consistent and sustained writing on all things chiropractic to date. The articles became core chapters of Vol. 1.

Gaucher-Peslherbe suggested that D.D. Palmer's outpouring of writing in 1905 was inspired by the publication of Davis' *Neuropathy*, also in 1905. Davis' first book, *Osteopathy Illustrated*, was published in 1898, a short time before he became D.D. Palmer's second graduate. *Neuropathy* claimed to teach chiropractic. This inspired D.D. Palmer to clarify and elucidate his own theories. D.D. was also actively sparring in the pages of *The Chiropractor* with other former students and colleagues as well like Smith, Langworthy, and Carver.

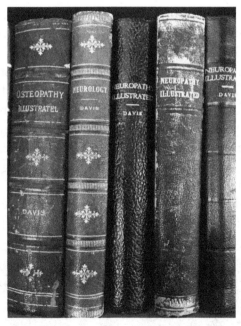

First editions of Davis' books

The content of D.D. Palmer's writings from 1905 provide an in-depth view of his theory and practice. For example, in the January 1905 issue, he wrote that chiropractic was "non-therapeutical" and that chiropractic should not "mix in portions of some other systems." Chiropractors adjust 300 articulations of the body and especially the spine. D.D. also included brief thoughts on epilepsy as it related to his theory on nerves and heat in the body, as well as the importance of adjusting the cause for mumps.

The March 1905 issue included his new article called *Chiropractic*, printed alongside a full page photo of the discoverer and developer of chiropractic. The article sums up his thoughts on disease, vertebral subluxation, and the ways in which spinal structure may affect body function. For example, he writes, "nearly all diseases are caused by subluxations of the vertebral column which impinge nerves." He referred to subluxations as "luxated joints" for the first time. He writes, "When these luxated joints are replaced and the pinched nerves freed, there is no longer abnormal sensation." Abnormal sensation related to his practice of nerve tracing, which was central to his methodology to "locate and verify with definite precision the apparently slight luxations which cause abnormal functions." To accomplish this the chiropractor needs to know the pathological variations of the spine and how to digitally trace the sensory distortions, which may be swollen, inflamed, or sensitive, from the foramen to the part that is affected.

In the last two paragraphs of the *Chiropractic*, D.D. Palmer gave his most comprehensive explanation of the spine to date. He viewed the spinal column as the central axis supporting the head, ribs, and extremities. The spine transmits forces through the articular processes. He referred to the elastic nature of the bodies and discs and how flexion, extension, and rotation have normal limits. When the vertebrae go beyond the normal range, the intervertebral and articular cartilages separate, which displaces the vertebra. This leads to narrowed foramen and impinged nerves, which leads to abnormal function.

He concluded that chiropractic was rational because it was based on natural law. He writes, "The inevitable conclusion is that the laws of natural philosophy apply to the backbone of the human body."

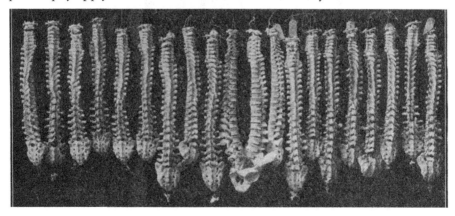

Idiosyncrasies of the Backbone, *The Chiropractor*, Volume 1, Number 4 (March 1905)

The 1905 issues of *The Chiropractor* are the foundation of the first chiropractic Green Book and the theoretical foundation of the chiropractic profession. Each issue is an invaluable source of chiropractic history and offers a richer understanding of early chiropractic theory.

D.D. Palmer's 1905 Writings on Mixing

In an article called *Suggestion,* published in February 1905 and republished in Vol. 1 and also in D.D.'s 1910 book, he wrote some new and interesting thoughts about chiropractic.

He responded to a letter from his friend and lawyer, Willard Carver. The letter was published several months before Carver earned his chiropractic degree from a student of D.D.'s named Charles Ray Parker. Carver wanted D.D. Palmer to include the practice of suggestive therapeutics as part of chiropractic. D.D. replied that such a merger was not appropriate. Any system that is a "therapy" and treats effects should not be combined with chiropractic. He wrote that "suggestion" treats effects, which does not allow for the natural to come through after the abnormal is changed to normal. Chiropractic does not use remedies because it goes to the cause. Palmer writes:

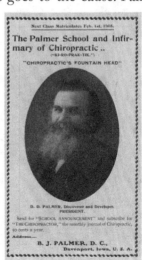

It is surprising to learn that every friend of Chiropractic thinks that his method of treating diseases is just the one that ought to be used in connection with the adjusting of the cause. All practitioners come to learn Chiropractic in order to add it to their mode of healing. Each person finds that the more Chiropractic he takes in, the less need he has of his former mode of treating symptoms. The person who understands the principles of Chiropractic thoroughly, has no need for remedies.

Next Class - Feb 1ˢᵗ 1905

According to D.D. Palmer, when effects are being addressed, then the practitioner does not know the cause. He wrote, "No thank you; we do not mix; we take Chiropractic straight. If it were adulterated with all the systems offered it would soon lose its identity."

D.D. Palmer's Philosophical Ruminations in 1905

In August 1905, D.D. replied to Carver again. The reply is also included as a chapter of Vol. 1 and in his 1910 book. Carver wrote a letter dated February 15, 1905, which was in response to D.D.'s article in the February issue. Palmer's reply is an important glimpse into his philosophical thinking. He reproduced Carver's letter with commentary throughout ten pages of text.

Palmer's responses were more casual than many of his other writings. Perhaps due to their familiarity, the two were old friends. Carver recounted in his autobiography in 1936 that he used to deliver eggs to the Palmers in the early 1880s in What Cheer, Iowa, when B.J. was a baby. He also said that D.D. Palmer sent him a letter in 1895 about the new method he discovered.

First, Carver wrote that D.D. was a materialist whose writings only included mechanics. Palmer agreed. He was indeed focused on the material joints impinging on nerves causing material injury and deranged functions. For Palmer, chiropractic is simply about "keeping the articulatory processes of the organism in proper position." D.D. Palmer was writing about displaced articulations rather than bones out of place.

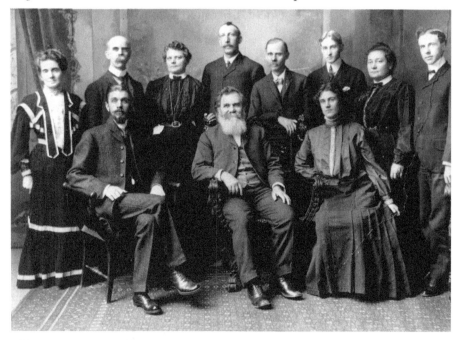

Class picture: Fron left to right sitting are B.J. Palmer, D.D. Palmer, Mabel Palmer. Those standing are Brake, Darnel, Oas, Hananska, Evans, Danetz, Doetz, and C.R. Parker. Photo taken Feb. 23, 1905. *The Chiropractor*, Volume 1, Number 3.

And yet, D.D. Palmer also used the occasion of his reply to write about the non-materialist aspects of his philosophy. He writes:

> When I go into the realms of ethereal and spiritual, which cannot be demonstrated, but must be accepted on belief, then I am not in the field of Chiropractic.

In his reply to Carver, D.D. Palmer expanded on his Innate theory. He used several synonyms for Innate Intelligence: mind, soul, spirit, nature, instinct, intuition, and subconscious mind. He also referred to life as a living principle that could vacate if enough disarrangement made the body uninhabitable.

According to D.D. Palmer, Innate has always existed and is transmitted from the mother in all "animated beings." It accommodates and changes to fit into its environment. He writes:

> It starts in the new being with a knowledge gleaned from an experience of a life, the length of which we have no conception. It has as full a comprehension of all its functions, which it runs as intelligently on the day of its birth as in adult life. It is infinite, unlimited in time and accomplishments.
>
> The Educated Intelligence knows nothing of running the human machine of which it has the outward care. Its education has to be acquired by years of experience.

He concluded that Educated Intelligence should not dictate to Innate, which he referred to as Educated's "superior." These philosophical insights were included as part of his overall approach.

Also in the article, D.D. Palmer referred to disease as disordered functions. "Inharmony" is the "heterogeneous condition of parts which are not in proper apposition." The chiropractor uses Educated Intelligence to remove the pressure on the nerves that Innate has not been able to handle on its own and will never be able to.

Palmer's reply to Carver also included other tidbits of chiropractic theory and practice, such as the notion that a perfect system does not need to include many modes of healing, that impinged nerves cause insanity, and that pernicious habits could be cured by adjustment. He also suggested that the Educated Intelligence should study kinematics and be able to use the spinous processes as levers or fulcrums. In his first known use of the term nervous energy, he writes that the adjustment frees the impinged nerves, then "they can supply nervous energy to their twig ends."

D.D. Palmer's Writings on Innate Intelligence in 1906

In February 1906, D.D. Palmer published an article called *Immortality*, which expanded on his philosophy of Innate Intelligence and explored the spiritual and ethereal elements of his philosophy. The article was significant enough to D.D. Palmer that he promoted it in the December 1905 issue, just after his wife, Villa, died. Waters suggested that it may have been written as a eulogy to Villa. In January 1906, *The Chiropractor* included a note about the article as part of the birth announcement of Dave Palmer. He writes:

Our Youngest Patient

Born to Dr. and Mrs. B.J. Palmer, Jan. 12, '06, a boy. Named Daniel David Palmer, Junior, a grandson and namesake of D.D. Palmer. It is needless to say that this advent, in a measure, accounts for the lack of the Immortality article in this issue.

He was adjusted for constipation when only four days old. The vertebra had been slightly displaced at birth. It was replaced by one Chiropractic adjustment, relieving the pressure on nerves, which caused a partial paralysis of the bowels.

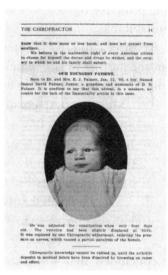

The Chiropractor Volume 2, Number 2 (1906)

In *Immorality*, which was reproduced in Vol. 1, D.D. Palmer updated his theory of Innate to include a broader philosophical perspective. Prior to 1905, his primary writings on Innate Intelligence were from 1902 and 1903 describing Innate and Educated nerves and an inherent biological function of growth, repair, and adaptation transmitted through the nervous system.

Immortality is only three pages long but it is one of D.D. Palmer's most profound, poetic, and philosophical writings. He acknowledged his own 35 years of spiritual work and how he dove into the mysteries of life and death. He wrote that his own spiritual knowledge had become material, "an expression of consciousness by all of my five senses." This spiritual insight included claims that he made in 1872 about the ability for the spirit or intelligence to leave the body in trance and exist beyond death. (Appendix 1)

D.D. Palmer described Innate Intelligence as the eternal part of man's duality. Educated Intelligence was the ephemeral part. Innate is passed on from the mother and leaves the body at death but it is immortal. Palmer used a grafting metaphor, which probably goes back to his early days as a beekeeper and raspberry farmer, to explain how Innate comes from the mother like a scion from the original plant stock. It is part of the intelligence that pervades the universe and branches off. D.D. viewed Innate as an immortal branch of Universal. He writes, "Immortality is the life entered by Innate at its birth." D.D. felt that he was describing a distinctly chiropractic answer to an ancient question. Man was a duality or a dual entity: physical and spiritual.

D.D. Palmer described Innate Intelligence using similar synonyms as he had in August with an emphasis on how Innate functions with Educated. He suggested that they have mirrored senses: interior and exterior. One looks after the interior and the other to the outward. Innate handles functions and Educated handles external needs.

He added several new attributes to his Innate Theory. Innate has its own consciousness independent of the body. It is invincible and invulnerable. It is not the mind but behind the mind. "Thot expresses itself thru it... The brain is a medium thru which Innate manifests itself." Thus the functions of the brain are governed by Innate and receives educated impressions.

D.D. Palmer viewed mind as a quality of the brain and Innate as the director of intelligence. He writes, "The brain does not create the mind any more than the rose does its color and odor." These ideas were a unique integration of everything Palmer had learned through decades of study, clinical practice, and living life.

Historian of 19th-century American healing and spiritual practices, Robert Fuller, suggested that Palmer's central theory was unique. D.D.'s view that the nervous system was the vehicle through which spirit and matter interacted was a new integration of ideas from magnetic healing, Spiritualism, and neurophysiology.

D.D. Palmer recognized the novelty and power of his approach. He writes:

> I do not pretend to fully comprehend any one of these questions; but Chiropractic has opened the door of intellectual reasoning, that will eventually enlighten the world on these important subjects.

Immortality contains his first known written use of the term "universal intelligence." He used lowercase letters and told the reader they could substitute "God" if they chose.

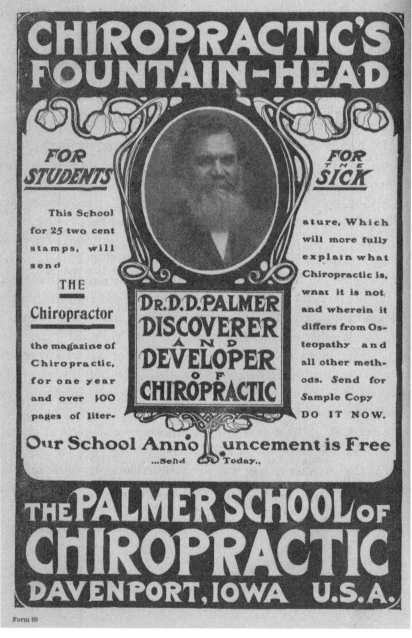

Chiropractic's Fountain-Head, *The Chiropractor*, Volume 2, Number 2 (1906)

Chapter 3
D.D. Palmer's First Two Books

D. D. Palmer only published one book during his lifetime, *The Science, Art, and Philosophy of Chiropractic* in 1910. As previously noted, his first book was Vol. 1 of the chiropractic series, which was initially published with him listed as the main author in 1906. It was comprised mostly of his writings and was originally planned by him and B.J. together. B.J. published it without his final input. These first two books of D.D. Palmer's represent a development of his thought and offer a first-person account of the historical emergence of the chiropractic paradigm.

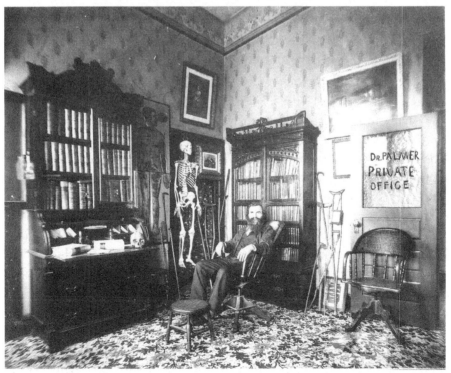

Dr. Palmer Private Office - From *The Chiropractor's Protégé*

The First Green Book

The new book, *The Science of Chiropractic*, was announced as forthcoming in January 1906 in the midst of a chaotic three-month period. D.D.'s wife died, he remarried, B.J. and Mabel's son, David, was born, and D.D. was awaiting his trial for the charges of practicing medicine without a license.

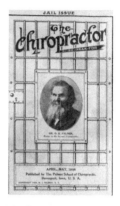

The Chiropractor, cover (April-May 1906)

In the January 1906 issue of *The Chiropractor*, two advertisements appeared. The first advertisement was for *The Science of Chiropractic*, a book of 200 pages. It was included in the table of contents as "Chiropractic Book," listed on page 8.

CHIROPRACTIC BOOK.

We have had so many urgent demands for a book on Chiropractic that we at last offer to the public a work, "The Science of Chiropractic." It contains 200 pages, is well bound, and contains much on this new science. It is the only one which explains vertebral luxations, and what we mean by replacing them.

Is used as text book and is the only complete work dealing exclusively on Chiropractic. Is the recognized authority, principles advocated are standard and endorsed by all Chiropractors who use pure and unadulterated Chiropractic.

$5.00 a copy. If sent by mail, add 25 cents for postage.

The Science of Chiropractic, 200 page book,
The Chiropractor (Jan 1906)

The small outlined announcement was set in the middle of a page of text discussing A.P. Davis' book, *Neuropathy*. The Davis book was advertised as "the only book on the market explaining how to apply the Chiropractic method." The second advertisement for the new Palmer book describes 285 pages. The full-page ad comprised the entire page 23 towards the back of the issue.

According to the advertisement, the 285 pages included 85 half-tone illustrations. When the book was eventually published, it included 108 illustrations. It appears that some of the additional images were created with D.D. Palmer's involvement after January 1906. The illustrations included pictures of the Palmers with students; images of the osteology collection; the rooms, offices, and library of the school and clinic, as well as pictures of D.D. and B.J. demonstrating adjusting with Morikubo as the subject; and a group photo in front of the school with B.J. laying on his side in front and D.D. in a chair off to the right. Based on the book, *The*

Chiropractor's Protégé, we know that some of the pictures in Vol. 1 were from The Palmer Chiropractic School at Santa Barbara, taken in 1903. In July 1906, after D.D. Palmer had already left Davenport, B.J. advertised that the book had 102 illustrations. The new illustrations, added by B.J., probably included several full-page portraits, compilations of student portraits, as well as group photos in the new classroom.

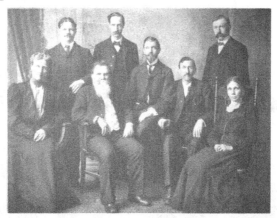

Class Group—The PSC from Vol. 1 (1906)

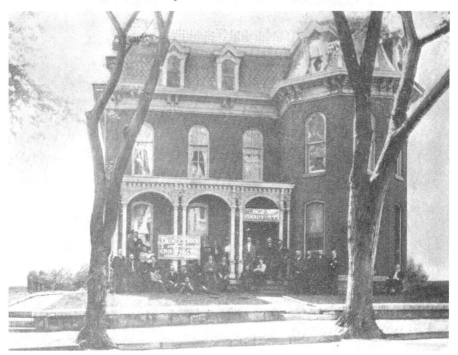

Group photo from Vol. 1 of the Palmer School and Infirmary of Chiropractic (1906)

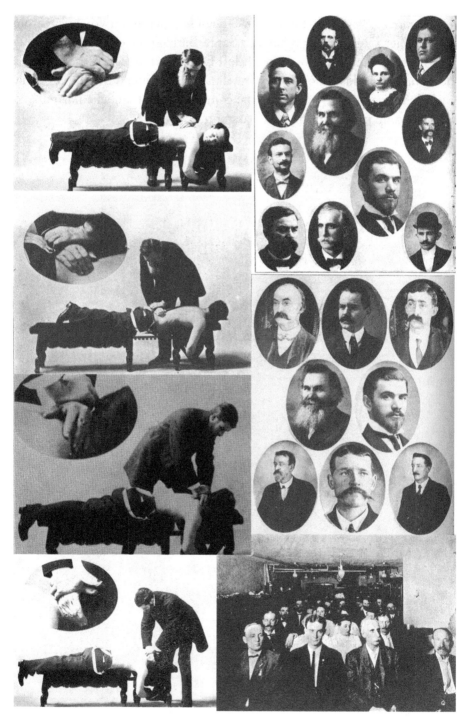

Illustrations from Vol. 1 (1906)

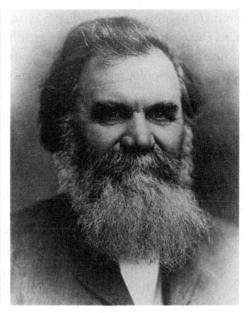

"The Science of Chiropractic"

Explains and Illustrates
Its Principles...

A 285 PAGE BOOK

By Its Discoverer and Developer

85 Half-tone Illustrations

Is used as text book and is the only complete work dealing exclusively on Chiropractic. Is the recognized authority, principles advocated are standard and endorsed by all Chiropractors who use pure and unadulterated Chiropractic.

Remit today, NOW, $5.00 per copy, postage 25 cents extra. First edition limited.

All orders from subscribers mentioning *The Chiropractor* will receive as a frontispiece a mounted photograph and autograph of the author, Dr. D. D. Palmer.

Form 91

The Science of Chiropractic, 285 page book, *The Chiropractor* (Jan 1906)

D.D. Palmer, Founder of Chiropractic

Even though both advertisements included information for purchasing and postage, the book did not get published as quickly as planned due to the events that unfolded that year. On March 30, 1906, D.D. Palmer was taken into custody at the district court in Davenport. He was found guilty of violating the law by professing to cure diseases in his magazine called "The Chiropractor." After his release on April 21, D.D. Palmer moved to Medford, Oklahoma, and opened a grocery store. In the early fall of 1906, B.J. went to print with the book while D.D. was living in Oklahoma. In the October issue, B.J. announced that he started shipping orders of the 400-page book, *The Science of Chiropractic*.

The book is mostly comprised of D.D. Palmer's writings and also includes writings from B.J. Palmer, E.E. Schwartz, Howard Nutting, and selections from the osteopathic literature. The 400 pages of articles were mostly taken from the issues of *The Chiropractor*, which included a few older essays. The chapters were organized by topic. B.J. Palmer hired Professor S.B. Harvey of Hillsdale College, Hillsdale, Michigan, to proofread the text.

None of the chapters or articles by the Palmers listed author information. According to D.D., 40 of the articles were written by him. The only way to differentiate between B.J.'s and D.D.'s writings within the book is to compare them to earlier and later writings. For example, even at this early date, some of B.J.'s unique ideas are distinguishable from his father's such as his views on the sympathetic nervous system and reflex mechanisms. B.J. felt that terminology about neuroanatomy and physiology should account for the intelligence and the integrated wholeness of the system. He disliked "sympathetic" and felt "reflex" ignored the intelligence. A careful reading of the 1906 text may help to determine the authorship of most chapters.

D.D. Palmer was bitter about being imprisoned, losing his school to his son, and having his book published without him as editor. In a letter to John Howard, written in 1906, D.D. writes that he felt robbed of his belongings and that B.J. added too many pages to his book. He writes:

> I see that he has on last outside page "400" pages of literature. When my wife died we had 106 pages. Altho I was to be the editor, he had, against my wish, put in 400 pages. I would have then left, but he changed to 100. He has not a few pages over 200.

Oddly, this complaint to Howard actually refers to an advertisement published in *The Chiropractor* from June 1906 for a collection of the issues. The "last outside page" was not an advertisement for the book at all. D.D. may have written the letter in haste and frustration while he was visiting his wife's family and moving from Davenport to Medford, where his brother T.J. lived. He may have mistook B.J.'s mention of "400 pages of literature" for the book. It is also possible that D.D. was aware the book was going to be published without him and with more than 400 pages. After all, in July 1906, B.J. advertised it as "a 500 page book," with "115 half tone illustrations."

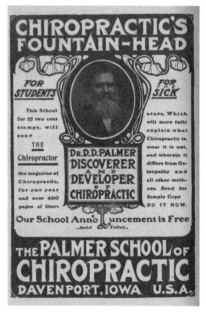

The Chiropractor (July 1906)

D.D. Palmer complained of these and other issues to B.J. in private letters. On April 28, 1907, he wrote to B.J. on stationary from his store, The Fair, in Medford, which listed M.H. Palmer as proprietor and D.D. Palmer as Manager. D.D. writes, "A fine thot came to me today to add to my book, but I do not know that I shall ever see its manuscript again." The book had already been published since the fall. Perhaps after months of the grocery business, he was finally getting ready to reenter his field and contribute to his chiropractic theories but was not able to add to his book. D.D. had been running his new grocery store, which opened on January 1, 1907, for several months. He found that the simplicity of running a store, like he once did in the 1880s in What Cheer, Iowa, was a respite from being in the school business and dealing with legal and professional complexities. After a few months of that, he wanted to get back to his book.

In the December-January issue of *The Chiropractor* (1906), B.J. published twenty-one endorsements of the book. These were in response to his request from the October issue, in which he writes:

> I would esteem an expression of appreciation from each purchaser of THE SCIENCE OF CHIROPRACTIC. It is the first book that scientifically demonstrates THE cause of a single disease. Therefore it is valuable. A copy should be read by every member of a sick family. Chiropractors cannot afford to be without one. The books have sold "like hot cakes." The third edition is now being bound.

The earliest date of the endorsements was October 20, 1906. The endorsements came from all over the United States as well as two from England and France. Some of these were written by historical figures from chiropractic's early days such as Samuel Weed, "Uncle Howard" Nutting, and Leroy M. Gordon, who became D.D. Palmer's partner in the D.D. Palmer College of Chiropractic in Portland, Oregon.

Interestingly, while the endorsements were universally positive, there was some critical feedback about the style, the writing, and the arguments. For example, Gordon noted he was "more than pleased," but also, "While it might not stand on its literary merits, its principles are true and homliness of language cannot destroy them." Morikubo's review of the book was titled *A Stray Thought on the Science of Chiropractic*. Morikubo considered the contents of the book crystal diamonds found while searching for gold, even with its crude logic, simplicity, and grammatical errors.

Also in the December-January issue, B.J. advertised that each of the chapters were available for purchase individually and also as phonographic recordings to be played for patients in the waiting rooms, or for lectures. There are no known copies of these recordings. The advertisement for the book in the back of that issue listed B.J. as collaborator.

In 1910, D.D. Palmer published several criticisms of B.J.'s original publication of the book. He writes, "I did not sanction its publication, as I then said, I did not know enough of Chiropractic to write such a book on the science, philosophy and art of Chiropractic as the subject demanded." He included a separate rebuke for B.J.'s second edition of the book, published in 1910, without D.D. listed as author. D.D. Palmer writes:

> B.J. represents himself therein as being the author of forty of my articles, as being "the fountain head" of all it contains and it was he who performed the many cures mentioned therein... All credit is taken unto himself. He has mutilated my writings and misrepresented facts, laying himself liable to the United States courts for a $100 fine for each article of mine appropriated by him... Much has been cut and mutilated in order to plagiarize that which belongs to another. By so doing he has been able to replace principle with principal.

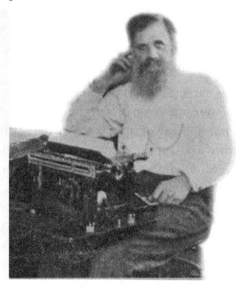

Revised Vol. 1

Vol. 1 will be ready for delivery on March 10th, 1910

The entire book has been torn to pieces. Much has been "cut"—much "new matter" added—in fact the body is so new that, if it wasn't for a few of the old articles and the old volume number, we could have announced it as a new book.

NOW is the minute to send your check—yes, in advance, we need it. As soon as this book is paid for—then comes the balance of those books.

Price
$2.20 Postpaid

The Chiropractor, V6, N2 (1910)   D.D. Palmer (1910)

We will never know what really happened between the two or why B.J. de-cided to drop his father's name from the revised book. A careful analysis of his edits might shed some light on the issue. B.J. Palmer was the copyright holder of all issues of *The Chiropractor*. He continued to credit his father for the remainder of his life as the revered founder of chiropractic, even though he developed his own theories, practices, and was the primary early force behind chiropractic's emergence as a recognized profession.

The Science of Chiropractic: Vol.1 (1906)

In Vol. 1, D.D. Palmer proposes that chiropractic was founded on anatomy, physiology, pathology, mechanical adjustment, nerve tracing, which was his method of determining the location of the subluxation in relation to the symptom by palpating the inflamed and sensitive areas, as well as "the reparatory plan," or making right the "cause of wrong doing." He also wrote that chiropractic is founded on laws "as old as the vertebrata of the animal kingdom." Central to the book is his model of vertebral subluxation and his theory of disease.

Displaced Articular Surfaces

D.D. Palmer's model of vertebral subluxation did not emphasize the bone-out-of-place theory, rather he focused on the joint. He defined vertebral subluxation as "a displacement of the articular processes." For example, he writes, "A Chiropractic luxation is a partial separation of two articular surfaces, which are readily replaced by the hands of a Chiropractor." Furthermore, he writes:

> Chiropractic is a combination of two Greek words, which mean done by the hand, a hand practitioner, one who repairs, one who adjusts; as used by Chiropractors it means replacing of articular surfaces that have been slightly displaced.

D.D. Palmer proposed that the subluxation affects physiological and psychological disease processes throughout the lifespan.

In the book, D.D. Palmer also contrasts his theories with those of osteopathic authors. For example, he writes that "the lesion theory of the Osteopaths, is not that of subluxation of the Chiropractor." For D.D., the lesion was secondary and the vertebral subluxation was primary.

D.D. Palmer's Theory of Disease

Vol. 1 expanded on D.D. Palmer's theory of disease as an intelligible condition. He writes, "The cause of disease is intelligible." Disease follows a certain progression.

D.D. Palmer viewed Innate Intelligence as complete but its expression could be interfered with. He theorized that the Innate Intelligence tries to carry out growth and repair but it cannot do so when the body is out of order.

This is primarily because the structures are disarranged, especially the spinal structures. He writes:

> Disease is a material derangement and must have a material cause. Innate of itself is complete and perfectly capable of running the body. Disease being the manifestation of the interference.

Slightly displaced bones or subluxations cause nerves to get impinged, which leads to abnormal physiological functions. He writes:

> Disease is the result of anatomical abnormalities (bones slightly displaced by various accidents) which cause physiological discord, and abnormal functions.

Disturbed functions lead to excessive or insufficient performance, or disease. He writes:

> Disease is excessive or insufficient performance of functions... Disease is but disturbed functions... The cause of disease is in the one afflicted.

Since the cause is within the individual, as is the cure, the adjustment corrects the wrong that is producing the cause by allowing the impulses to be carried to the intended organs. Thus, disease is intelligible and determined by ascertaining the neural involvement. Locating the excessive or hindered functions and their relationship to displaced vertebra was the key. Here are a few quotes that sum up his theories. He writes:

> We are in health when the innate and educated nerves are free to act. Disease is but abnormal functions. Innate nerves control all the vital functions. Nearly all diseases are caused by vertebral subluxations which impinge nerves.

> Remember that disease is function performed in excess or not enough.

> The cause of every form of disease is the inability of Innate to express her wonted mental functional abilities to a certain organ by means of impulses that are carried and deposited and then placed into action to perform the character of the impulses as given. If hindrance occurs, disease is the result. The character of the disease depending entirely upon what functions are being hindered and to what extent.

D.D. Palmer's Portland Writings

In October 1908, D.D. Palmer moved to Portland, Oregon, started a journal called *The Chiropractor Adjuster*, and opened a school. The second issue of the journal announces: "The D.D. Palmer College of Chiropractic will give you Chiropractic unadulterated—no mixing." The first and only class of students concluded after one year. A two-year program was designed but was not completed because he had a falling-out with his partner, John LaValley, in 1909. After the partnership dissolved, LaValley opened his own school, which has roots to Western States Chiropractic College. D.D. Palmer moved his school to his home at 490 Morrison Street and continued writing.

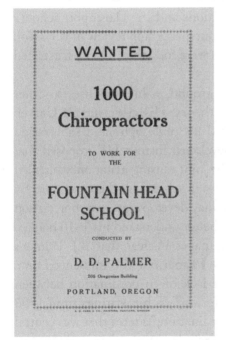 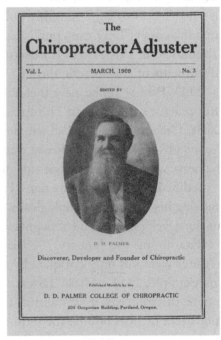

The Chiropractor Adjuster, Vol. 1, March, 1909, No. 3

Six issues of the journal are preserved in the Palmer archives. Numbers 2, 3, 4, 6, and 7 were published between January and December 1909. Number 8 was published in February 1910. Correspondence published in issue Number 2 indicates that Volume 1, Number 1 was published prior to October 16, 1908. The issues are filled with articles, letters, and critiques of other chiropractor's theories, especially those of his son. On page 4 of the January 1909 issue, he writes:

The Adjuster will be the mouth-piece of the original adjuster. It will present Chiropractic normally just as it should be, as it was originally intended to be by the discover. It will adjust all abnormalities found in Chiropractic literature, that right is inherent. This adjusting will be done on crippled literature, with the same pleasure, satisfaction and good feeling as we would that of an injured person.

The many articles and correspondence published during this period were edited and included in D.D. Palmer's 1910 text.

By the time D.D. Palmer moved to Oregon, B.J. Palmer published his own lectures as Vol. 2 and Vol. 3. B.J.'s students in Portland must have shared copies with D.D. because he critiqued those volumes specifically. He also had access to B.J.'s monthly publications and the Davenport school's announcements. D.D. even published a four-paragraph review of B.J.'s Vol. 5, published in 1909. All of B.J.'s writings were fodder for D.D.'s frustrated adjustments of chiropractic theory.

D.D. Palmer broke new theoretical ground in his responses to other chiropractor's ideas about chiropractic theory. His criticisms of Carver, Davis, Gregory, and B.J. Palmer, clarified his philosophy and subluxation theory. His impingement theory was developed further. He proposed that the nerve was impinged on one side of the joint causing irritation, which led to modified physiological functions. He also developed his theory of tone. By studying his writings chronologically, we may develop a greater appreciation for the development of his thoughts and better understand his 1910 book.

Examining the January 1909 issue makes it clear that B.J. Palmer's writings were not only critiqued by D.D. Palmer but also influenced him. For example, D.D. writes, "Disease is a lack of co-oordination between Innate, the source of power and its expression." In his writings from 1906 and earlier he does not use the term "coordination," a term that was central to B.J.'s Vol. 2. However, D.D. Palmer included the new terminology to expand upon his own theories. This was an innovative strength throughout his chiropractic career. He used the ideas that he learned, criticized what he disagreed with, and then used the same terminology to evolve his own ideas. For example, he adopted B.J.'s metaphor of Innate as "the controller," a term he hadn't used before, and writes, "To study functions without Innate—the controller—is like studying creation without a creator."

In his writings of March 1909, D.D. introduces a new viewpoint on Innate. He refers to "Innate's desire" and "the will of Innate." He writes:

The first Chiropractic Adjustment was given Harvey Lillard in September 1895. The principles upon which Chiropractic is based lie in that first vertebral adjustment given by D.D. Palmer. For years he had questioned M.D.s and others asking what difference there was in two persons who were similarly situated, that caused one to have a certain ailment and the other not. That important question was answered by the discovery that displaced (sub-luxated) vertebrae impinged nerves, which are but tubular cords of the same substance as that composing the brain and spinal cord, the functions of which are to convey impulses and sensations to and from the nerve centers. This pressure, caused by projections, modifies the force of Innate's desire, therefore, disease is but aberrated impulse, increased or decreased from that of normal; if it was so in deafness, why not in other diseases? Disease is nothing more or less than functions performed in too great or a less degree than normal; if in natural amount as desired by Innate, we have health. Pressure on nerves causes irritation and tension—result— deranged functions. Why not release the pressure? Why not adjust causes instead of treating effects? Why not?

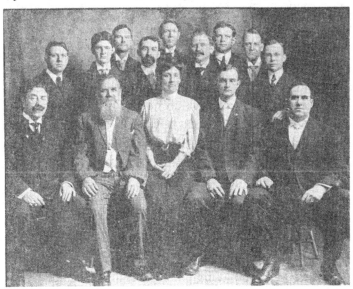

Left to right sitting: Geo S. Breitling, DC; D.D. Palmer; E.L. Farnung, DC, L.M. Gordon, DC; A.N. Briggs, DC. Left to right, standing: Geo Eckerman; L.A. LaJole, DC; F.H. Armstrong; J.E. LaValley, DC; O.H. Scheetz; J.E. Marsh, DC; N.C. Hampton; W.E. Slater; V.K. Tindra, MD. *The Chiropractor's Adjuster* (Jan 1909)

By using terms like "desire" and "will," D.D. Palmer makes Innate theory even more organic and teleological. It gives it qualities that might be described in terms of an intelligent morphic field pushing and pulling the form and function into normality. He writes that the desire itself is normal and cannot be otherwise because it is natural. Later that year, in September, he referred to every vital energetic impulse of Innate as faultless.

Also in March 1909, D.D. Palmer published one of his most iconic passages about man as a "physical and spiritual epitome of the universe." He reasoned that because the spiritual manifests through the physical and controls it as a "conscious intelligence," it is our moral duty to "keep the corporal frame in proper alignment," and:

> become acquainted with the osseous and nervous makeup, that we may intelligently adjust any displaced portion of the skeletal frame so that Innate (that portion of Universal Intelligence usually known as spirit) may manifest itself through and take in a correct knowledge of the material world as the spiritual does of the psychical.

A few years later, he developed this into a full lecture, which was published as part of his final book in 1914, after his death.

In May 1909, D.D. critiques B.J.'s concept of decreased function, and that the transmission is interfering with the flow or current leading to various types of paralysis. He writes, "If a lack of Innate impulse is the cause of disease, then functions would always be below normal in all ailments." B.J. may have responded to this critique in the second edition of Vol. 2, published in 1913, in which he includes a chapter titled *Excess of Function—How?* In the chapter, B.J. offers a rationalization for how decreased transmission may indirectly lead to increased function of other systems. However, even though B.J. built upon these ideas for years, the majority of his writings emphasized decreased function and a spectrum of paralysis in relation to vertebral subluxation. For D.D., disease is always defined as too much or not enough function.

Also in May, D.D. Palmer expanded on his philosophy of mind and Innate. He wrote that mind controls intellectual functions but behind the mind, its source, is the Innate Intelligence. He also concluded that the soul is "life guided by Innate" and "the life principle."

In September 1909, D.D. Palmer critiques an article by Joy Loban, published in *The Chiropractor*. Loban was the head of the philosophy department at PSC Davenport at the time. D.D.'s criticisms are fascinating because it is the first time, that we know of, where he introduces his theories of vibration. D.D. writes, "Molecular vibration as the kinetic energy as the means used by Innate to transmit its impulses, vital functions, the energy of life." Vibration became a central element of D.D. Palmer's theory. His initial writings on the topic in 1909 were in response to writings by B.J. and Loban. This is another case of D.D. using new ideas in the literature to expand and develop his own theories. The vibration theories of D.D., B.J., Loban, and Howard, were related but distinct.

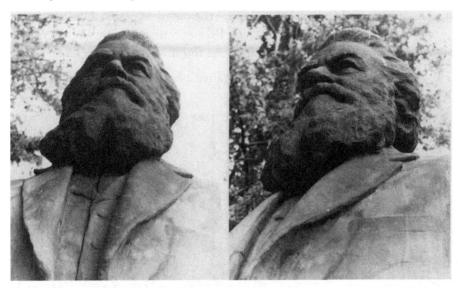

Memorial to D.D. Palmer

Another important contribution to D.D. Palmer's theory of Innate was published in the December 1909 issue. B.J. Palmer may have republished D.D.'s old essay on Innate Intelligence, or D.D. Palmer may have gotten inspired to critique his own earlier writings for other reasons. Perhaps he was still angry because B.J. included the essay in Vol. 1 or that B.J. still listed "Innate Intelligence" for sale by the hundreds in most issues of *The Chiropractor* as *Form 41*. It was listed for sale at least since March 1905. Whatever D.D.'s motivations were, in this issue he updates his own theory, paragraph by paragraph using the same basic style he used when critiquing others. This is the first explicit account in the literature of D.D. Palmer systematically developing his Innate theory. He now considered that Innate retains all knowledge across lifetimes like an ancestral and organic memory passed from one generation of life to the next. He writes, "Innate

knowledge is acquired during life of the species, life of the vertebrata."
Through the "untold ages of adaptation, knowledge and skill in running
vital functions," Innate learned all there is to know about living. In contrast,
Educated begins life without knowledge of the past and acquires it during
life. The commands from Innate are expressed in the vital functions. Innate
is the inherent force that furnishes the mental impulses with energy.

As a precursor to his future writings, using his theories to make the
legal case that chiropractic has a religious foundation, in December 1909
he writes:

> Innate Intelligence embodies the religious plank of the foun-
> dation of Chiropractic. D.D. Palmer was the man who hews
> out that plank and fitted it in the framework of chiropractic.

He viewed this approach as an alternative to the legal strategies of B.J.'s
United Chiropractor's Association.

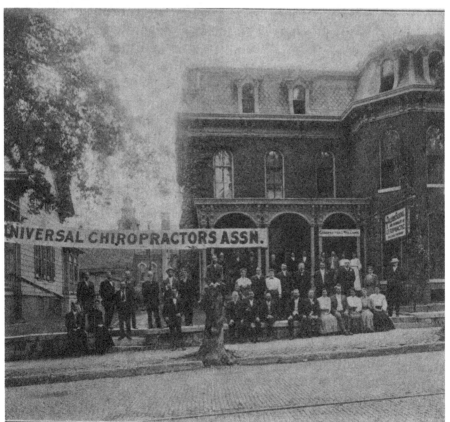

Universal Chiropractor's Assn. *The Chiropractor*, Vol. 3, No. 2 (October 1907)

D.D. Palmer's Second Book (1910)

The last known issue of the journal, *The Chiropractor Adjuster*, is Vol. 8, published in February 1910. This may be because D.D. Palmer spent most of 1910 writing his book, *The Science, Art, and Philosophy of Chiropractic*, or *The Chiropractor's Adjuster*. Many of the articles he published while in Portland were edited and included in the text. Some of the chapters include revisions of older writings. In the book, he expanded on his many theories. For example, in the six issues of *The Chiropractor Adjuster*, he used the term "Innate" 145 times. In the 1910 book he used "Innate" 468 times.

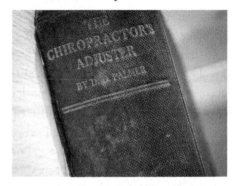

The Chiropractor's Adjuster (1910)

In 1910, D.D. Palmer completely rewrote his 1905 article, *Immortality*, and renamed it *Innate*. This provides us with another public update to his Innate theory. He proposed that the Impulse was a "spontaneous emotion originated by Innate, the spirit." The impulses direct the energy, but it is the vital force, the Innate, or spirit, that runs the body and provides the energy for the impulses. The Innate is behind thought because it produces the thoughts or "thots," which D.D. viewed as "entities." Impulses move thots by vibration or nerve force. The "force of thot rouses energy to action." Energy is the inherent capacity to perform functions. He concludes that Innate cares for the body for as long as "the soul holds spirit and body together."

In 1910, D.D. Palmer also expands on his subluxation theory, his theory of disease, and introduces some new concepts like tone and neuroskeleton, both of which he would develop in his final years. His goal was still to correct or "adjust" misconceptions about what chiropractic is and is not. He critiqued medicine, osteopathy, and various chiropractic luminaries of the day. Like in the articles of 1909, he saved his most incisive critiques for his son, B.J.

D.D. "adjusted" B.J.'s theories in many places. For example, he wrote, "In disease, mental impulses are not impeded, hindered, stopped or cut off—they are modified." And, "I wish that all Chiropractors could take in this basic principle of our science—that too much or not enough energy is disease." This quote contrasts with B.J.'s theory that subluxation leads to decreased quantity flow and decreased function. D.D. also considered that, "The determining causes of disease are traumatism, poison and autosuggestion." This contrasts with B.J.'s theory about subluxations caused by concussions of forces. However, it is not evident that D.D. fully understood all of B.J.'s writings. Reading their texts side-by-side is the best way to research this issue. For example, D.D. writes, "A luxation, or displacement, may be the result of a concussion of bodies—not forces." He felt that the adjustment too, was a concussion of bodies, not forces.

D.D.'s theory of tone was central to the book. On the front page he states that chiropractic was "Founded on Tone." Later in the book he writes:

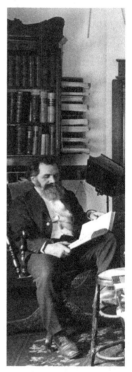

The science and philosophy of Chiropractic is built on tone. The source of every Chiropractic principle, whether physiological or pathological, is founded upon tone. That one word means much to a Chiropractor who desires to comprehend the basis of Chiropractic in its scientific or philosophical phase.

Tone is that state or condition of a body, or any of its organs or parts, in which the organic or animal functions are performed with due vigor.

The tone or tension of muscles and organs depends upon the tonicity of the nervous system.

Tone, in biology, is the normal tension or firmness of nerves, muscles or organs, the renitent, elastic force acting against an impulse. Any deviation from normal tone that, of being too tense or too slack, causes a condition of renitence, too much elastic force, too great resistance, a condition expressed in function as disease.

In the text, D.D. Palmer demonstrates a mastery of the literature on surgery, anatomy, physiology, and pathology of his day. Historians have noted

D.D. Palmer (1903)
-from *Protégé*

that his use of references went above and beyond what the average medical student was studying within a 100 miles of Davenport, Iowa. D.D. Palmer was a self-taught expert in anatomy, physiology, pathology, and all things chiropractic.

Chapter 4
D.D. Palmer's Final Book

Several months after D.D. Palmer's death in 1913, his widow published his revised lecture notes as a small book titled *The Chiropractor*. These lectures contain his final explanations of chiropractic. Appendix 2 establishes that the book was indeed a later version of his teaching notes from 1912 at the Ratledge Chiropractic College and a revision of his notes from the summer of 1913, when he delivered 22 lectures at several chiropractic schools in Davenport. In the book, he develops the concept of neuroskeleton, and expands his theories of tone, Innate, and subluxation. He also explores the legal issues in terms of morality, ethics, and the subjective religious elements of the philosophy.

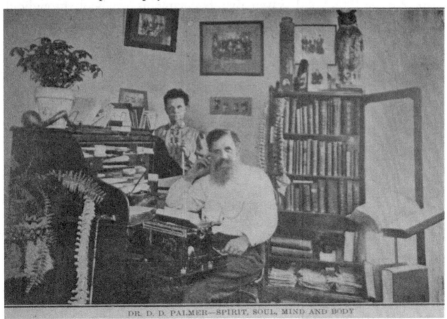

DR. D. D. PALMER—SPIRIT, SOUL, MIND AND BODY

D.D. Palmer and Mary Palmer in Portland
"Dr. D.D. Palmer—Spirit, Soul, Mind and Body" (1910)

Unlike his 1910 book, there are very few direct attacks on B.J. or other chiropractors. Instead, each lecture strives to present the ideas in a straight-forward manner. However, he does include several critical comments. For example, he critiques B.J.'s theory of "direct mental impulse" and contrasts it with neuroanatomy "known by all anatomists." He also includes a few indirect barbs such as, "I originated nerve-tracing and taught it to my early students while the pseudo fountain head was fishing for tadpoles." All in all, these lectures are less contrary than previous writings and more designed to teach. Wherever he briefly mentions the theories of other chiropractors, he does not detract from his focus on his own ideas as the founder, developer, and originator of chiropractic science, art, and philosophy. And rightly so.

Of his previous book, he writes, "In my work on the *Science, Art and Philosophy of Chiropractic* I have given an extensive explanation of the laws of life and nature of disease." Throughout *The Chiropractor* he refers his students to specific pages of the 1910 book, such as his discussion of spinal nerves on page 515, neuralgia on page 472, and his list of references about luxations on pages 189-225, which was titled *Chiropractic Beams of Light*. That chapter was originally published as *Chiropractic Rays of Light* in June 1905 in the PSC journal also named *The Chiropractor*. It was published as a chapter in the 1906 Vol. 1 as well. By referencing his own book throughout the lectures, he makes it evident that these lectures were meant to be supplemented by the textbook. He acknowledges this fact in relation to his discussion of diseases when he writes:

> You will find a brief description of, and where to adjust for, the above diseases in the Adjuster. I prefer to give you some ideas of value not found in the *Science, Art and Philosophy of Chiropractic*. These lectures are intended as an appendix to the *Adjuster*, not a Mail Course, not a Correspondence Course, nor a Post Graduate Course.

It is statements like this that provide further indications that D.D. was planning these lectures as a second book.

Since the lectures were shaped into a book posthumously, not every chapter seems complete, a few of the sentences or paragraphs come across as choppy, and the lectures are not organized in the order D.D. Palmer originally delivered them. For example, at the start of the chapter called *Impulse*, he writes, "In our last lesson we learned that intuition is a knowing without reasoning." That statement is in the lecture on nerve tracing, which comes after *Impulse* in the book. Also, not only is the sequence out-of-order but some of the chapters may have added topics towards the end. For example, the chapter on *Impulse* concludes with several paragraphs about abnormal functions, morbid tissue, biological principles, nerve-tension, vertebral luxations, adjusting, as well as poisons affecting nerves, and various types of nerve pressure. These paragraphs seem to have been tacked onto the lecture or were used at the end of the talk to sum up major chiropractic theories. There is no attempt to tie those ideas in with the main topic of the chapter. Overall, the theories and practices discussed in the book are quite coherent and represent D.D. Palmer's most mature thought.

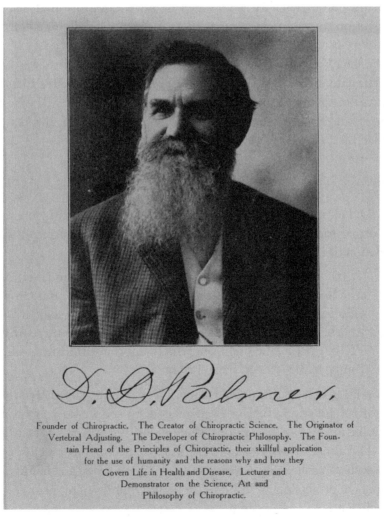

Founder of Chiropractic. The Creator of Chiropractic Science. The Originator of Vertebral Adjusting. The Developer of Chiropractic Philosophy. The Fountain Head of the Principles of Chiropractic, their skillful application for the use of humanity and the reasons why and how they Govern Life in Health and Disease. Lecturer and Demonstrator on the Science, Art and Philosophy of Chiropractic.

The Chiropractor, Author page (1914)

Each chapter of *The Chiropractor* is organized by the lecture's topic. Topics include the art of chiropractic such as palpation, nerve tracing, and vertebral adjusting; lectures on the science including function, impulses, nerve vibration, the nervous system, and a lecture on normal and abnormal spinal movements; also, lectures on philosophy, biology, life, death, disease, and health, as well as lectures on trauma, toxins, and auto-suggestion, and also on the moral and religious duty of a chiropractor. He had several lectures on pathophysiological processes such as Inflammation, Rachitis or Rickets, Neuritis, Arteritis, Rheumatism, Fever, Constipation and Costiveness, Catarrh, Pyorrhea Alveolaris, and Spinal Pathogenesis. Rather than follow the chapter order, which was arranged by his widow, this brief discussion will focus on the main chiropractic ideas of the book with an emphasis on the evolution of his theories.

The language that D.D. Palmer used to define his terms was specific and articulate. Because of that we have decided to explore his theories by contextualizing several important quotes in a logical order. The best way to understand his meaning is to read his words directly. For this reason we included his *Brief Review* lecture as Appendix 3.

Tone

D.D. Palmer first wrote about tone in relation to healthy organ tone and normal function in 1896 and 1899. By 1910, he declared it was the foundation of chiropractic. In 1914, he writes:

> Its science is based on tone. Tone is the standard from which we note the variations of structure, temperature, tonicity, elasticity, renitency and tension; it is the standard of health; any deviation therefrom is disease. Tone is the BASIC PRINCIPLE, the one from which all other principles, which compose the science, have sprung.

The condition of a healthy organ is tone, which relates to normal physiology and normal function. Tension is regulated by the neuroskeleton and is observable in the tone and vigor of the tissues.

D.D. Palmer's theory of tone is still relevant today. A recent paper by McDowall and colleagues suggests tone could be used as an identity for the chiropractic profession as an interface between philosophy, neurology, and biomedicine.

Biological Principles

D.D. Palmer felt it was essential for "scientific chiropractors" to understand the principles of chiropractic. He writes, "The principles which compose the science of chiropractic have existed as long as animals have had backbones." He concluded that physiology was the best way to describe the principles of living organisms. Furthermore, any discussion of biology should focus on physiological functions, "the processes, activities and the phenomena incidental to life." In that regard he found that chiropractic was the study of functions not the study of anatomy or structure only.

In relation to principles he writes:

> Chiropractic is a science and an art. The philosophy of chiropractic consists of the reasons given for the principles which compose the science and the movements which have to do with the art.

This view of the philosophy of chiropractic as the exploration of principles, related to the science and art, was central to his approach. The philosophy was also viewed as the explanation of health and disease according to biological principles.

Health and Disease

D.D. Palmer viewed the nerve impulses as conveyors of thoughts or commands. Health results when these impulses "are carried over nerves" that are under normal tension, structure, renitency, and firmness, or normal tone. He felt that this view of health allows us to understand that disease is not an entity but a process. He writes:

> Disease consists of a change in structure, position or function. Disease is a disturbed condition, functions performed abnormally, in too great a degree or not enough; it is not something foreign to the body which by some means enters it; it is not a thing of enmity which we have to fight.
>
> Disease does not involve any new functional expression which it did not already possess. Disease is a manifestation of too much or not enough energy. Energy is liberated force; in the living being it is known as vital force.

Disease is "a deviation from tone" because of the abnormal structure and the consequent result of too much or not enough energy, which is a condition favorable to the proliferation of other pathological processes.

Normal living tissue is a coexistence of quality and functionating or the living act of functioning. In this sense, disease may be understood as "abnormal functionating and morbid tissue." Thus, health is normal physiology and pathology is physiology modified. He writes:

> Pathology is modified physiology. Pathological operations are physiological acts modified. Processes which are pathological are but modified functional movements. Physiological impulses may become pathological in their expression.

Also, he writes, "behind all abnormal functions, is the change in the structure of nerve tissue and an increase or decrease of nerve vibration." When the impulse is normal, the force of the impulse, which is related to the rate of vibration, is normal. Energy is then utilized normally. This is intelligent action, which D.D. simply defines as life.

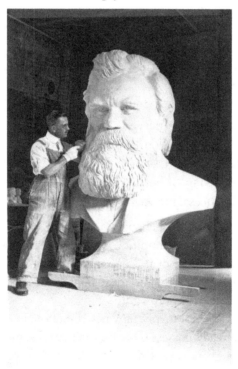

Sculpting the D.D. Palmer bust

Life and Death

The Chiropractor is clearly a culmination of a lifetime of contemplation and research guided by clinical practice. D.D. Palmer writes, "My ideas concerning health, disease, life and death have been greatly modified by years of careful research." These lectures summed up his final thoughts on all things chiropractic, central to which were his views on life and death. After all, he defined chiropractic as "the science of life," because it answers the question, "what is life?"

He defined life as "actions guided by intelligence" and death as the result of natural law. Of death he writes that it is "a situation wherein action has ceased to be controlled by intelligence." For decades, Palmer graduates referred to death as when the body ceases adapting to the environment. Vitality is the active principle that life depends on.

Vital Force and Energy

D.D. Palmer viewed life in terms of the flow of forces and energies. His viewpoint is congruent with his other theories about normal and abnormal functioning. The resources the body has available in health or disease are of paramount importance. He writes:

> The body is incapable of creating new forces. Force is that which originates or arrests motion. Vital force is the energy which gives life or action to an organism, the vital power which distinguishes living matter from dead. Organic force is the inherent vigor latent in an organ. Nerve force is the power or ability to conduct impulses. Reserve force is the energy which is stored in an organ or organism that is not required for normal functionating. Intelligent actions are the expressions of the sum total of life. This intelligence is able to accumulate and store energy derived from without. Certain fixed and definite conditions release this energy.

This idea that the body derives energy from the environment and utilizes it for organic functioning, storing a reserve, and releasing the excess, was also described in detail by B.J. Palmer in 1909. This may be another instance where B.J.'s research and theory influenced D.D. Palmer. Also, this is a viewpoint that is congruent with late twentieth-century theoretical biology such as the theory of Nobel Laureate Ilya Prigogine, who demonstrated how the living system utilizes the energy from the environment to further its own self-organization as a nonlinear, far-from-equilibrium, dissipative structure.

For D.D. Palmer, vital force is the energy utilized by living processes inherent to each organ. Energy is an internal power and the product of functional activity. It is aroused by impulses.

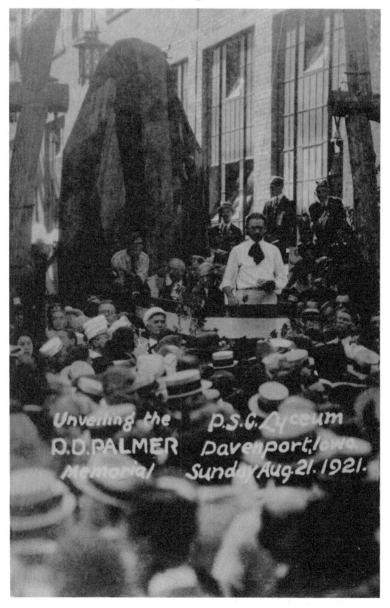

B.J. Palmer at the podium dedicating the D.D. Palmer Memorial (1921)

Impulse

According to D.D. Palmer, the impulse was crucial because it is what incites the action that characterizes living. He viewed impulses as distinct entities, thoughts created by intelligent beings. Impulses are transmitted by nerve vibration in response to a normal stimulus, "furnished by Innate, the spirit, a segment of Universal Intelligence." The impetus of the impulse, its force, is dependent upon the tension of the nerve itself. So the impulse is directly affected by too much or too little tension and the nerve's ability to transmit the nerve-vibration.

D.D. Palmer classified impulses as sensory or motor, which, he said, was in contrast to B.J.'s lumping all impulses into one category as "mental impulses." Motor impulses are controlled by the will (Educated) and sensory impulses are controlled by the spirit (Innate), which also controls functions of organic processes. A sense impression is made from the environment, "it is no more or less than a recognition of nerve vibration, which is set in motion by the force of a sensational impulse." This theory is very similar to B.J. Palmer's Normal Complete Cycle, from Vol. 5, which D.D. Palmer briefly reviewed in 1910. This may be another case of how D.D. built on the ideas of others to further develop his own theory.

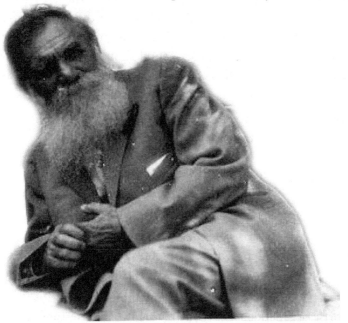

D.D. Palmer visiting Davenport (1913)

D.D. Palmer's impulse theory was central to his theories of life, function, and chiropractic. He writes:

> Life (intelligent action) is the response to an impulse. This is true of the voluntary and involuntary functions. The former are those of the human will, the latter are those of the spirit. The impulse in transit is the thought sent out, it always remains the same in its requirement and command; however, its force may be augmented or decreased, owing to the amount of nerve vibration.

Impulses cannot be obstructed or hindered, only modified. Nerve tension modifies impulses.

Neuroskeleton as a Nerve-tension Frame

D.D. Palmer first used the term neuroskeleton in his 1910 book to refer to the endoskeleton, "the backbone," and the way in which "normal tension is extended to the nervous system by its attachment and extension to the neuroskeleton." His neuroskeleton model combined with his theory that the transmission of impulses is modified by tension, may be viewed in the same context as Alf Breig's neurosurgery paradigm of the late twentieth century. Breig demonstrated that the biomechanics of the central nervous system, due to the attachments of the cord at both ends of the spine, may lead to a decrease of the transmission of neural signals because of adverse mechanical tension pulling on the cord and the dural sleeves of the spinal nerves. D.D. Palmer writes:

> Physicians and surgeons knew of and have taught nerve-tension; neurectasia, nerve–stretching and nerve vibration. They have used, and so have osteopaths, the stretching of nerves as a therapeutical agent for many years. I was the first to assume that the neuroskeleton was a nerve tension-frame.

In his 1910 book, D.D. Palmer cites Landois as his source for understanding how nerve-stretching was used as a therapy. He concluded that Landois' theory was congruent with chiropractic principles. He writes:

> Landois' statement agrees with one of the earliest principles of Chiropractic, viz., that a light impingement increases tension with an increase of functional activity; whereas, a heavy pressure causes a lack of tension and tonicity, a condition we name Paralysis.

According to Landois, the stretching acts as an irritant. Light stretching led to increased activity and "stronger stretching" diminished activity and eventually led to paralysis.

Chiropractic vertebral subluxation theorists from the 1930s to the 1960s linked these ideas of D.D. Palmer's to the theory of A.D. Speransky. Speransky's extensive research established a theory of medicine based on neurodystrophic processes of abnormal patterns that were self-perpetuating in the nervous system and thus neuropathic. Several chiropractors concluded that Speranksy proved the basic neurological principles that chiropractic was based upon.

D.D. Palmer also wrote of his knowledge of the medical literature on nerve-pressure. He writes:

> The different kinds of nerve-pressure have been known to physicians and surgeons. I have added nothing new on pressure. However, I am the first to state that displacements of the joints of the tension-frame cause nerves to become more tense than normal, thereby creating disease.

He viewed the neuroskeleton as a "regulator of tension" when the articular surfaces "have not been forcibly displaced, separated from their normal bearings." He concluded that articular processes "not in normal contact, partially displaced are disease producers." This was the core of his vertebral subluxation theory.

D.D. Palmer (1890s)

Vertebral Subluxation

In his lecture called *Vertebral Luxations*, D.D. Palmer describes the chiropractic focus on the incomplete luxation, with the "articular surfaces slightly displaced" in relation to each other. When these displacements of the vertebrae occur, nerves are impinged upon, or stretched, leading to irritation. He referred to this as a "contraction of nerve tissue" and tension. He writes:

> Tension, more or less than normal, causes an increase or decrease of vibration, which means a greater or less force of an impulse and a corresponding amount of heat.

Too much or not enough tension changes the renitence of the tissues, the ability to "bound back" is affected. This leads to "deranged function" because the nerves convey the impulses that "create functions." Restoring the vertebra to the normal position leads to normal function.

Any of the 200 bones, mainly of the spine, could put pressure on nerves. He felt that 95% of all disease was directly caused by subluxated joints of the spine and the other 5% related to other joints. He writes:

> About 95 per cent of all diseases are accompanied by slightly displaced articulations the vertebra is not displaced—the sliding movement of the articulations are increased beyond the normal—consequently, increasing the size of the foramen on one, or the foramina on both sides.

Based on his mastery of the literature, he concluded that he was the first to correct vertebral subluxations by replacing the articular processes. He writes:

> Vertebral luxations have been known for many years. I was the first to affirm that slightly luxated joints, those in which the articular surfaces had exceeded their normal limit of movement and there becomes fixed, was quite common...
>
> To D.D. Palmer rightfully belongs the credit of replacing displaced vertebral articulations.

To relieve the tense nerves from the impingement was the central practice of chiropractic and the focus of its philosophy. He writes, "Chiropractors philosophize on the art of relieving abnormal conditions by adjusting displaced bones." When the impingement is released, Innate is freed up to transmit and receive the impulses in a normal fashion.

Pinching versus Impinging

D.D. Palmer concluded that other chiropractors who had previously relied on the "pinching model" of vertebral subluxation were adopting his use of the term "impingement" incorrectly. He had used the term since 1897 but only in his final years did he clearly differentiate it from the pinching terminology. One term refers to being pinched between two objects and the other term refers to being impinged upon. It is the difference of against versus between. Nerve tension, or the stretching of nerves was due to vertebra pressing against them not pinching them.

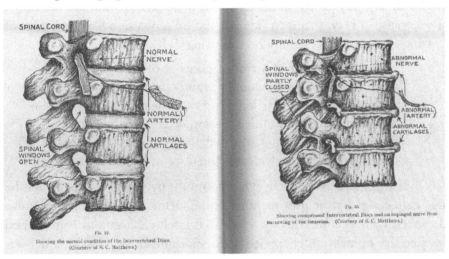

D.D. Palmer referred to these illustrations, especially Fig. 33 from Gregory's 1910 book, *Spinal Adjustment*, to demonstrate Gregory's error. D.D. corrects Gregory by stating, "The spinal nerves and their branches may be impinged upon or against, or stretched because of displaced vertebra, but not pinched."

D.D. Palmer's definition of the vertebral subluxation as a displacement of articular surfaces and his theory of stretched and impinged nerves were directly related. He writes:

Nerves are never pinched or impinged upon in the foramina. Foramina are never narrowed. WE DO NOT ADJUST THE VERTEBRA. The vertebra itself, so far as a chiropractor knows, is never displaced, dislocated or subluxated.

Any extreme movement of the articular surfaces enlarges the foramen or foramina, causes the nerves and blood vessels to become stretched, irritated, increasing its carrying power.

Nerves are never shut off by the closure of the foramina. There are no dams or obstructions that restrict. Impulses are never interrupted.

Reducing the luxated intervertebral articulation; diminishing the displacement of the articular processes, replacing the two articular surfaces, returns the enlarged foramen to its normal size, removes tension and irritation. Irritated nerves cause muscular contraction. The location and amount of disturbance depends upon the portion of the nervous system involved.

D.D. Palmer was focused on the open side of the articulation not the closed side because only on the open side was there a protrusion like the bridge of a stringed instrument pushing on the strings. He writes:

The arch or bar of a violin, guitar or other stringed instrument, which gives permanency to and causes the wires or strings to be tensely stretched, do not prevent the passage of vibration. An impingement modifies tension, it changes the amount of vibration, but does not obstruct the course of an impulse; it simply augments or decreases the force of an impulse.

In this regard, by defining what he meant by vertebral subluxation he was correcting the theories of other chiropractors, especially B.J. He also disagreed with B.J. on etiology, whereas B.J. felt subluxations were caused by excessive or awkwardly applied concussions of forces, D.D.'s model was more complex. He considered not only trauma but also the role of poisons and thoughts.

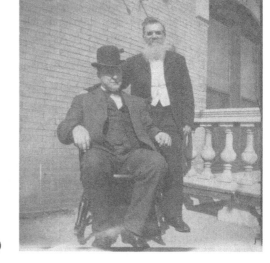

Palmer and Gregory (1908)

Trauma, Toxins, and Autosuggestion

D.D. describes three different etiologies of vertebral subluxation: trauma, toxins, and autosuggestion. He writes:

> Trauma the cause of disease, increasing or decreasing function, is direct in displacing osseous tissue. Poisons as causes are indirect, they act on nerves, nerves on muscles, their combined action draw vertebrae out of alignment.
>
> Autosuggestion may be therapeutical, curative, or morbific, causing hysteric paralysis, contraction of muscles, impairment of vision, convulsions, sensory disturbances and psychic manifestations. A change of thought is restful, but a constant continuation of the same thought, using the selfsame nerves, causes nerve disturbance and some form of insanity, and yet there is no discernible lesion of the nervous system.

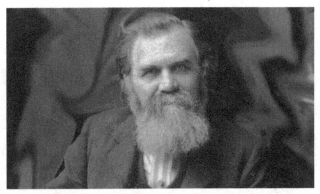

D.D. Palmer (1902)

He felt that traumatism was a direct cause because it displaced the bones immediately. Poisons and autosuggestion were indirect. In those cases, vertebra are drawn "out of alignment by the contraction of nerves and muscles."

His theories of etiology impacted the profession in various ways because his students like Carver, Ratledge, Drain, and Cooley led the profession for decades. Chiropractors, starting in the 1950s, linked D.D.'s theories to Selye's stress model. By the 1970s Selye's theories were thoroughly integrated into vertebral subluxation theory. In the 1980s, chiropractic theorists and researchers linked stress theory to morphological changes of the spinal cord by combining the chiropractic paradigm with Breig and Selye. Some even suggested the stress response led to an inflammatory reaction of the meninges, exacerbating the vertebral subluxation patterns.

Inflammation

Inflammation was an important concept to D.D. Palmer. He considered it to be a result of disturbed function, which led to "modified physiological processes." He wrote that he first recognized the relationship between vertebral subluxations and inflammation in terms of nerves heating the blood, on July 1, 1903, at his Palmer Chiropractic School at Santa Barbara. That school was short-lived. His article on the discovery was published in the 1906 Vol. 1 and in his 1910 book. He proposes that inflammation is involved with most diseases and possibly all of them. In his 1910 book he included photos of the class he was teaching in 1903 alongside the story.

In the 1914 book, D.D. Palmer proposed that neuritis, or the inflammation of nerves, involves increased sensitivity of the skin. He notes that microscopic studies demonstrate swollen myelin sheaths and a changed structure of nerves. The change in tissues decreases the vibration and "the carrying quality of impulses." This type of morbid change in the tissues is always related to "abnormal functionating." He found that the skin sensitivity presents clinically as a lengthwise contraction that is hardened and "enlarged diametrically."

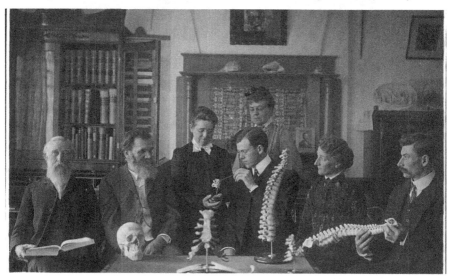

D.D. Palmer with students in Santa Barbara, 1903
- From *The Chiropractor's Protégé*

Palpation and Nerve Tracing

Chiropractors examine the position of vertebra and use palpation to physically diagnose "the condition and pathway of subdermal nerves." It requires a "discriminating touch" by sensitive, practiced fingers. The art of nerve tracing and palpation requires practice.

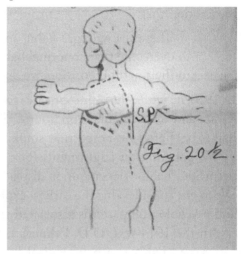

Nerve Tracing diagram from O.G. Smith's unpublished vade mecum, titled *Chiropractic*, page 135. (1899) Demonstrating a sore throat coming from an injured nerve at S.P. (From the Smith papers.)

D.D. Palmer concluded that nerve tracing, which he developed, is distinct from older medical approaches of determining "the condition of subcutaneous organs." He writes:

> The chiropractor should trace sensitive, swollen, longitudin-ally contracted nerves, for the purpose of locating their imp-ingement and tension. By palpation he determines the one or more spinous processes which project posterior of the normal outline. The projection of the displaced spinous process is in the direction of the bend; in the cervical it is an anterior, in the dorsal posterior and ventral in the lumbar. In a practice of twenty-five years I have only known one case of reversed kyphosis and lordosis which I relieved by adjusting the twelfth dorsal. There is no better way to locate the cause of disease, or demonstrate to a prospective patient how bones and nerves are related to each other and why such relationship accounts for health and disease, than by palpation and nerve-tracing.

This practice allows the chiropractor to determine the affected organ and the subdermal innervation related to it. The sensitivity to touch is a sign that there is an abnormal condition.

Habit Grooves of the Nervous System

D.D. Palmer first wrote about habit in relation to chiropractic in January 1897, in relation to the first care plans. He wrote that he did not know how long it would take for patients to be cured. Some may take a treatment or two, others may take weeks or months. The key factor was a recognition that:

> There is a wrong, a habit, an error, and how long it will take to overcome that abnormal habit and get the parts accustomed to their natural position, we don't know.

In 1910, he wrote that "chiropractic is able to cope with insanity, pernicious habits and other mental conditions." He also wrote that he adjusted for habits only after he noted that smoking and liquor were sometimes quit by the patient after adjustments for other conditions. He concluded that pernicious habits "depend upon displaced vertebrae for their continuance." We might consider this the earliest explanation of structural, physiological, and psychological patterns associated with vertebral subluxation.

In the 1914 text, D.D. Palmer's theory of habit is developed further. He viewed habit as a neurological function. He proposes that biological functions as well as inherited predispositions in regards to health are simply habits. He writes:

> Hexiology is the science of habits. A habit is a tendency to perform the same spontaneous action under similar circumstances. Habit applies to individuals, instinct to ancestors. Habits acquired through our ancestors are known as instinct.
>
> Organic habits may be acquired by the physical organism during the life of an individual or of a race. The system of bodily processes of the physiological organism has been acquired through past generations.
>
> Constant practice, frequent repetition, habitual custom, confirms habit until it becomes a function. Mental or organic habits are acquired through the education of the nervous system.

He refers to Sherrington's 1905 theory of reflex action, without citing the reference, and suggests chiropractors should comprehend it. He defines reflex action in terms of "bounding back" of impulses. This is the essence of renitency or tone. He writes, "The amount of function depends upon the renitency, the impulsive force obtained by the bounding back, the reflex action." He also writes, "habits are really acquired reflex actions. Habit trains certain nerve centers." He expands on this theory when he writes:

> Every time we think, each time we act, a record is made. Each repetition of a thought, each performance of an act deepens the groove of habit, mental or physical; it renders the next similar impulse or movement more automatic until in time the nervous system becomes like a phonograph disk; without apparent consciousness we find ourselves guilty of repetition. Habits become our master and we its slave.

Palmer's intent was to develop an alternative explanation for hereditary disease processes. In doing so, he developed a pioneering neurological habit model. D.D. Palmer's habit theory shares similarities with Ukhtomsky's theory of *the dominant* developed at his research center in St. Petersburg, and also with physiological models of dynamical attractor basins such as Goodwin's theory of life and Sheldrake's theory of morphic resonance, especially in relation to the patterns of the past.

D.D. Palmer also extends his theory of habit to right living. He writes:

> Pure air, clean water, unadulterated food and thoughts free from error and vulgarism will form cleanly habits of mind and body.

Good habits lead to health and pernicious habits weaken the individual physically and morally. He writes:

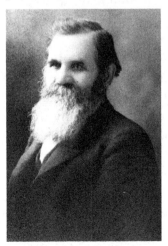

> In biology our environments are the aggregate of all the external conditions and influences affecting the life and development of an organism. In a measure we regulate our surroundings, giving but little thought of individual and organic habits. Pernicious habits may become fastened upon the human will, weaken vitality and bore tunnels through the reservoirs of force and character. Self-respect and restraint of passions are as essential to longevity as prophylaxis, the science and art of retaining the health.

D.D. Palmer (1906)

Organism and Environment

Central to D.D. Palmer's paradigm is that the organism successfully adapts to the environment when in a state of normal health. He writes:

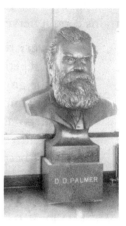

> Through the nervous system the intellectual receives all impressions and appreciation of the outer world. Nerve vibration is associated with consciousness. By and through it thon adapts itself to thon's environments.

The function of interacting with the environment is controlled by waking consciousness; the Educated Intelligence.

D.D. Palmer bust

Consciousness

Educated has its own senses; feeling and sensation, which derive impressions from the body's senses. Consciousness or "conscious intelligence" perceives the stimulus from the environment. Educated is conscious of the impressions. This conscious observation of the interaction with the environment involves "perception, apprehension, recognition, understanding, discernment and appreciation of our physical surroundings." And, according to D.D. Palmer, these objective observations of subjective experience are "increased by occult intuition and spiritual instinct." Intuition and instinct are described as "the ability of knowing and the power of acting without the assistance of reason."

He is describing three levels of Educated's awareness. The first level is the sensory impression of feeling and sensation. The second level uses reason to understand the impressions. Thus the conscious intelligence observes the sense impressions from the environment not only from a first-person experiential perspective but also from a third-person objective perspective. The third level, involving instinct and intuition, involves two types of knowing that are unrelated to reason but are still utilized by the Educated Intelligence, the conscious mind.

Instinct is described as an "inward unconscious principle" and intuition as a result of "inward consciousness." D.D. Palmer describes intuitive knowing as the innate tendency to act based on ancestral organic habits.

Additionally, D.D. Palmer posits that intuition is affected by the health of the body or the "variations of tone." Furthermore, a modification of the senses associated with intuition impacts the "actions of instinctive consciousness." He writes, "Intuitive knowing and instinctive action are determined by organic habits and unconscious sensation without thought or volition." His theory of consciousness was set in the context of his theory of Innate.

Innate

Intelligence is everywhere in the body because of the nerves. D.D. Palmer writes:

> Do not forget for one moment that all organic functions are the characteristic work of organs or an organism directed by an intelligence known as spirit. This intellectual being transmits its impulses, its commands, over the nervous system by molecular vibration.

Innate not only runs the body and keeps the living system organized but it is that which keeps the organism alive. He writes:

> What is that which is present in the living body and absent in the dead? It is an intelligent force, which I saw fit to name Innate, usually known as spirit. It creates and continues life when the vital organs are in a condition to be acted upon by that intelligence.

He refers to the two intelligences as; Innate and Educated; spirit and mind; creator and created.

His theory of Innate became the central way he expanded on the philosophy and summed up his many theories. He writes:

> Innate is embodied as a personified part of Universal Intelligence, therefore, co-eternal with the all creative force. This indwelling portion of the Eternal is in our care for improvement. The intellectual expansion of Innate is in proportion to the normal transmission of impulses over the nervous system; for this reason the body functions should be kept in the condition of tone.

Viewing Innate as a co-eternal creative force, the embodiment of Universal Intelligence, took on greater importance in his final writings.

On The Revelation and Inspiration

D.D. Palmer says that chiropractic was "revealed" to him so that he could enlighten the world. He writes:

> It is not surprising that those who have given to the world its greatest and grandest thoughts have been, more or less, connected with those who had passed into the spiritual existence.

He specifically states that an "intelligent spiritual being" named Dr. Jim Atkinson, who practiced in Davenport fifty years ago, provided him with "the underlying principles of Chiropractic." In the 1910 book, *The Chiropractor's Adjuster*, he writes of frequent communication:

> Dr. Atkinson has frequently informed me that replacing of displaced vertebrae for the relief of human ills had been known and practiced by ancient Egyptians for at least 3000 years.

Adding to these mysterious claims from D.D. Palmer, is this statement, published in the 1914 book:

> The method by which I obtained an explanation of certain physical phenomena, from an intelligence in the spiritual world, is known in biblical language as inspiration. In a great measure *The Chiropractor's Adjuster* was written under such spiritual promptings.

There are several ways we might interpret this claim based on historical facts in the context of psychological and sociological interpretations.

In terms of historical facts, we now know, based on a recent article by Foley, that an actual Dr. William Benjamin Atkinson practiced in Davenport in 1854. We also know from D.D. Palmer's private letters that he didn't only describe such experiences in public lectures and writings but also in private letters and conversations.

In letters to John Howard, written in 1906, D.D. Palmer wrote of his "spirit friends" guiding him and how he discussed this with his brother T.J. On June 4, 1906, he writes about his and B.J.'s falling out, "My spirit friends prophesied our dissolution, of which I told T.J." In another letter he writes, "My spirit friends told me, a short time before my wife died, that B.J. and I would not hold together." He also wrote that he felt he was being led "for what or where I do not know." These letters help us to understand that D.D. Palmer believed his inspirations came from the spiritual world.

These interior experiences were related to D.D. Palmer's beliefs and his philosophy. This was explored in *Secret History* and *Traveling Library* in relation to the Spiritualist culture and modern psychological interpretations.

Interpreting D.D. Palmer's claim of a "revelation" from the spirit realm, from historical, psychological, and social viewpoints, makes it more complex, and yet, perhaps it should remain so. For example, D.D. Palmer was a Spiritualist and a magnetic healer for two decades prior to adjusting Harvey Lillard. He collected many books on these topics starting in the 1880s, some of which are preserved in the Palmer archives. It was a common rhetorical strategy for authors of books on magnetic healing to give credit to "spirits" of famous doctors of the past. One book preserved in the archives was Andrew Stone's *The New Gospel of Health: An effort to teach people The Principles of Vital Magnetism: Or, How to Replenish the Springs of Life Without Drugs or Stimulants*. The copy in the archives includes the following inscription on the front page, "Dr. D.D. Palmer's, Davenport, Iowa. Aug.6.1888." He wrote small numbers in the margins on some of the pages. The preface to the book begins when Stone writes:

> We desire to be brief and explicit in narrating in what way and manner we are connected with this book. Some five years since, we received, through a medium of known integrity and ability, a communication, purporting to come from Sir Astley Cooper and Sir Benjamin Brodie, informing me that they, in connection with my Spirit-Band, numbering some eighteen or more physicians, who had stood at the head of their profession when in earth-life, desired to communicate some twenty short sections upon different medical subjects, for me to publish.

Perhaps D.D. Palmer was inspired by authors like Stone. And, perhaps authors like D.D. and Stone interpreted their own spiritual experiences and inspirations from the perspective of their cultural worldview; Spiritualism.

Another curious historical fact related to D.D. Palmer's revelation was published in *Protégé*. D.D.'s partner in the Santa Barbara School was O.G. Smith. After they left California because of legal troubles, they moved to Chicago to start a school in 1904. Smith noted on the back of one of his essays that D.D. Palmer wanted to practice close to the state line so that he could flee the jurisdiction. He also noted that D.D. was considering a religious legal strategy by viewing himself in the same light as the founder of Christian Science. A decade later, D.D. Palmer crafted this into an argument for a future legal strategy.

Proposed Religious Legal Strategy

In the first chapter of the 1914 book, D.D. Palmer describes a moral and ethical vision for chiropractic; and also proposes an alternative legal strategy to the one advocated by his son and the U.C.A.

At the start of his presentation on the moral and religious duties of the chiropractor, D.D. notes that this lecture often received more applause than any other but only after misconstrued criticism. He writes:

> The following has been sharply criticized by a few chiro-practors... A part of this criticism was based upon rival jealousy, the balance because of wrong impressions. That which was on account of a lack of information discontinued as soon as the would-be critics were well informed. I have received greater applause at the close of the following lecture from my classes than from any other. Every important chiropractic idea that I have advanced has been bitterly assailed, yet, although some-what discouraged at times, I have not turned from that which I knew was correct.

In the lecture, he describes his new ideas about morality, ethics, duty, and personal religion.

The lecture begins with a brief treatise on the U.S. Constitution's clause that "Congress shall make no law respecting an established religion, or prohibiting the free exercises thereof." He then cites medical laws from states such as Kansas, Virginia, Washington, and Illinois, in which medical practices are limited from discriminating against the practice of religion. He emphasized his home state's California Medical Act of 1913, with its clause against religious discrimination.

D.D. Palmer proposes that since chiropractic unites the physical and the spiritual, laws preventing chiropractors from removing nerve tension are an "unmitigated crime against humanity," because it prevents "physical, mental and spiritual develop-ment." He viewed chiropractic as a subjective religion or a "religion of chiropractors."

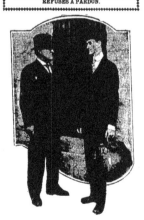

FIGHTING FOR PRINCIPLE, CHIROPRACTOR REFUSES A PARDON.

Dr. T.F. Ratledge, at right, going to jail with Deputy Sheriff Ehring

The case against Ratledge started in 1913. He spent 90 days in jail in California rather than receive a license as a drugless practitioner. *The Fort Wayne Sentinel* (May 18, 1916)

Spiritual But Not Religious

D.D. Palmer felt that believing in mysterious, supernormal, supernatural, and occult forces was a distortion, which developed from personal experience, the direct knowledge of the Divine. He referred to religious beliefs as "the morbid outgrowth of subjective religion." Today, this type of distinction is referred to as being spiritual but not religious. Individuals have direct experiences that are religious or spiritual without being associated or affiliated with traditional religion.

D.D. Palmer concluded that cultivating spiritual experiences was a systematic development of knowledge. He referred to it as "scientific religion" because it was based on personal evidence not on faith or belief. He felt that "knowledge is superior to faith and belief." He defined faith as the unification of trust and belief. Belief is more intellectual and requires acceptance of some truth beyond personal experience. Knowledge is based on direct and personal evidence, which may be different between two people.

According to D.D. Palmer, chiropractic is based on principles, practices, scientific facts, and moral obligations. Based on these, he considered that chiropractic consists of a "subjective religion" as opposed to a traditional "objective religion."

He distinguished between objective religion, which includes rituals and practices associated with magic, theology, superstition, secret forces, and Deity worship; and "subjective ethical religion," which is concerned with "the existence, character, and attributes of God, the All-pervading Universal Intelligence." He writes:

> Subjective religion includes the moral and religious duty, the inner intellectual feeling, the science which treats of the existence, character and attributes of God and His laws regarding our duty toward him.

This form of religion deals with ethical practice and phenomena that can be known. People of any religion may be upstanding practicing chiropractors.

Since chiropractors assist individuals to experience the union between spirit and matter, they perform a subjective ethical religious duty. Because chiropractors are also assisting the sick to get well, which transforms this life and the hereafter, they have a moral obligation to practice chiropractic.

By understanding the basic principle and also the "philosophy of the science and art of vertebral adjusting," chiropractic practice may be understood as a moral obligation and a religious duty, which transcends all beliefs and faiths.

Chiropractic as a Moral Obligation and a Religious Duty

The moral duty of the chiropractor is distinct from the science, art, and philosophy of chiropractic. He concludes that "The practice of chiropractic includes a moral obligation and a religious duty." Knowledge of chiropractic science is the essential step to "comprehend these responsibilities."

It is also a moral duty because we carry with us into the next life all that we find necessary in this life. Thus it is our duty to care for our physical bodies. D.D. Palmer writes:

> The philosophy of chiropractic teaches the Universality of Intelligence and that its aim is always onward and upward toward perfection. This truth makes the practice of chiropractic a moral and a religious duty both in theory and in fact.

Also, he writes:

> Morally, chiropractors are in duty bound to help humanity physically. Religiously, they are required to render spiritual service toward God, the Universal Intelligence, by relieving mankind of their fetters, adjusting the tension frame of the nervous system, the physical lines of communication to and from the spirit… By correcting the skeletal frame the spirit is permitted to assume normal control, and produce normal expression.

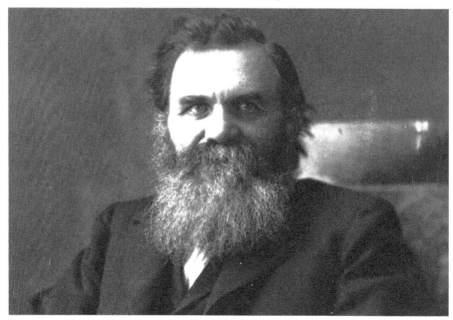

D.D. Palmer's Doctrine

D.D. Palmer writes:

There is no living religion without a doctrine; a doctrine however elaborate, does not constitute a religion. The doctrine of our principles, faith and knowledge are as follow:

I believe, in fact know, that the universe consists of Intelligence and Matter. This intelligence is known to the Christian world as God. As a spiritual intelligence it finds expression through the animal and vegetable creation, man being the highest manifestation. I believe that this Intelligence is segmented into as many parts as there are individual expressions of life; that spirit, whether considered as a whole or individually, is advancing upward and onward toward perfection; that in all animated nature this Intelligence is expressed through the nervous system, which is the means of communication to and from individualized spirit; that the condition known as TONE is the tension and firmness, the renitency and elasticity of tissue in a state of health, normal existence; that the mental and physical condition known as disease is a disordered state because of an unusual amount of tension above or below that of tone; that normal and abnormal amounts of strain or laxity are due to the position of the osseous framework, the neuroskeleton, which not only serves as a protector to the nervous system, but, also, as a regulator of tension; that Universal Intelligence, the Spirit as a whole or in its segmented parts, is eternal in its existence; that physiological disintegration and somatic death are changes of the material only; that the present and future make-up of individualized spirits depend upon the cumulative mental function which, like all other functions, is modified by the structural condition of the impulsive, transmitting, nervous system; that criminality is but the result of abnormal nervous tension; that our individualized, segmented spiritual entities carry with them into the future spiritual state that which has been mentally accumulated during our physical existence; that spiritual existence, like the physical, is progressive; that a correct understanding of these principles and the practice of them constitute the religion of chiropractic; that the existence and personal identity of individualized intelligences continue after the change known as death; that life in this world and the next is continuous—one of eternal progression.

The doctrine concludes with:

> The controlling intelligence is everywhere present, manifesting through the nervous system its desires for advancement, making use of these nerve centers as receiving and distributing stations.

> The founder of chiropractic has located the spirit in man, found its abiding place to be throughout the entire body, a position from which each and every nerve ganglia may be used for receiving and forwarding impulses.

> Therefore, inasmuch as the light of life was revealed to me in order that I should enlighten the world, and as our physical health and the intellectual progress of the personified portion of the Universal Intelligence depend upon the proper alignment of the skeletal frame, I feel it my right and bounden duty to replace any displaced portion thereof, so that our physical and spiritual faculties may be fully and normally expressed, thereby not only enhancing our present condition, but making ourselves the better prepared to enter the next stage of existence to which this earthly existence is but a preliminary, a preparatory step.

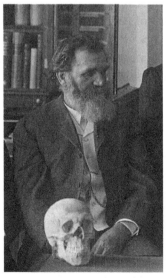

> By correcting these displacements of osseous tissue, the tension frame of the nervous system, I claim that I am rendering obedience, adoration and honor to the All-Wise Spiritual Intelligence, as well as a service to the segmented, individual portions thereof — a duty I owe to both God and mankind. In accordance with this aim and end, the Constitution of the United States and the statutes personal of California confer upon me and all persons of chiropractic faith the inalienable right to practice our religion without restraint or hindrance.

D.D. Palmer (1903)

Social and Cultural Impact

D.D. Palmer felt that chiropractic offered a form of salvation. Of the many patients he saw over the years, he felt that chiropractic was "making them physically, mentally, and spiritually invigorated and whole."

He considered the impact of chiropractic not only in terms of body, mind, and spirit, but also in relation to society and culture. For D.D. Palmer, a scientific understanding of how humans are a "segmented, personified portion" of Universal Intelligence, will "lesson disease, poverty and crime, empty our jails, penitentiaries and insane asylums and assist us to prepare for the existence beyond the transition called death." It was a new idea. This wider viewpoint included not only the physical and the spiritual, but also the cultural impact of the ideas as well as the social impact each adjustment might have on the world.

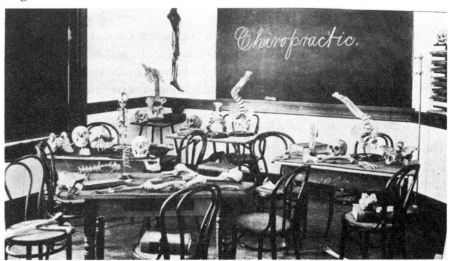

Palmer Chiropractic School at Santa Barbara (1903)

In relation to the culture, Palmer's thinking was at the transition between rational and post-rational thought. Post-rational thinking characterized the leading edge of the late twentieth century's cultural and scientific movements such as civil rights, women's rights, ecological thinking, the integration of systems science, and attempts to bridge the gulf between materialist and non-materialist worldviews. D.D. Palmer was a pioneer of a new perspective and a more complex way of thinking. It is impossible to know just how his paradigm, which was integrated into small towns throughout the world by chiropractors, helped to transform the culture.

Individual Greatness

Based on decades of clinical practice, D.D. Palmer expanded the Innate theory. His original quest in the 1880s was to figure out why one person got sick and another stayed well. In his final lectures, D.D. Palmer viewed Innate in terms of greatness and included the full spectrum of human development within its domain. He writes:

> It explains why all persons are not equal, mentally and physically; or if born alike, why some become superior or inferior to others similarly situated, why certain individuals are not able to express themselves as intelligently as others, why some persons are not mentally and physically alike at all times.

He provides a case study for this in describing a 17-year-old hemiplegic boy who had not spoken and had the mental maturity of a 3-year-old child. He writes:

> Six weeks of chiropractic adjusting caused the distorted sixth dorsal articulation to become normal in shape and to occupy its normal position, releasing a stretched condition on the sixth pair of dorsal nerves, creating a normal tension of nerves and muscles, the usual force to impulses, arousing the normal amount of energy, consequently, the normal expression of ideas.

The boy normalized in all areas. D.D. Palmer also gives another account of a 21-year-old man who was crippled and "an imbecile." He too was restored to normal.

In both cases, D.D. Palmer viewed his service as a moral and a religious duty and tied that in with his overall view of Innate, health, and disease. He writes:

> I had performed a moral duty, as well as a religious duty. It points out the conditions upon which both health and disease depend. It explains why and how one person becomes affected with disease while his associate or neighbor, apparently living under the same conditions, remains well. Furthermore, it makes plain the reason why one, or more, of the bodily functions are performed in an excessive or in a deficient degree of frequency or intensity, either of which condition is a form of disease.

D.D. Palmer built upon this expanded Innate theory to emphasize the role of chiropractic for the betterment of mankind in this life and the next.

The Great Advancement

D.D. Palmer included his spiritual perspective as a central element of his philosophy. For example, he considered death as one step on the "road of eternal progression" and thus, chiropractic shined new truth on the cause of disease and the life beyond. He writes:

> In time it will lift the veil of superstition which has obstructed our vision of the great beyond. In time, a spiritual existence will be as well-known and comprehended as that of the physical world.

He felt that chiropractic includes the science of life "in this world, and the recognition of a spiritual existence in the next."

The principles that comprise chiropractic are tied into human progress He writes:

> They originate in Divinity, the Universal Intelligence, and constitute the essential qualities of life which, having begun in this world, are never ending.

Intelligence and matter comprise man, the mortal and immortal, one everlasting, the other transitory. Intelligent action, life, is the way in which this duality is expressed. Living is how the intelligence is advanced.

Chiropractic is viewed as an "educational, scientific, religious system" because earthly experience is the pathway to "supreme spiritual existence." Chiropractic brings the spiritual and the physical together and so it enlightens mankind. Chiropractors play a role in this "great advancement." He writes:

> Chiropractors, especially, are aiding in this great advancement by adjusting the osseous structure, the position of which has to do with determining normal and abnormal tension, for in whatever part function is abnormally performed tonicity is either lacking or excessive — Creative Intelligence is prevented from expressing itself normally. Many a child has been injured at birth by a vertebral displacement which caused an impingement upon one or more of the spinal nerves, as they emanate from the spinal canal, the fibers of which are distributed to certain organs. The result of this excessive tension is physical or mental debility; often both; which, from a lack of pathological knowledge, may be lifelong; the mental defect extending even into the next world. For we retain only that which has been

acquired during this earthly, preparatory existence. By properly adjusting the neuroskeleton, these unfortunates may be enabled to acquire sufficient knowledge, rightfully due them, to become useful members of society and enjoy life in this world and the one to come. The chiropractor who can accomplish the above desirable results and refuses to do so, as a religious duty, should be compelled to perform it as a moral obligation.

Even though D.D. Palmer included a non-materialist spiritual perspective on chiropractic and life, he wanted chiropractic to be viewed as a science. He writes, "I have succeeded in making displaced articular surfaces adjusting practical. Why not make it definite, specific, scientific?"

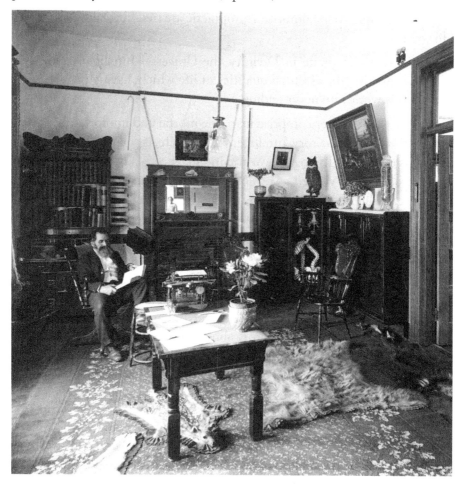

D.D. Palmer in his offices, Santa Barbara, California (1903)
- From *The Chiropractor's Protégé*

Chapter 5
B.J. Palmer's First Five Books: Vols. 2-6

In his first five books, Vols. 2-6, B.J. Palmer developed the philosophical approach he would follow for the next fifty years. His new ideas were based on clinical observation of hundreds and thousands of patients at the PSC clinic between 1906 and 1911. Lecturing forced him to refine his ideas in order to teach the growing student body.

B.J. Palmer used photographs and diagrams to instruct his students. By 1908, he presented thousands of slides during his lectures using the stereopticon lantern projector. All lectures were transcribed and published as books including the images from the lectures.

B.J.'s lectures were characterized by many new innovations of theory and practice. His new insights about the creation, transmission, and expression of brain impulses was his central inspiration. The intense development of theory and practice during these years fueled B.J.'s decades-long odyssey. In the ensuing years he helped to launch the new profession by printing

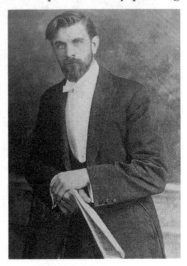

thousands of books and millions of pamphlets, speaking extensively throughout the United States and the world, eventually broadcasting lectures on radio in the 1920s and television in the 1950s. The profession of chiropractic would never have reached the level of success in its early years without B.J.'s tireless efforts. Understanding his first five books helps us to appreciate the ideas and excitement behind those efforts.

In the preface to Vol. 4 in 1908, B.J. explains that "Vols. 1 and 2 tell why adjustment is preferable to treatment. Vol. 3 tells you how to palpate and adjust. Vol. 4 tells

B.J. Palmer, DC, PhC (1909)

you where to adjust." Soon after, he published another book on "why" as Vol. 5, and another book on "where" as Vol. 6.

B.J. Palmer's First Book: Vol. 2 (1907)

Vol. 2 or *The Science of Chiropractic: Eleven Physiological Lectures*, was the transcript of B.J.'s second series of talks after his split with D.D. Palmer. The first series was in the fall of 1906, on twelve disease processes. The new lectures on physiology were presented to the students at the PSC on Wednesday evenings in January, February, and March of 1907. In these talks he introduced his new model called the circle of life.

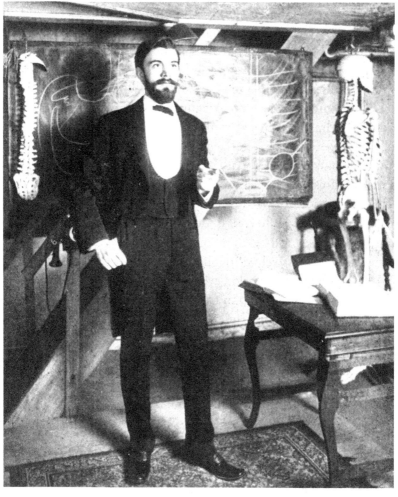

B.J. Palmer, Vol. 2 (1907)

The circle of life was a metaphor designed to capture the cycle that begins with the moment when the intelligence is transformed into the brain impulse. The impulse is then transmitted to the tissue cell as intelligent action and expressed as function. The other side of the circle starts with the impression from the environment, which is transmitted to the brain for interpretation. The vertebral subluxation interferes with transmission of impulses. Correction of vertebral subluxation restores transmission so that normal function may be expressed as health.

In B.J.'s estimation, these new "thots" were to:

> Raise the standard of specific, pure, unadulterated, phil-osophical Chiropractic which is destined to revolutionize therapeutics to non-therapeutics; chemics to mechanics; superstition to knowledge.

The book included B.J.'s additions to subluxation theory, as well as his thoughts on neurophysiology from the holistic perspective of Innate. In this sense, it is evident that he felt the current language in the literature, splitting the nervous system into various parts such as sympathetic and parasympathetic with its separated ganglionic centers and reflex mech-anisms, was too mechanistic. That linguistic way of describing the nervous system did not capture the integrated wholeness of the system, the over-arching guidance of a central controller, and the embodied intelligence that was behind involuntary and voluntary actions, functions, and brain impulses.

According to B.J., vertebral subluxations are caused by wrenches, falls, jerks, and strains. This was consistent with D.D. Palmer's etiology of subluxation, although in later years D.D. also wrote of chemical and mental/emotional causes.

B.J. Palmer developed his vertebral subluxation model based on the premise that it causes pressure on the nerves. Obstruction at the IVF could affect quantity and quality of an impulse and impede the impulse's expression. Nerve impingement leads to less transmitting capacity, which leads to less expression. This impedes brain impulses and reduces the quantity of nerve supply, which ultimately causes a partial expression of life. This condition presents as a lack of harmony or "in-coordination." Disease is proportional to the pressure on the nerve. Health is normal coordination of functions because impulses are not impeded by subluxation.

One of B.J.'s innovations in this text was the introduction of minor subluxations. He explained that this discovery came about from observations at the school clinic. The increased volume of patients offered a wider variety of patient presentations. Based on this clinical experience, B.J. concluded that Harvey Lillard's subluxation was very obvious for D.D. Palmer because it was prominent. If it was a minor subluxation, according to B.J., D.D. might not have noticed it. This innovation was one of the first developments of subluxation theory based on empirical observation from a busy chiropractic clinic.

In Vol. 2, he builds on other D.D. Palmer theories. B.J. proposes that Innate uses the brain as a medium to send impulses. He also suggests that it is the intelligence and inherent power that guides embryonic development and then takes over functions at birth. A child is born with two brains; an innate brain in charge of building the body, and an educated brain that learns throughout life. The innate brain governs the interior functions and the educated brain the voluntary functions, which involves the interface of

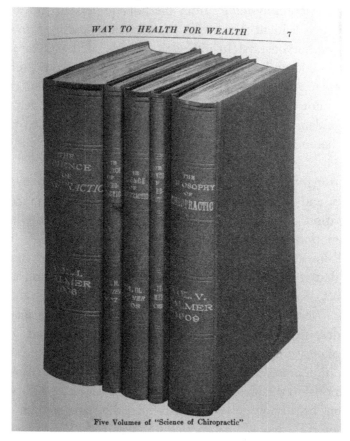

Advertisement for Vols. 1-5

the organism with the environment. B.J. also writes, "By studying innate you investigate that power which has always lived." D.D. Palmer believed that Innate brings with it memories of the species from ages past, all lives of all vertebrata.

B.J. wrote that in the last few years he worked 18 to 20 hours a day, which led to the further development of the philosophy. This is evident, not only with his circle of life, but his own version of the Innate philosophy. Over the next fifty years, he would continue to develop his view of Innate as an intelligent source of inspiration, power, and energy, in and around us. He writes:

> When many grand movements are in the bud, some men are endowed with peculiar faculties. Their every move is controlled by a something which exists in and around them. You have noticed some persons who seem to receive help from what appears supernatural beings.

Later on in the book he also refers to Innate as that power within and surrounding us. He writes:

> Remember that, in and around us, all the time, is this intelligent power in contact with physical, and our mental mind, thru brain, receives and places it through a transformation—brain impulse.

This was one of his major early innovations of chiropractic theory. The intelligence, which is everywhere, becomes personified in the brain impulse during a moment of transformation.

Additionally, B.J. felt that conscience was an Innate sense. Even though the Educated Intelligence often tried to drown it out, one could learn to listen to the Innate senses. He writes:

> That is why I daily urge upon you boys, 'Let your innate sway your entire internal and as much of the external as you can,' and you will not lose. That Innate knows thousand times more than you and I ever will. Follow the appetite and inward desires and you cannot go wrong.

This was also a development from D.D. Palmer's idea that one day Innate and Educated would communicate to each other. This theory and the methods to achieve it were refined and developed as central components of B.J.'s teachings in his final books, decades later.

B.J. Palmer's Second Book: Vol. 3

Vol. 3 or *The Philosophy and Principles of Chiropractic Adjustments* was published in 1908 as 24 lectures. In the book, B.J. introduces several new concepts such as currents, creation, resistance, innate recoil, and concussions of forces. He also expands on D.D. Palmer's theories about the integration of spirit and matter in relation to the chiropractic adjustment. The book teaches how to palpate and adjust every type of subluxation.

B.J. Palmer hypothesized that the brain impulse was a current flowing over the nerve from the mental to the physical. This built on a metaphor he introduced in Vol. 2, describing the innate power in terms of electricity. He concluded that subluxation is not the cause of disease. The cause of disease is the lack of current. He also considered subluxation as the physical representation of the cause and that the etiology of subluxation was a concussion of forces. He writes:

> When we have two bones coming together so as to make a pressure upon a little fibre, then we have the physical representation (subluxation) of the cause of disease. Concussion of forces is cause of the subluxation.

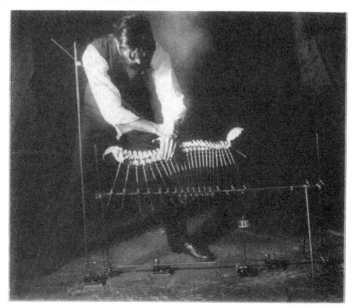

B.J. Palmer demonstrating adjustment. Vol. 3

Viewing subluxation as a "physical representation of the cause of disease" is found in the writings of his students, J.R. Drain and J.N. Firth, years later.

The chiropractic adjustment restores the flow of current, therefore, restoration of the current completes the circle of life so that life may be more fully transmitted. He writes:

> Adjustment—the connecting of Innate Intelligence into thorough and unhindered relation: restoring mental co-ordination with the physical elements to make one unit; the name given to what a Chiropractor does when he restores equilibrium between the above two essential principles— creation, ethereally and expression, physically.

This equilibrium between creation and expression of function at the tissue cell is health.

The concepts of resistance, Innate recoil, and concussion of forces were at the core of his subluxation theory and his Innate philosophy. He writes:

> Subluxations are caused by concussion of forces, excessively and awkwardly applied. The interruptions to the normal flow of Innate mental impulses is the cause of all diseases. When conditions are made possible, and gap created, Innate can, will and does reverse the order and uses the same means, but in different direction and degree.

These theories built upon D.D. Palmer's model that Innate would rebuild the health of the body once the impingement was corrected. It also lays the foundation for the theory of retracing, also developed from D.D., which posited that the restoration process involved a systematic return to normality. During this process the body may re-experience old traumas. B.J. coined the term "retracing" as it related to the chiropractic adjustment a few years later. It was a central component of chiropractic theory in most schools for decades.

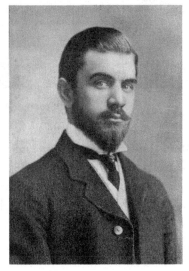

B.J. Palmer (1906)

B.J. proposed that the philosophy bridges the gap between the spiritual and the material and that man was a "psychophysical unit." Chiropractic philosophy integrated mind and body. His early students, Morikubo and

Loban, used the same phrase, "psychophysical," when summing up B.J.'s teachings. Expanding on this, B.J. writes, "The work of a Chiropractor is to allow God full expression in man the physical and mental man." This viewpoint is found throughout the writings of both Palmers. However, each specified they were referring to the God of all religions and both preferred the term Universal Intelligence.

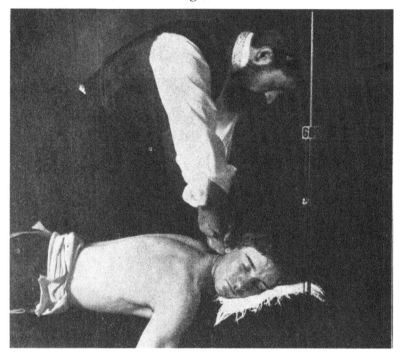

B.J. Palmer demonstrating on Joy Loban, Vol. 3 (1908)

B.J. viewed the whole universe as psycho-physical and that all living systems are "products of one mind, therefore one common creation, transmission and expression." He referred to chiropractic as a "materialistic application of an art" for an "immaterialistic reason." He proposed this philosophical perspective could be applied to studying textbooks. One should begin with the Intelligence, then the forces, and then the anatomy and physiology.

The second edition of Vol. 3 was published as 38 lectures with an additional 400 pages and more than 100 new images. In the second edition he writes that chiropractic is, "the first non-therapeutical theological philosophy." Both editions cover a wide range of philosophical, scientific, and clinical topics.

In the 1911 edition, B.J. offers an early history of ideas in chiropractic. He suggests that the philosophy has taken on new dimensions. The first three years, chiropractic was an art, the next seven years chiropractic developed a science, and in the last five years, a philosophy. By 1911, he had already published Vols. 4-6 and thus he was mainly referring to his contributions to the philosophy.

B.J. Palmer's Third Book: Vol. 4 (1908)

Vol. 4 or *The Science of Chiropractic: Causes Localized*, was dedicated to Joy Loban. B.J. writes, "he is a companion such as gives backbone to a philosophy as good as this." The running title on the page headers reads "The Philosophy of Chiropractic" rather than the title, *The Science of Chiropractic*. The book was based on observations made from the PSC clinic, which was now seeing 200 patients per day. B.J. supervised every case. Of the 107-page book, B.J. writes, "The brevity of this book is its beauty." The book introduces the meric system.

Vol. 4 gives the "where to adjust" for a wide variety of disease processes. The first 15 pages provide definitions of various disease processes from Abscesses to Worms. The next 54 pages includes listings for each vertebra from Atlas to the Coccyx, with disease processes that might arise from subluxations at each level. He included abbreviations such as; 1st cervical = At. P., lower lumbar as L.P.P., and coccyx = C.C.P. He also includes some of his unique terminology. Here are a few examples:

> Inco-ordination—A term used to express lack of ease between the mental creation of life and its physical personification by expression in any instance commonly known as disease, diseases in any degree or character in any tissue.
>
> Nerve—Nerves are mediums of transmission of Innate mental impulses from the brain to all tissues in the body. The only abnormality possible is lack of function.
>
> Reflex—A thing impossible to a living physical—where the Innate does not receive "message," does not interpret their value and does not "reply" as her judgment thinks best, therefore a shadow of a substance that Chiropractors are not desiring to spend valuable time on.
>
> Symptom—Any function not being performed coordinately with its mental equivalent; symptoms are endless and but

express conditions that are in no two alike and points as an index to cause which teaches the observant to adjust it, rather than treat the effects.

The short book includes 23 pages of advertisements at the end, which provide a great deal of information about the PSC, early chiropractic, and the Green Book series.

One interesting aspect of these advertisements from 1908, is how B.J.'s new terminology was being integrated. For example, his advertisement for the 1906 book, *The Science of Chiropractic*, Vol. 1. The book was still in its first edition and comprised mostly of D.D. Palmer's articles. The advertisement does not include D.D. Palmer's name. Furthermore, B.J.'s new ideas like in-coordination, concussion of forces, and expression of intelligence in the tissue cell, are used to describe the book. The cause of disease is described as, "inco-ordination between Innate Intelligence and her physical medium, the human body." None of those new ideas are actually in the 1906 text.

Also in the advertisements, B.J. proposes that Vol. 5 is "along deeper lines" developed in Vol. 2. He writes that:

> Dr. B.J. Palmer's discovery of the complete, direct Cycle of Life and its forces, gives to man a philosophical completeness which unlocks the door of mystery and makes every known function, whether performed normally or abnormally, clear as daylight.

The term "philosophical completeness" is also used in the writings of his students, Morikubo and Loban.

The advertisement for the non-yet-published Vol. 5, mentions B.J.'s rambling lecture style. The pre-order date for the book was December 1, 1909. The ad reads:

> To observe Dr. Palmer when lecturing is to see a man lost to his surroundings. With head bent low, thots emit faster than the word can give utterance. For a space of time the deepest logic, bearing upon new discoveries, will issue, then without warning, perhaps the subject uncompleted, his mind will switch to some of the follies of medicine, in connection with his subject, then again the theme is taken up and finished. To omit these erratic interjections from these lectures would be not to listen or read one of "B.J.'s" lectures.

> While appearing verbose, yet this is the only way this lect-
> urer, author, and writer can bring forth what is necessary to
> develop new thots.

Most of the texts follow his meandering approach to lecturing. This
lecturing style was transcribed and is one reason why B.J.'s books are
sometimes difficult to read.

B.J. Palmer's Fourth Book: Vol. 5 (1909)

Vol. 5 or *The Philosophy of Chiropractic* was based on B.J. Palmer's lectures from the winter of 1908, with at least one lecture from 1909, the year
it was published. The book includes 24 lectures. Vol. 5 was B.J.'s second
philosophy text. It was written as an update to Vol. 2. An advertisement
comparing the two reads, "If that book was a 'rouser,' then Vol. 5 will be
another along deeper lines."

The main topics of Vol. 5 include the union of mind and matter,
power, and cycles, which was an expanded theory of the cycle of life. In
Vol. 5, B.J. codifies many of his central chiropractic theories such as current,
interpretation, Innate mind, Innate brain, and impression. He also develops
his theory of vibration, and introduces his new model called the Normal
Complete Cycle (NCC).

The book demonstrates a dramatic evolution of his ideas. And yet, his
new ideas are consistent with the chiropractic paradigm. For example, he
writes, "Chiropractic, is the science of the cause of symptoms." Chiropractors do nothing for disease, they adjust the cause.

B.J.'s biographical information at the front of Vol. 5 is a good example
of how his new ideas made him feel as though he was onto some genuinely

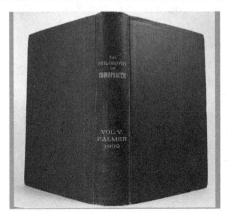

Copyright, 1909,
B. J. PALMER, D. C., Ph. C.
DAVENPORT, IOWA, U. S. A.

Philosophy of Chiropractic Vol. 5
(copyright 1909)

new breakthroughs, not only for chiropractic but the history of health practices and human culture. Vol. 5 states the following:

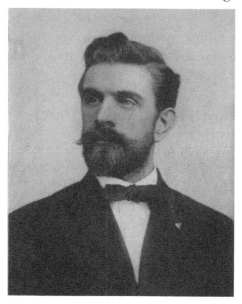

From Vol. 5 (1909)

B.J. Palmer, DC, PhC

Student, Author, Lecturer and Teacher on any phase of Chiropractic Philosophy, Science or Art, anywhere at any time.

President and Proprietor of The Palmer School of Chiropractic ("Chiropractic's Fountain Head"), Davenport, Iowa, U.S.A.

Developer of the Philosophy, Science and Art of Chiropractic. Author of Volumes I, II, III, IV and V of The Science of Chiropractic and many other lectures.

Secretary and Philosophical Counsel for The Universal Chiropractor's Association.

Counsel for The P.S.C. Class and Clinic Record Club.

Manager and Assistant Editor THE CHIROPRACTOR.

Therapeutical Idol Shatterer. Destroyer of Superstitious ideas regarding Creation, transmission and expression of life, in any form and replacer of impractical with practical studies, etc. etc.

Considering how D.D. Palmer responded to B.J.'s use of the title "developer" in 1907, one could only wonder how D.D. might have viewed his son's new biography page.

Vol. 5 is one of the most complex and difficult of the Green Books. It covers a wide spectrum of ideas, which may be explored in three broad categories: mind and matter, power, and the Normal Complete Cycle.

Mind and Matter

The main area of inquiry for the book is the philosophical knowledge of cause and the unification of soul and body. He viewed the mental and physical as emanations from Universal Intelligence and the foundation for the "philosophical physiology" described in Vol. 2.

B.J. suggests that viewing mind as a function of the brain is incorrect. Instead he proposes that consciousness is a property of matter. From this perspective, mind and being are fully integrated. For example, he suggests reversing the phrase, "as a man thinketh so he is," to "as he is so he shall think." From his perspective, this approach is more philosophically correct.

He used Vol. 5 to critique the materialist culture and criticize what he viewed as hypocritical medical doctors who also had a faith or belief in God. B.J. writes, "He does not see a God but mythically believes in one. His religion is still a faith, not a reality." He wrote about this cultural clash between materialist and non-materialist worldviews in many of his later books.

For B.J. Palmer, the chiropractic adjustment of the vertebral subluxation in conjunction with an understanding of this non-materialist viewpoint were crucial in changing the world for the better. He proposed that the chiropractic adjustment transforms the individual so dramatically that they are no longer embedded in the materialistic cultural norms. He taught this to students as a way to develop the self. He writes:

> Students... are taught to think, reason and live the practical Chiropractic life. While here they receive adjustments and many is the man or woman that entered a servant of the masses because, physically they could not do better, that leave the master, because their functions are fully expressed. Their functions have been fully restored; they no longer are at the beck and call of the many, but stand on pedestals created for the few that energetically think and unreservedly do.

In a chapter on *Insanity*, B.J. covers the topic from the perspective of the intelligences. The discussion begins with a definition of mind as an embodied consciousness. B.J. then proposes there are two types of insanity: Type 1 is when God and the brain are not connected and Type 2 is when the brain and body are not connected. He related Type 1 to subluxations of C1 and C2. Type 2 has to do with a lack of oneness between brain and body. Any abnormality is a type of insanity of the tissues.

B.J. proposed that Universal Intelligence is the first premise and Innate is the second premise. Health is when the universal power from Universal Intelligence moves through the brain down to the body and out to the tissue cells.

Power

Vol. 5 is the first book where B.J. relies on references such as Morat's textbook on neurophysiology, specific articles from *Encyclopedia Britannica*, as well as a few other books on philosophy and healing. In Morat, B.J. found a kindred spirit, also searching for the missing link between mind and matter. He referenced Morat throughout his many books over five decades. In the *Encyclopedia*, he found the latest scientific theories.

His references to Morat and Britannica demonstrate his awareness of several scientific concepts about neurophysiology, electricity, energy, and physics; including the law of conservation of energy. From the articles in the encyclopedia, written by college professors in the United Kingdom, he developed several theories relating to cycles of current, free flow of energy, and power in living systems.

As B.J. integrated these scientific models with Innate philosophy, he was awestruck by the insight that humans had never made such connections before. He writes, "We open our eyes in wonderment and stare at such monumental ignorance." He felt that chiropractic philosophy was making significant contributions to human health and knowledge.

In the lectures on *Power*, B.J. proposed that the brain is a concentrator of power. Environmental energies are transmitted through the physiology from the afferent system. The brain draws these energies from the environment and concentrates that energy throughout the brain tissue. He writes:

> The significant function of the brain is to suck inward through process of osmosis, those immaterial units of force that exists in the atmosphere in countless numbers and put them through the material.

He proposed that when the inner and outer meet, the vibrations from the environment register at the sensory system. Those vibrations are converted to an impression, or a force/energy, that travels to the brain. The raw energy is then transformed into something the body can use as power. The brain acts like a dynamo that transforms the ethereal power for bodily use. Life is the expression of this universal power.

The transformation process is when the brain takes these raw units of force, what he termed "foruns" or "force-units," from the environment and imbues them with intelligence. Thus, he distinguishes two kinds of power, intellectual power (the body's energy) and non-intellectual power (like electricity). The new transformed unit can be transmitted as an impulse to the tissue cell and expressed as power in action. He writes:

> The sum total of individualistic mental impulses each of which is composed of multitudes of intellectual and material units of energy after they have been received at the brain and transformed for the need of the body.

This is the afferent efferent circuit, the key to life. He continues:

> The mental impulse current starts from the brain dynamo, goes to the nerve's wires, from there to through the controller and only when normal in shape and size the IVF to the tissue cells, the motors, from there it's returned to the brain where it completes its cycle.

B.J. was fascinated by this transformation, which occurred at the juncture between the afferent and efferent cycle.

After the impression of the vibration from the environment was interpreted by the intelligence, then a new thought was created. He viewed this as an act of creation itself, made by the creator, the intelligence, which is a part of the ocean of Universal intelligence, and hence, sacred, holy, and thoroughly amazing.

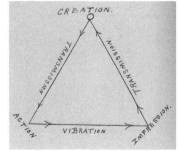

Cycle of Life Vol. 5 (1909)

B.J. was so enamored with the model of creation, transmission, and expression, that he emphasized the efferent side of the cycle because the creation of the mental impulse and the interference to transmission were vital to the expression of life.

Normal Complete Cycle (NCC)

B.J. hypothesized that chiropractic was a practical application to healing and living, which centered on three primary principles of life: creation, transmission, and expression. Connecting the three phases into "one scientific or philosophical completeness," establishes a triune or "a tri-unity."

To B.J., this was a major philosophical breakthrough for human thought, a solution to Cartesian dualism, and "the conundrum that has never been solved until this lecture places the solution before you." It is clear from these first volumes that B.J. sincerely thought he had broken through to new ground, not only from his father's ideas but from the history of philosophy and science.

The NCC was first defined during his lectures in 1908 and published towards the end of Vol. 5. The NCC is an elaboration on the cycle of life, introduced in Vol. 2. First, he defined the simple cycle, later referred to by Stephenson as the safety pin cycle. Then, B.J. expanded upon the cycle theory and proposed how Universal Intelligence, Innate Intelligence, and Mind, enter into the physical as the mental impulse. Finally, B.J. described and formalized 31 steps of the NCC as well as many variations of cycles, or ways the NCC is affected by vertebral subluxation. According to B.J., when the creation, transmission, expression cycle is unobstructed, normal function or the normal cycle ensues. When it is obstructed various types of paralysis manifest.

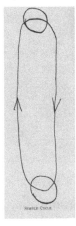 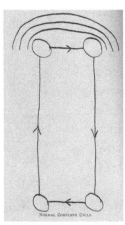 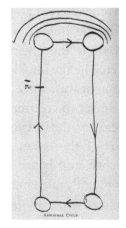

Simple Cycle	Normal Complete Cycle	Abnormal Cycle
	Vol. 5 (1909)	(with subluxation as step 12)

The Spectrum of Paralysis

The vertebral subluxation sets the parameters for a spectrum of paralysis. Partial pressure causes a lack of expression, which leads to partial paralysis. This could relate to muscle systems or decreased function of organ systems. Paralysis could occur at any stage between full life expression and death. He writes:

> If transformed power is unimpeded and freely courses through nerves, then actions will be free and paralysis cannot exist. The expressions in tissues will be exactly as transformed at brain. This is the man of ability, mental and physical, that we admire in executive positions. He will be able to think perfect thoughts and express them freely—that man is one with manhood.

Expression is the personification of the intelligence, the fullness of the transformation process, and the embodiment of the creation in action.

The other end of the spectrum of paralysis, where life's full expression is impeded, may present as pathophysiology of tissues and also as limited functioning in life. Pathophysiology, dis-ease, and types of insanity may be found between the poles of the spectrum. He continues:

> Observe that shuffling, shifting, evading, agitated, equivocating common person and he represents paralysis in the functions of tissue cells, one lobe or several lobes of the brain or some other physical tissues. Instead of his being the keen thinker or active doer, he is the parrot like repeater of what others ask or command. He is the servant of the masses to be sandwiched between. He never rises above his bodily inability.

B.J. wrote about this type of person for decades. He even developed this viewpoint into his later philosophy of genius, listening to Innate, and a spectrum of greatness. He continues:

> There are men of great and small abilities. The first has free and open channels through which to express unlimited vitality; the other has the thought but has closed channels so that a limited power is put into execution. The latter man's functions are paralyzed.

Power being transformed into the expression of life's intelligence, as an act of creation, was the most profound philosophical truth for B.J. Palmer.

The Chiropractic Vision

B.J. envisioned how chiropractic adjustments may affect the future. He writes:

> I am advancing ideas which will not be realized until chiropractic has been utilized for several generations; after adjustments have been given to the present and the younger generations and to their children, we will then begin to see the new growth in future personifications that man's physical beings erected after the image of their makers. Then the world will be decidedly better for having had chiropractic.

This type of epigenetic vision is echoed in later Green Books by his faculty, other chiropractic visionaries, and also by B.J. himself in future books. The idea is rooted in D.D. Palmer's singular vision that chiropractic will help the world to evolve.

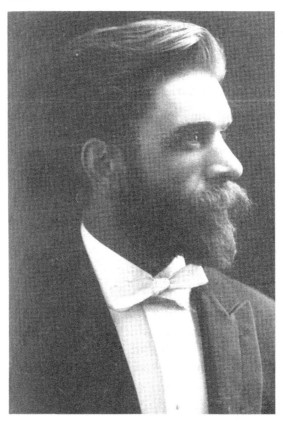

B.J. Palmer, Vol. 6 (1911)

B.J. Palmer's Fifth Book: Vol. 6 (1911)

Vol. 6 or T*he Philosophy, Science, and Art of Chiropractic Nerve Tracing: A Book of Four Sections*, was published in 1911. The header on each page reads "Study 31: Lesson 1." The dedication is to Mabel Palmer, to whom B.J. writes, "M.H. Palmer, DC, that tireless, constant and truest friend any worker could desire—his wife, is this book dedicated."

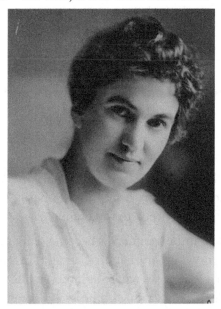

Mabel Heath Palmer, DC

The book codifies the chiropractic practice of nerve tracing, which was D.D. Palmer's original method of chiropractic analysis. However, the book does not mention the founder as the originator of the method. Instead, B.J. describes it in relation to his own theory of cycles.

Vol. 6 is a unique contribution to the series. It is written more as a manual than a text. The 800 pages contain 735 photographs of nerve tracing. There are only about 42,000 words in all of those pages, most of which are descriptions of the photographs, listed as illustrations. According to B.J., the book cost $14,000 to produce. In 2018, that equates to $381,137.

Vol. 6 did not go into a second edition. By the 1930s, nerve tracing was abandoned by the PSC due to the new innovations of thermography and the upper cervical technique. Nerve tracing was carried on in other schools started by students and faculty from this era like Drain's Texas Chiropractic College; and Firth, Vedder, and Burich's Lincoln Chiropractic College.

Theory of Nerve Tracing

Vol. 6 is divided into four sections with a twelve-page introduction called *Nerve Tracing*, which is the only philosophical part of the text. In the introduction, B.J. suggests medicine is based on ancient myths, superstitions, and practices. He contrasts this with chiropractic as, "The first completely revolutionary idea that has been presented to the world of therapeutics for ages." The introductory pages cover B.J.'s views of the nervous system from an Innate perspective and lays the foundation for an exploration of the topic of nerve tracing, which he defines as:

> The process of tracing from the physical representative of the cause to where effects are known to exist, objectively or subjectively.

The practice of nerve tracing is:

> The actual, physical, manual palpation by which we trace a nerve from its emergence from the spinal cord to its peripheries or nerve endings, or trace from the peripheries to their entrance into the spine to proceed to the brain.

According to B.J., impinged nerves become tender and swollen. This is detected by placing pressure on that area, eliciting a tender sensation. This practice is only possible in cases where light nerve pressure has not affected the ability to feel, such as in cases with heavy pressure. B.J. concludes:

> I should say unquestionably every Chiropractor should use nerve tracing in all cases that come to him in which it is possible to do so.

Nerve tracing provides the chiropractor with the location of the subluxation, and thus, where to give the adjustment. It also lets the patient understand the relationship between the periphery and the subluxation, the cause of the incoordination.

Method of Nerve Tracing

The practice of nerve tracing is considered by B.J. to be one of the three main branches of the chiropractor's analysis, the other two are analysis and adjusting. Becoming a good nerve tracer requires an ability to clearly differentiate palpation findings through refined interpretations of sensory input from the finger tips. There are two methods. The first one is to use three fingers on the spine to locate the subluxation. Next, is to locate individual tender spots with the finger tip. The second finger (tracing finger) is reinforced by the thumb and forefinger.

Section One demonstrates the method using 180 illustrations with step-by-step explanations on one case. For example, illustration number 179 demonstrates the course of the tender areas related to a left superior vertebral subluxation at the 3rd thoracic. Crosses are marked for non-tender areas and dashes for areas of tenderness:

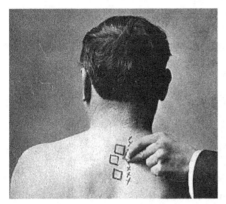 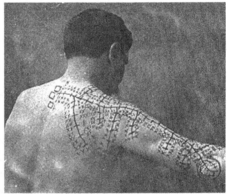

Illustration No. 5. Hunting for the main nerve of the trunk as it leaves the spine & No. 179. Complete nerve tracing showing the line and all divisions, Vol. 6 (1911)

B.J. describes the process of nerve tracing in terms of a cooperation between chiropractor and patient. As the chiropractor drops the finger into different depths of the tissues, perhaps as deep as an inch, the patient reports whether the quality of tenderness is the same. Two things are important in this regard: to make sure the patient understands what you are doing, and also to be able to distinguish "the muscle contraction along the course of the nerve which is an evidence that you have crossed the nerve." But central to the practice is working in unison with the patient. He writes:

> Nerve tracing is careful work, it requires the normal intellectual interpretations of your patient as well as yourself. It is that condition wherein your patient must use his intelligence linked with yours to the entire absence of anything surrounding you. You two must be conjointly working to a common end.

According to B.J., nerve tracing is the "key-note of our work." In fact, he felt that it was proof of his theories about the nervous system in terms of a direct flow of current from the brain to the tissue cells. His approach was to clinically determine how the tender sensations and symptomatology presented and then disappeared after the adjustment.

Section Two demonstrates the nerve tracing method from the effect to the cause. For example, in one case he uses 118 step-by-step illustrations for a case with tender areas around the chest:

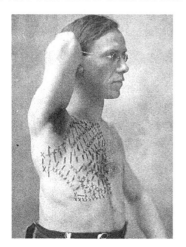 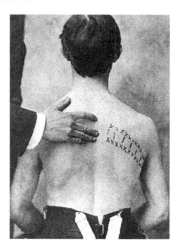

Illustrations Nos. 280 & 296. - Three fingers on same vertebra during palpating showing right inferior position subluxation. Vol. 6 (1911)

Section Three includes 156 simple, completed tracings. The illustrations demonstrate many types of tracings. B.J. felt that "nerve tracing eliminates any possible error in connecting cause with effect or effect with cause." Section Four includes more complex tracings, requiring "an artist with his hands." Confidentiality of the subjects in the photos is kept by employing face-masks and blindfolds.

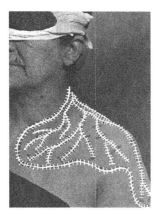 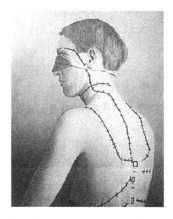

Illustration No. 366 (Mrs. G.) & No. 311 (Mr. D.). From Section 3, Vol. 6 (1911)

The Chiropractic Standpoint

In Vol. 6, B.J. coined the phrase "the Chiropractic standpoint." He describes a viewpoint that could be applied to biology, chemistry, botany, zoology, and other sciences. He refers to this as the big revolutionary idea.

The phrase, "the chiropractic standpoint," was used by Firth and Craven in the titles of Vol. 7 (1914) and the second Vol. 3 (1924). The phrase was also used by Vedder in regards to physiology in Vol. 8, Craven's writings on the expression of life in the second edition of Vol. 5, Thompson's writings on x-ray analysis in Vol. 10, and by Stephenson in regards to cycles in Vol. 14. It was also used by D.D. Palmer in his 1914 text but we have no evidence that he read B.J.'s Vol. 6, so D.D.'s usage may be unique.

The Chiropractic standpoint is one way of capturing the perspective of the chiropractic paradigm. It is a perspective on the living organism that considers the organismic point of view. By viewing all subjects in relation to what Innate is trying to accomplish through the nervous system and how that relates to even wider questions about the Intelligence inherent to the universe, chiropractic brings forth its own perspective. This is evident in the entire Green Book series.

B.J. Palmer's Updates to the First Green Books

The second edition of Vol. 2, published in 1913, included the full text of Vol. 4, and an expansion of B.J.'s latest theories about power and cycles, as well as his views of the sympathetic nervous system, reflex action, and serous circulation.

A chapter called the *Meric System* was also included in the second edition of Vol. 2. This was an attempt to systematize nerve tracing by taking into account the embryologic development of the body's layers.

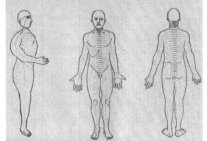

Meric System, Vol. 2 (1913)

In 1913, he also proposed five theories of excess function related to subluxation, expands on his nine primary functions, and develops a complex diagnostic system called "Equations" based on in-creased or decreased function.

In the preface to the second edition of Vol. 2, B.J. describes the future of the book series. He writes:

> At the present time, some ten other books have been written, compiled, and the lectures finished although not published. We hardly feel that Chiropractic has advanced in public favor sufficiently yet to warrant us putting forth too many books at once. Inquiry will elicit the fact as to whether others have been published since this.
>
> No one book, of this library, will encompass all the hasty reader will care to peruse. They have not been written for that purpose. Desiring to spread the work, we have purposely made no one book a general discussion, but taking each and doing it the justice it deserves. We trust that only students will study these pages, for they are the only ones who can best distribute the value we herein aim to give.

Besides new editions of these first books in 1916 (Vol. 5), 1917 (Vol. 1), and 1919 (Vol. 2), and the publication of a technique manual with his faculty in 1920 (Vol. 13), B.J. Palmer's next solo-authored book was not until 1934 (Vol. 18). However, during those intervening years he published dozens of pamphlets, some of which became chapters of future Green Books.

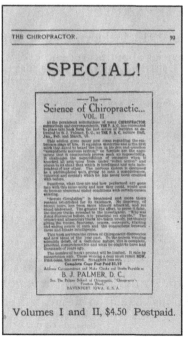
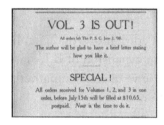
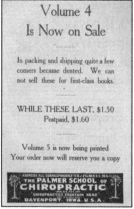
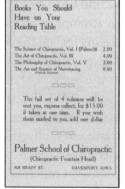

PUBLIC LECTURES

24 Lectures to be Delivered at The P. S. C. this Winter.

Beginning with the first Wednesday in October' 1907, and continuing each Wednesday evening for six months, B. J. Palmer, D. C., will deliver a series of 24 lectures at THE P. S. C. LECTURE HALL, 828 Brady St., Davenport, Iowa. Each subject will be on some disease.

EVERYBODY IS WELCOME. If strangers are in the city, we shall be glad to welcome them. Our correspondents are always invited to partake of further insight into the detail of this broad philosophy.

DAY OR NIGHT STUDENTS now matriculated or who will this winter Have An Advantage over summer classes.

TO HAVE THESE TALKS ELUCIDATED and demonstrated is well worth the many points of knowledge gained. Some of these lectures will, from time to time, be reproduced in THE CHIROPRACTOR. *All of them will be bound in book form* to add another volume for *The P. S. C. Chiropractic Library.*

COME AND BRING YOUR FRIENDS. This invitation is broad and includes all who have a further interest in uplifting mankind from the depths of superstition to the substantial platform of facts.

The following are the topics:

1. Hernia and Prolapses,
2. Tuberculosis.
3. Insanity.
4. Rheumatism.
5. Kidney Diseases.
6. Paralysis.
7. Stones, Renal, etc.
8. Catarrh.
9. Cancer and Tumor.
10. Neuralgia.
11. Skin Diseases.
12. Contagious Diseases.
13. Diseases of the Alimentary Tract.
14. Alcoholism.
15. Meningitis.
16. Poisoning.
17. Diseases of The Senses.
18. Appendicitis.
19. Excessive Heat.
20. Female Diseases.
21. Diseases of the Heart.
22. Epilepsy and Apoplexy.
23. Abnormalities.
24. Haemorrhages.

Attend the lecture every Wednesday evening, 8 P. M. at *The P. S. C.*, 828 Brady Street, Davenport, Iowa, U. S. A.

100   THE CHIROPRACTOR

About Volume 5

The P. S. C. aims to keep faith with its friends anywhere and everywhere, but once in a while we overshoot our mark. So it is with the above book. We promised delivery before this, we know you have a good right to be expecting the issue, and when it don't come on schedule you have a good reason, to be unreasonable. Do you know why it was not out on time? Because we was adding more material, at the same cost to you (altho more to us.) Never mind, you have been patient, very much so, we appreciate your thotfulness. We have had hundreds of requests within the last two months and I am glad to state that

Volume 5 leaves the P. S. C. Saturday, May 22, 1909

If your copy does not come in due process of mail delivery, let us know and we will know the reason why.

This is the first time we have given you a definite date for delivery. I know that this date is correct. Orders will be filled on that day—all of them.

Price $2.50 Postpaid

570 pages of solid "type matter." Solid philosophy, answering those everlasting questions of "WHY?" of this or that.

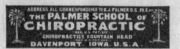

---

40   THE CHIROPRACTOR

One Complete Book on Nerve Tracing Vol. 6

Page 367 of the 1911 P. S. C. School Announcement speaks of the above named book containing "600 half-tones." "Over 200 cases are recorded." "These books will be published in three parts." "Part I contains a full set of half-tones showing how to trace from effect to cause, and another set showing how to trace from cause to effect." "Part II contains complete sets of views of actual diseases, traced with a complete history of the tracing." "Part III contains the same as number II, only on an entirely different set of views."

The publishing of the above, we figured conservatively would cost $8,000. That work has required one department constantly. The effects and subluxations have been recorded by the hundreds, the nerve tracer has put in thousands of hours, the photographer has used over 1,000 plates, etc.

We have now compiled ALL THREE BOOKS INTO ONE BOOK. It will be the largest book The P. S. C. has published. Will contain 875 half-tones; the book will be over 800 pages and will have complete histories of over 450 distinct effects traced. 90% of these half-tones are full page. The half-tone bill for this book was over $5,000. In point of size, number of half-tones, explanations, value, etc., it will exceed Volume 3.

THIS BOOK IS BEING PRINTED. We are not calling for advance orders, but should you care to place your order in advance, then remit special price and save $2.00. Volume 3 was unavoidably dragged; This is not occurring with Volume No. 6.

The 1911 P. S. C. "S. A." lists the three books at $15.00. ALL ORDERS PLACED WITH THE P. S. C. PREVIOUS TO OCTOBER 1st, 1911, mailed at $6.50 post paid.

Regular price for Volume 6 (nerve tracing) $8.50 post paid, after October 1st, 1911. We guarantee delivery on or before that date or refund order.

Remit through P. L. M. O., Express Order or bank draft. Direct all correspondence to THE PALMER SCHOOL OF CHIROPRACTIC, "Chiropractic Fountain Head," Davenport, Iowa. U. C. A.

THE CHIROPRACTOR   61

Volume 3

We have sold more Volume Three's than all other books, per the same space of time. We see the need for this book—therefore the revision of Vol. 3 is now going on—it will contain at least 100, and possibly 200, more views. The text matter will be much improved and considerably added to. We propose to thus increase the size and value of each and every revised edition to such an extent, that every person who bought one of the first edition will find it to his advantage to buy a second. We know that, "if it were the same," you would not buy, and if you did it would be us that were sold, not the book—hence we shall make it so much better, that you would gladly pay twice its cost to get it.

Volume 3 Ready for Delivery April 1st, '10

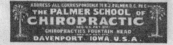

VOLUME 1 (REVISED)

Complete Copy, $2.00

Postpaid,$2.20

Ready for Delivery March the 1st.

1909 Bound Chiropractors

Every year we bind (only) 25 complete sets

While they last, $2.00 Complete

You pay the postage

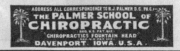

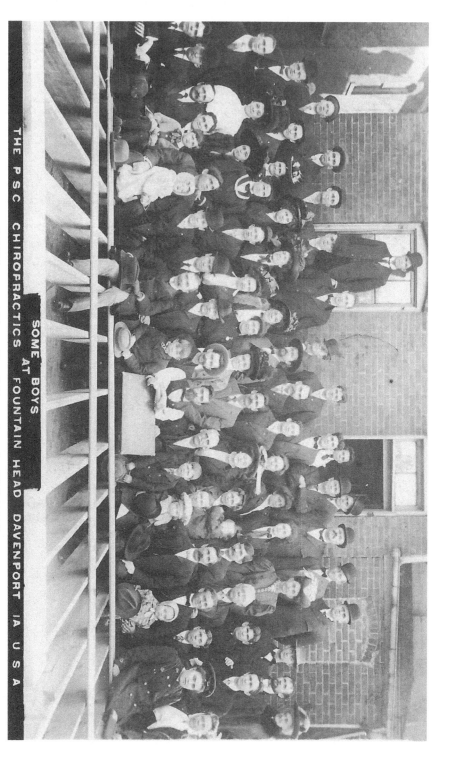

SOME BOYS AT
THE PSC CHIROPRACTICS FOUNTAIN HEAD DAVENPORT IA U S A

B.J. Palmer and "Some Boys" Expanding the PSC (1909)

Chapter 6
The Chiropractic Textbooks: Vols. 7-13

Between 1914 and 1919, six new volumes of Green Books were published. These books were published as teaching texts for the classroom by the full-time faculty at the PSC. The books shared a common perspective, the chiropractic standpoint. Even though the topics included symptomatology, physiology, anatomy, gynecology, chemistry, spinography, and technique, they all viewed the organism through the lens of the Innate philosophy, included the centrality of subluxation as a major cause of human disease processes, and built upon the core theories and models developed by B.J. Palmer in Vols. 2-6.

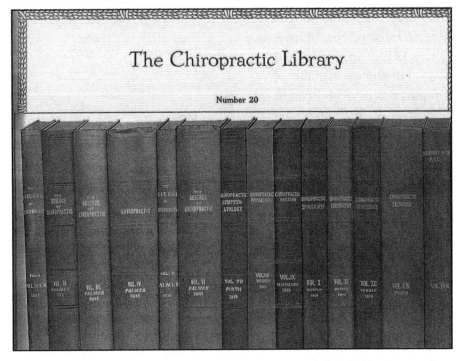

Advertisement for Vols. 1-14 from the PSC Catalog (1922-25)

Firth's Chiropractic Symptomatology: Vol. 7 (1914)

James N. Firth, DC, PhC, published *A Text-book on Chiropractic Symptomatology; or, The Manifestations of Incoordination Considered from a Chiropractic Standpoint* in August 1914. The publisher was Driffill Printing Co., in Rock Island, Illinois.

Firth was the first of the Palmer School faculty to write a book for his students. It may be the first text exclusively on diagnosis from the chiropractic standpoint. It was also the first to apply B.J. Palmer's theories and equations of excess or inhibited function introduced in 1913.

Jim Firth was born September 16, 1886, in Sterling, Michigan. According to Rolf Peters' book, Firth became Principal of the Public Schools of Saganing, Michigan, from 1907 to 1909. He enrolled at the PSC in July 1909 and graduated on July 18, 1910. He practiced in Manistique, Michigan, after graduation. Firth was listed as an examiner in Symptomatology at PSC on March 27, 1911, and officially joined the faculty in August 1911. Firth was one of the best loved instructors. He resigned from the PSC in 1925 and founded Lincoln Chiropractic College (LCC) in 1926 with Vedder, Burich, and Hendricks, all former PSC faculty. Firth served as president of LCC from 1941 to 1954. He died on June 24, 1964, in Indianapolis, Indiana.

By 1912, Firth was listed as head of the department of Symptomatology. He taught all courses on Pathology and Nerve Tracing. He also taught the clinic "pit" class alongside B.J. Palmer for many years.

In February 1913, the PSC listed Firth's articles about infantile paralysis and spastic paralysis for sale by the hundreds, along with articles by B.J., Mabel Palmer, and Harry Vedder. Firth published a series of articles in *The Chiropractor* on various topics from *Gall Stones* to *Diabetes*.

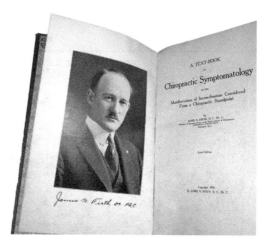

Firth's Symptomatology: Vol 7
(Second edition, 1923)

Of Firth's book, B.J. Palmer writes:

> Little do you and I know what the small thot and action of today may grow into. Little does the acorn realize that within its shell is shade for the hot, rest for the weary; food for the squirrels and furniture for the men; the potential possibilities are great.

B.J. endorsed the book and praised Firth as a star pupil while also explaining that the PSC did not publish the book. He writes:

> Little did we think, some years ago, that when we "took on" one James N. Firth to our Faculty Body that in a few short years he would Be Ye Editor and publisher. The P.S.C. has not been in any way connected with the same. It is written in such a manner that it is applicable to be used in any other Chiropractic school in the U.S. Nothing would please Dr. Firth more than to see it a standard in all standard schools.
>
> It is a masterful production of a masterful student; it comes as the result of years of thotful production; only one who has gone as deeply into his subject could have equaled it—I consider the work the only worthy book dealing with symptomatology, Chiropractically considered, on the market.

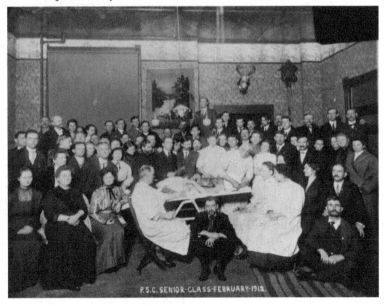

Jim Firth on B.J. Palmer's left, Harry Vedder standing behind table
PSC dissection class (1912)

B.J. also added that the faculty voted to stop using Butler's *Diagnostics of Internal Medicine* and adopt Firth's Symptomatology. B.J. writes:

> --and above all impress the public that books of our own take care of our own teachings in our schools.
>
> I am in receipt of the 1st volume, autographed, from which I thank you, Dr. Firth, very much. I appreciate it from all angles and I can only with the publication the universal use that it merits.

The book was copyrighted by Firth on August 4, 1914. During Firth's time at the PSC the book went through two editions, one supplement, and six printings. After he left PSC, the book changed title to *Chiropractic Diagnosis* in 1929.

In one advertisement for the book, it was marketed as the only book on the subject and as a way to increase business "by being posted on diseases chiropractically." An endorsement in that ad from Dr. Lewis Scott, of Des Moines, Iowa, he writes:

> It is a clear-cut statement of the things every Chiropractor should know, expressed in good English and printed in clear, bold type, thus, for the Chiropractor. It is the book of books.

Firth's dynamic approach to symptomatology from a chiropractic standpoint is one of the first attempts to apply the chiropractic paradigm to systematically explain diagnosis. Chapters included topics such as diseases of the digestive system, the respiratory system, the circulatory system, the blood and ductless glands, the kidney, the nervous system and constitutional diseases.

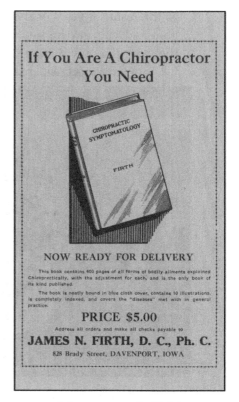

Advertisement for Vol. 7

The book focuses on function. Abnormal function is defined as a lack of expression of the mental impulse in the tissue cell. Firth writes:

> The kind of disease produced depends upon the quantity, quality or combination of abnormal expression of function that occurs in the part diseased, for it is found that different nerves convey mental impulses which, when expressed give rise to different functions. There are certain nerves that have to do with motor function, involving the tonicity and immovability of muscle. There are other sets that have to do with sensory function. Still other nerves called trophic nerves, which have to do with the nutrition. Summing them all up, we find that there are nine primary functions. Every disease, regardless of its character, can be analyzed as an abnormal expression of one or some combination of... nine functions by its lack of expression.

The nine functions were coined by B.J. Palmer in Vol. 5 and expanded upon in the 1913 edition of Vol. 2.

According to Firth, chiropractic analysis determines the normal or abnormal expression of function, which leads to where to adjust the vertebral subluxation. The focus is determining the cause of abnormal expression. Analysis is conducted through symptomatology, palpation, nerve tracing, and history taking. The case history always begins with questions about possible birth trauma.

Firth provided novel insights into the disease process from a chiropractic viewpoint. For example, he expanded on the medical concept of diathesis. He writes:

> A diathesis is a constitutional disposition to certain forms of incoordinations. This predisposition, however, is caused by vertebral subluxations, which, to a greater degree, are capable of causing the diseases to which the body is predisposed.

According to Firth, the restoration process and the body's return to health is a process of adjustment, which consists of gradual, daily changes or alterations to the character of symptoms. It takes time for the body to adapt. Retracing, and other phenomena related to the change of symptoms could take weeks of regular adjustments to resolve.

Firth also wrote about the philosophy and theory of chiropractic. Specifically, he wrote of mind force, which he viewed as synonymous with brain force and Innate Intelligence.

Vol. 7 applies many of B.J. Palmer's new chiropractic theories such as nerve tracing, retracing, momentum, equations, nine functions, and cycles. Firth's book integrated B.J.'s cycle theory. The brain receives the impression from the sensory system and then determines the quantity and quality of mental impulses that are required. The brain then furnishes the power to the organ. The mental impulse is generated in the brain and transmitted to the tissue cells where it is expressed as the power of the Innate Intelligence. The vertebral subluxation impairs the transmission, which leads to the organ not receiving its proper quantity or quality to perform its normal function. The chiropractor relieves the impingement at the IVF by "proper adjustment of the partially displaced or subluxated vertebra."

Firth was in Davenport in 1913 when D.D. Palmer visited and lectured at the PSC. He may have also attended D.D.'s 22 lectures at the Universal Chiropractic College in Davenport. According to his student, R.J. Watkins, Firth did attend the famous homecoming parade that year.

The second edition of the book, published in 1919, included 100 pages of new material on topics such as skin, eyes, hernia, and hemorrhoids. A third edition of the book was retitled as *Chiropractic Diagnosis*. Overall, Firth provided a template for other faculty to follow: apply the chiropractic standpoint to your topic and publish your lectures as a text.

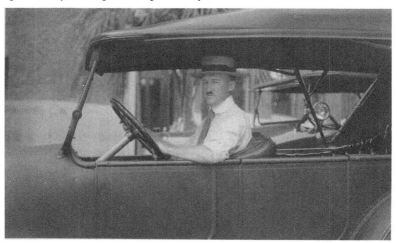

Firth at the Wheel (1920)

Vol. 7 had nothing to do with musculoskeletal complaints. The emphasis was on Type O disorders and the whole spectrum of abnormal expression of any of the nine functions. It was a text on assessing the pathophysiology of the body as it relates to the chiropractic vertebral subluxation.

Vedder's Chiropractic Physiology: Vol. 8 (1916)

Harry E. Vedder DC, PhC was born on March 26, 1891, in Hudson, Michigan. He enrolled in the PSC in January 1911 and graduated in January 1912. He joined the faculty even before that, in September 1911. Vedder wrote textbooks on physiology, gynecology, and advertising.   He published them as Vol. 8 in 1916, Vol. 12 in 1919, and Vol. 16 in 1924. Vedder resigned from the PSC in 1926. Rolf Peters provides some insight about Vedder's resignation, interspersed with Vedder quotes. He writes:

> Being a well-liked and capable teacher, he was considered an authority on chiropractic physiology and gynecology. On 19 July 1924 he predicted that "Chiropractic is facing a period of storm, which will last for the next three to five years" and that "the Chiropractic profession has been flooded with practitioners who look at Chiropractic as a business rather than a profession." He also noted, "I do not always agree with my co-workers in the decision of matters of policy pertaining to the Palmer School, and in sessions with my co-workers/fight for the principles which I believe to be right. Yet, if the majority is against me I realize that for the ultimate success of the institution, I must cooperate with them."

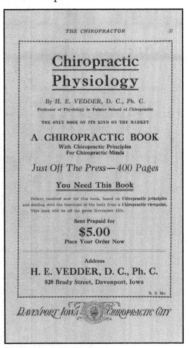

Advertisement for Vol. 8

Peters continues:

> Harry Vedder resigned from the faculty effective 15 May 1926, after 13 years as Professor of Physiology, apparently due to a conflict of opinion with B.J. Palmer.

Vedder founded LCC in September 1926, with Firth, Burich, and Hendricks. He served as the first President of LCC from 1926-1940. Harry Vedder died on July 27, 1949, in Hermosa Beach, California.

Vol. 8 or *A Textbook of Chiropractic Physiology* went into two editions and five printings. The book pioneered a theoretical approach to physiology

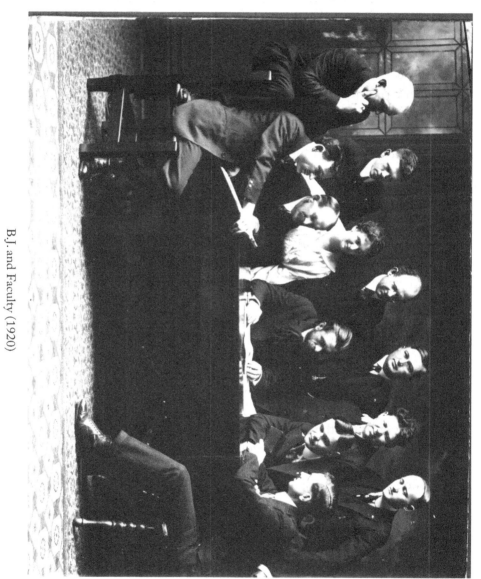

B.J. and Faculty (1920)

in the twentieth century with its emphasis on Innate in action. This approach to physiology in a textbook was unique. Rather than focusing on the physical aspects of the physiological systems, it emphasized the organization of the systems and the perspective of the organizer, the Innate. In the book, the term Innate is used 357 times. This kind of interior perspective of the body written into a physiology text was unheard of during this era. That type of approach wouldn't reach the mainstream of theoretical biology until the 1980s with Maturana and Varela's *Autopoiesis and Cognition*. They viewed the organism as cognitive and self-organizing. Vedder considered physiology as an expression of the living organism's intelligent self-organization.

The perspective of Vol. 8 views the physiology from the inside out. For example, instead of using the traditional term, "involuntary actions," Vedder includes B.J. Palmer's terminology, "Innate voluntary actions." This was a way to describe traditional involuntary actions by including the perspective from the body's intelligence. The voluntary or conscious actions were governed by Educated Intelligence. Vedder distinguished these as Educated functions and Innate functions. Functions were explained in terms of the overarching plan of the organism as a whole.

In the introduction he describes how this viewpoint sets the chiropractic perspective of biology apart from chemistry and physics. He writes:

> The Chiropractor assumes an entirely broader viewpoint. There is no question but that the laws of Chemistry and Physics are involved in the functioning of the human body. But, these laws of Chemistry and Physics are in turn governed and controlled by a higher power, an immaterial force which we have called Innate (inborn) Intelligence.

The chiropractic emphasis on "life" was what truly set it apart from traditional viewpoints that emphasized the components of the living system, not the intelligent wholeness of the system.

Vedder also wrote about consciousness. He proposed that the conscious and subconscious aspects of the mind are each "conscious to itself." He concurred with B.J. Palmer that the conscious Innate Intelligence derives its power from somewhere and transforms it in the brain for use in the body as physiological function.

To Vedder, the "immaterial something" was a "power" working through the nervous system. This power is the cause of living and reasoning. It is the same "great aggregation of power" that governs the universe and coordinates all of its parts.

Vedder adopted other terms from B.J. Palmer like Universal Intelligence and Mental Impulse. He preferred the term Universal Intelligence because, "it seems to express more fully the entire scope of its influence." He also chose "mental impulse" over "nerve impulse," because it captured the immaterial essence organizing physiological actions. He writes:

> In our opinion it establishes a closer connection between the immaterial Innate Intelligence which controls the cells of the body than any other term. What the nature of this impulse is we cannot say. Derived as it is from an immaterial, it undoubtedly is an immaterial itself, even though it may be recognized by material change along the course and at the periphery of the nerve.

Vedder's philosophy of physiology emphasized the human body's controlling principles. Physiology blends material anatomy with immaterial philosophy. Life is the application of the philosophy of chiropractic.

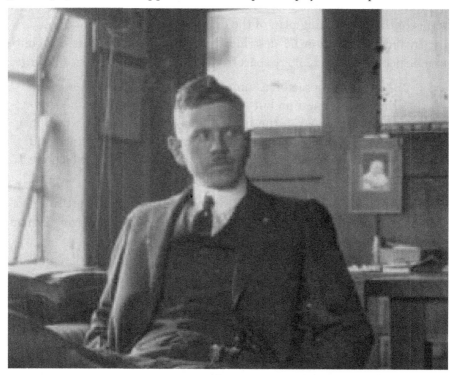

Harry Vedder, DC (1924)

Mabel Palmer's Chiropractic Anatomy: Vol. 9 (1918)

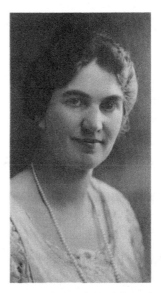

Mabel Heath Palmer, DC, PhC, was born on June 5, 1885, in Milan, Illinois. Mabel Palmer married B.J. Palmer on April 30, 1904. She graduated from D.D. Palmer's School in the class of 1905. Mabel was professor of Anatomy at PSC from 1909-1945, secretary of the Palmer Institute and Chiropractic Infirmary 1904-1906, and of the PSC starting in 1906. She was the mother of Dave Palmer, DC, who was born on January 12, 1906. She published Vol. 9 or *Chiropractic Anatomy* in 1918.

Mabel Palmer, Vol. 9 (1918)

The book went into five editions through 1923. She also published her world travels with essays about religion and women of the orient in the book *'Round the World with B.J.*, which was published in 1926. Her memoir was published in 1944 as *Stepping Stones*. Mabel died on March 30, 1949, in Tucson, Arizona. In Rolf Peters book, he writes:

> In September 1909, Mabel Palmer joined the faculty as Professor of Anatomy after her return from studying Anatomy under some of the best instructors in the United States. She also acted as private faculty adjuster for ladies. On 19 May 1914 Mabel founded the Sigma Phi Chi Sorority, the first Greek letter Sorority in chiropractic with 14 members. In 1918 Mabel Palmer published the first edition of *Chiropractic Anatomy*, which went through 5 editions and was used by most chiropractic schools. The book was still in use during the mid- 1940s… as she was still on faculty in 1945. Due to her soft, feminine side, she came to the aid of many students in a motherly fashion and was generally known as "the Sweetheart of the PSC."

On June 29, 1918, B.J. Palmer published an advertisement for Mabel's *Chiropractic Anatomy*. He wrote that Mabel had been working on the book for five years and that she had taught and studied the subject for ten years. Mabel saw "a crying demand for a book on this subject," one that would incorporate chiropractic research into every subject of anatomy. He writes, "She has studied deep into every Work on Anatomy, modern and ancient—34 all told." The advertisement was designed to encourage her to complete the book by taking pre-orders. He concludes:

> I have assured her the book would be welcomed because—
> 1st., there is nothing like it; 2nd., no other person is so qualified
> to produce it. She smiles this all to one side. Nothing can quite so
> strongly convince her as CONCRETE ORDERS BACKED
> UP WITH CASH... Come on Boys, writing a book for 5 years
> is some task. Let's give her a little encouragement.

Like Firth's book on symptomatology and Vedder's book on physiology, Mabel's textbook on anatomy takes the inside-out perspective. The structures of the body are considered from Innate's perspective. She described metabolism and body functions as directed by Innate Intelligence. The organism was viewed as intelligence personified in structures. The Innate portions of the text mostly emphasize physiological function and the ways in which vertebral subluxation diminishes the current and disrupts function.

Mabel intended to offer a chiropractic viewpoint on anatomy so that chiropractic may include a more scientific basis. Mabel's ability to describe core philosophical elements of the chiropractic paradigm is commendable. For example, she writes that the senses bring the mind "into relation with external objects." The sense organs were instruments of the mind. Her descriptions of muscle systems included those controlled by Educated and those by Innate.

The book includes B.J. Palmer's theory of creation, transmission, and expression of mental currents, and integrates his normal complete cycle. She writes:

> The brain, therefore, is the seat of all intelligence in the body
> the habitat of Innate Intelligence, which is the director of all
> functions in the body, from the time of birth to the dissolution
> of the physical and mental, which is death.

The brain is the place from which the mental currents, which control all functions of the body, emanate and flow to all parts of the body, to each tissue cell, the brain constitutes the beginning and the ending of the one great cycle, called life.

Innate adapts to the environment by protecting tissues and expressing optimal function. Mabel writes:

When no interference exists along the circuit, the brain works in completely harmonious order, for the fulfillment of the duty for which it was originally intended—a complete cycle—health.

Mabel Palmer wrote her anatomy text so that students and chiropractors in the field could have a text that would be useful for daily practice. The book is a compilation of nine years of her lectures. Her ultimate goal was to develop a book for chiropractors written from the chiropractic viewpoint.

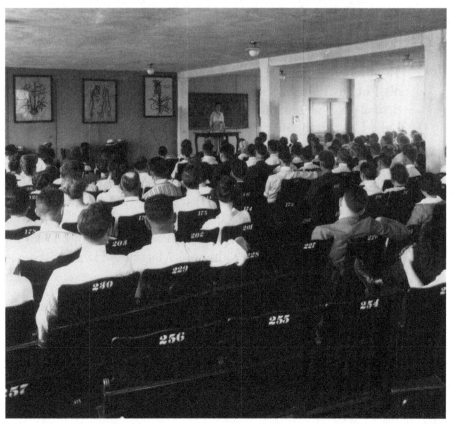

Mabel Palmer lecturing to Sophomore Class at the PSC (1920)

Thompson's Chiropractic Spinography: Vol. 10 (1918)

Ernest A. Thompson, DC, PhC, was born on March 8, 1891, in Chattanooga, Tennessee. He graduated from PSC on February 11, 1914, and joined the faculty in March. Thompson was head of the department of Spinography until August 1925. He died on October 15, 1970, in Baltimore, Maryland. In his book, Rolf Peters writes:

> Ernest Archibald Thompson, DC, a February 1914 graduate, was placed in charge of the Spinograph Department upon the departure of James Steele in March 1914. He had been an associate faculty member in Steele's department... He [had] lived in Rochester, New York, where he had been employed by the Mercury Manufacturing Company as a salesman. His assignment was to travel the Western territory. When he reached Davenport, he decided to change position and obtained a clerkship with a chain of cigar stores, which brought him into contact with chiropractic. He enrolled at Palmer and worked his way through school, working as a janitor and in a restaurant. Thompson became a prolific writer on spinography and gained his PhC in 1916. He severed his connection with the Palmer School on 1 September 1917, joining Dr. C.B. Johnson in Salt Lake City, Utah, but returned on 1 April 1918 and resumed his previous position. In 1919 he published *Text on Chiropractic Spinography* as Volume 10 of the Palmer Green Books. The text saw 4 editions and 4 printings. The fourth edition, published in 1923, was 4 times the size of the first edition. On 1 September 1922, under his directorship, Spinography was made a required subject in the curriculum. He left the PSC on 1 August 1925 to enter private practice in Baltimore, Maryland. He practiced for over 50 years until his death in October 1970.

Thompson's first writing on spinography was published in *The Chiropractor* in April 1914, as *What the Spinograph Does*. He suggested that spinographs are ideal for "stubborn cases" so that the chiropractor might see the positioning of the vertebra. He makes the case that spinographs get quick results on such cases because palpation alone does not account for spinal anomalies like bent spinous processes and a myriad of other conditions.

His articles provide a history of the growth of x-ray analysis in the early profession. Every few months he published articles about the value of spinography, and asked chiropractors to send their cases and provide case studies. In October 1914, in *The Value of Spinograph*, he mentions that spinography was taught at Lyceum and several were planning to buy private units. In January 1915, in *Chiropractic* and *The Spinograph*, he mentions that chiropractors were sending cases to Davenport for spinographs from as far away as Hawaii. In May 1915, in *What Will the Spinograph Do for Me?*, he promoted spinography as a way to increase the standard of the profession, improve chiropractic's reputation one chiropractor at a time, and get more business. Thompson writes:

> We all know that the science of Chiropractic is coming into its own very rapidly, and it is your duty as a Chiropractor, to keep it above all other methods of healing, and to keep it there you must obtain the results your patients come to you for. Every failure you have with a patient means a "knock" for you and Chiropractic also, while every result means more business and success for you.

Vol. 10 or *Text on Chiropractic Spinography* was published in 1918. B.J. Palmer wrote an eight-page *Introduction* to the second edition of Vol. 10, where he provides a history of chiropractic's integration of x-ray analysis since 1910. He writes:

> We take a pleasure in writing this introduction to this able and excellent work on Spinographic Technic. Dr. E. A. Thompson has been with us more years than any other teacher on this subject. He has unquestionably seen more work, read more plates, taught more students than any other man living, not excepting the author himself. It is because he is so eminently fitted for this peculiar line of work that his work on this question becomes a paramount, valuable addition to the world's scientific publications. Judge not this work by its size, but by the actual definite working knowledge it contains.

Thompson used the word "Innate" one time in the text. He was referring to ankylosis in acute rotations with chronic curvatures. He writes that it "clearly illustrates the adaptability of innate in building up a bridge work to strengthen the weakened area." This is exactly how D.D. Palmer originally used the term Innate Intelligence in 1902.

Thompson made several contributions to vertebral subluxation theory. He mentions "subluxation" over 275 times in the 1923 edition of the book. One contribution to subluxation theory was his finding that small spinous processes sometimes palpated as if they were anterior. This was especially the case with T10. Other innovations to vertebral subluxation theory comprise analysis and adjusting protocols. For example, Thompson suggested that if two adjacent vertebrae are rotated from the center, the chiropractor should adjust the greater rotation first because of the increased pressure to the nerve fibers.

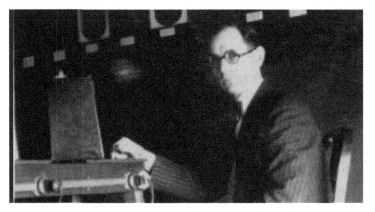

E.A. Thompson with x-ray reader (1925)

He also gave many tips on how and why to notate vertebral shapes and spinal curvatures. For example, in cases when the vertebra palpates the opposite of the actual listing, notating malformations and exostosis is especially important. On notating tipped vertebra it is important to assess rotatory conditions and curvatures. There will not always be subluxations in scoliotic cases. Great care is required to determine the apex of lateral scoliosis and rotatory scoliosis as the subluxation may often be found above or below the apex.

He also recommends the chiropractor "always list the axis first," before listing the atlas. In one instance he explains that axis subluxations often "carry" atlas and third cervical with it. This is important to consider when palpating a prominent atlas in the opposite direction from the axis. The atlas is usually adaptive to the axis. Correcting axis in such cases will also correct the atlas.

Thompson's book includes many types of analysis for chiropractors. It also covers basic terminology, theories, and the science of x-ray practice comprehensively for its time.

Burich's Chiropractic Chemistry: Vol. 11 (1919)

Stephen J. Burich, DC, PhC, was born on August 15, 1887, in Reedsville, Wisconsin. He graduated from PSC in May 1913 after he had already joined the faculty in March 1913. Steve Burich was head of the Department of Chemistry starting in 1913, and head of the Department of Neurology from 1922 until 1926. He was one of the founders of LCC with Firth, Vedder, and Hendricks. Burich died on February 3, 1946.

In his book, Rolf Peters writes:

> [Burich] attended common schools in Rockland Township and Milwaukee and graduated from the Whitewater High School in 1907. He attended Beloit College and taught Chemistry in Milwaukee for a year before attending Palmer. As head of the Chemistry Department, he established the laboratory in March 1913, and was listed as Professor of Chemistry and Microscopy, also teaching Histology and Psychology. A frequent contributor to *The Chiropractor*, he wrote *A Textbook of Chiropractic Chemistry* as Volume 11 of the Palmer Green Books in 1919. The book was reprinted 3 times. In 1922 Burich was placed in charge of the Department of Neurology. He resigned from the Palmer faculty effective 15 May 1926.

Burich published several articles in *The Chiropractor* between August 1913 and 1922. Topics included habits, curing, tonsillitis, sense organs, chemistry of digestive ferments, and the development of the mind.

Vol. 11 or *A Textbook on Chiropractic Chemistry* is the first book of its kind to integrate the Innate perspective and subluxation theory into the field of chemistry. The first edition of the book came out in 1919. Two more editions were published by 1921. Burich views Innate Intelligence as the "great supervisor" of chemical processes related to metabolism and function. A nervous system free from subluxation allows for this supervision to continue unimpeded. Normal function and health are the result. For him, Innate is the will behind function, action of the organs, and even influences enzyme formation.

The book defines a chemistry of life. According to Burich, Innate is able to act only when the elements of proper organization, such as oxygen and nutrition, are in place. Innate may then guide the coordination of functions, actions of the tissues, and expression of health. This theory was the precursor to his student Ralph Stephenson's theory of "limitations of matter," defined in Vol. 14.

In Vol. 11, Burich also relates subluxation theory to chemistry. He viewed subluxation as "the cause of all disease," due to nerve impingements. He writes:

> As long as no subluxations exist in the spinal column and there is no impingement upon the spinal nerves which emit through the intervertebral foramina, no incoordination exists, and the material which is taken into the body as food under these normal conditions is properly digested, absorbed and assimilated under the supervision of Innate Intelligence. In cases where no impingement obtains, just the right amount of fat, which is to be used in the metabolism of the body, is taken from the food. Under Innate's supervision there is no deficiency or surplus of fat ever present in the human body.

According to Burich, as long as there are no subluxations, Innate can direct, supervise, guide, and furnish mental impulses to glands and organs, which can secrete and regulate physiological chemistry and keep the vital processes under control.

Burich and Vedder both resigned from the PSC on May 15, 1926. In response to their resignations, B.J. Palmer writes:

Men have a right to differences of opinion and judgment, based upon their vision, but it is not to the best interest of any institution to attempt to compromise on vital principles. Conflicting instruction in proven fundamentals retards and destroys the process of constructive advancement. Progress makes way to those who will. The departure of friends always leaves its imprint upon the pages of memory.

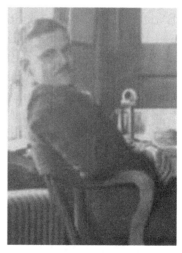

Burich (1924)

Vedder's Chiropractic Gynecology: Vol. 12 (1919)

Vol. 12 or *A Textbook on Chiropractic Gynecology* by Harry Vedder, DC, PhC, was published in 1919. The book went into five editions through 1929. It is a pathophysiology book written from the perspective of Innate Intelligence as it relates to the chiropractic subluxation and gynecological diseases. He writes,

> Chiropractic is, always has been, and always will be, based on the foundation of natural laws; the cause of disease being found in subluxations of the spine and relieved by the adjustment of those subluxations. That is Chiropractic in its simplicity...

According to Vedder, the simplicity of chiropractic should not include other methods and teaching texts should only include procedures that are chiropractic. Explaining the rationale for the book he writes:

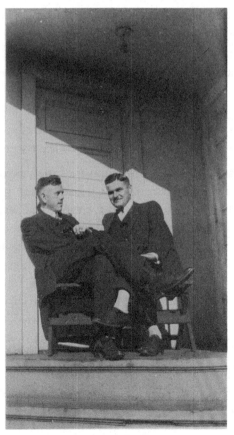

Vedder and Burich (1924)

The author has felt for many years that a strictly Chiropractic book on the subject of Gynecology was a real necessity. What other authors had written mattered little, because they had all left out the essential element that was necessary in a Chiropractic publication. Looking at the problem from the standpoint of the field Chiropractor and the student of Chiropractic, he saw that the essential elements required were a statement of the cause of the disease; a thoroughly Chiropractic explanation of that cause and the results that might be expected under adjustments.

These three factors have been incorporated in every disease considered, and it is with the sincere hope that this publication fills a long felt need in the Chiropractic world that this book has been produced.

Throughout the text, Vedder includes many references to Innate in terms of reparation of damage due to degeneration, coordinating adaptive measures to various conditions, the formation and branching of anatomical structures, maintaining normal tonicity of vessel walls and tissues, and sending out "mentality" via impulses 100 percent of the time for normal function.

Vedder refers to subluxation as the etiology of 78 disease processes from cysts to gonorrhea. In the latter, he even describes a holistic view of causation in terms of a weakened condition of the tissues. He writes:

This leads us to the conclusion that the microorganism is a condition in the course of the disease rather than a causative factor in its production. If this were not true, every individual who came in contact with the gonococcus would, of necessity, develop the disease. A subluxation in the lumbar region producing impingement on those nerve fibers which supply the generative tract is essential as well as a subluxation at K. P. which affects the general bodily elimination. As a result of these impingements, there is a generally weakened condition of the tissues and in consequence any toxin which comes in contact with the congested mucous membranes acts as an irritant which is productive of inflammation. In brief, the mere fact that the bacillus is present is not proof that it is the causative element.

The diseases themselves are described in terms of incoordination due to nerve impingement, mainly at K.P. and P.P. These abbreviations were started by D.D. Palmer. He referred to K.P. as Kidney Place in the 1890s. B.J. Palmer referred to P.P., for private place, in relation to ureters, bladder, and urethra in 1907 and used abbreviations extensively in Vol. 4 in 1908.

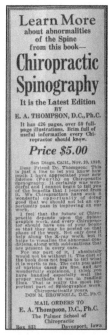

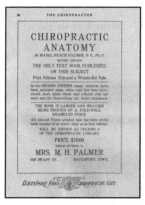

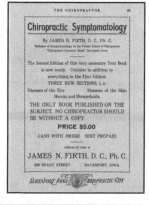

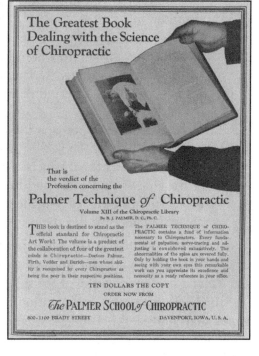

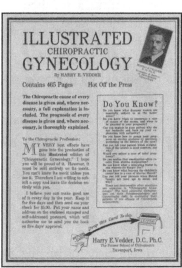

Advertisements for Vols. 7, 9, 10, 12, 13

B.J. Palmer's Technique Textbook: Vol. 13 (1920)

Vol. 13 or *A Textbook on The Palmer Technique of Chiropractic* was published in 1920. The bulk of the text is dedicated to teaching the student how to adjust using the toggle-recoil. Vol. 13 is a full-spine, toggle-recoil adjusting manual. B.J. Palmer was listed as the sole author. However, his dedication reveals that the book was developed by him, Firth, Vedder, and Burich. B.J. writes:

> On every subject, in every movement, with every progression, there must be a leader, but closely allied to him are always the several close and intimate helpmates from whom and about whom too little is known.
>
> Chiropractic is no exception to that rule. Drs. Firth, Vedder and Burich are three of those men who have been close to me and mine for years. In the classroom; in my home, at my table and in Sunday conferences, we have threshed over the thousands of angles until our ideas have so mutually blended that they are as one.
>
> When it came to getting out a book on this subject, I knew of no one set of men to whom I could entrust so much of its subject matter as these. And, as you review the work, realize with me, that I take very little of its credit. To them must go practically all of it.
>
> As a pioneer, I perhaps thought a bit; but, as a finished product in the text-book for the student, to them must come all appreciation of that which you see and read.
>
> To Drs. Firth, Vedder and Burich do I gladly dedicate this book. To those who have made it possible should go whatever credit and honor is due them.

Vedder collaborated with B.J. on the sections on palpation. Burich collaborated with B.J. on the section on nerve tracing. Firth's contribution was the sections on abnormalities of the spine.

The book represents a culmination of PSC methods by 1920. It integrates and applies B.J. Palmer's theories developed in Vols. 2-6, with the diagnostic and physiological approaches developed by his faculty as published in Vols. 7-12.

Vol. 13 applies the chiropractic perspective to practice. In this regard, the emphasis is on the "chiropractic analysis." The chiropractic analysis determines the abnormal expression of function, the manner of the abnormal expression, and the cause of the abnormal expression. To complete this analysis, the chiropractor takes a case history and uses palpation, nerve tracing, and symptomatology, methods pioneered by D.D. Palmer.

This determination of abnormal expression and the location of its cause is highlighted as a contribution to the field of diagnosis. Rather than just naming "a given specific pathological or diseased state," B.J. writes:

> In contradistinction, the Chiropractor in making an analysis, upon finding the existence of a diseased condition, immediately arrives at the conclusion that there is an abnormal expression of function. By further application of reason, based upon a knowledge of the body and its functions, he determines what function is abnormally expressed and in what way it is abnormally expressed to produce the specific condition present. By further reason and further examination he determines the exact cause of this abnormal expression of function.

Through palpation and nerve tracing, coupled to a knowledge of anatomy, physiology, and symptomatology, the chiropractor locates "the causative condition necessarily existent in the spine." According to B.J., this approach to analysis provides more than just an assessment of symptoms but a determination of the pathological condition, what we refer to today as pathophysiology. This is confirmed through nerve tracing. B.J. writes:

> Having determined the etiology of the effect, the Chiropractor employs a method distinctly his own which proves that his analysis is correct. This method is nerve tracing and by it the direct connection between the cause and effect is absolutely established. Thus it will be seen that nerve tracing is not only of inestimable educational value to the practitioner, in his field practice, but it is also one of the scientific features which differentiates Chiropractic from all other sciences

Three years after the publication of this text, B.J. started researching spinal thermography. Thermographic instrumentation and X-ray replaced the older practice of nerve tracing at the PSC. This shift in analysis and the focus of teaching at PSC may have played a role in B.J.'s split with his co-authors of this text, all of whom resigned from the PSC by 1926. A few years later, PSC would abandon the traditional focus on using symptoms to locate vertebral subluxation relying solely on objective measures.

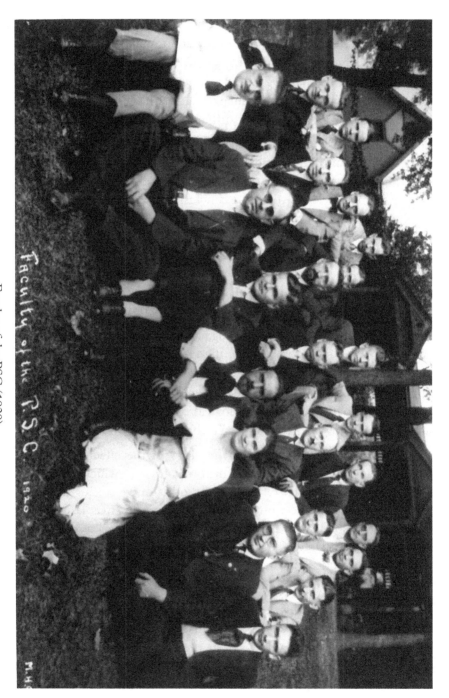

Faculty of the PSC (1920)

Chapter 7
The Humanities Green Books
Spirit of PSC, Advertising, and Malpractice

Between 1920 and 1924, the PSC published three Green Books that were not directly about the philosophy, science, and art of chiropractic. We are referring to these books as The Humanities Green Books. The first one published was James Leroy Nixon's *The Spirit of the PSC: Vol. 14*, the second was Vedder's *Chiropractic Advertising: Vol. 16*, and the third was Arthur Holmes' *Malpractice as Applied to Chiropractors: Vol. 17*.

These books capture different domains of chiropractic. Nixon's book covers personal, cultural, and social aspects of the early profession, just at the time when the PSC was booming and chiropractic was becoming part of United States culture. Vedder's book includes the business side of chiropractic, especially marketing and communications. Holmes' book covers the legal structures of the profession in relation to practice and the courts.

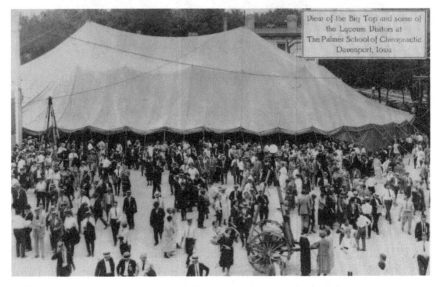

PSC Lyceum (1921)

Nixon's Spirit of the PSC: Vol. 14 (1920)

James Leroy Nixon was born on April 8, 1851, in Caton, New York. He graduated from the PSC on August 29, 1920. Nixon was an author and a newspaper man from New York. He went to Davenport to write a story about chiropractic because he was helped by chiropractic adjustments. He met B.J. and Mabel and decided to enroll in the PSC. Nixon died in 1933 in Caton.

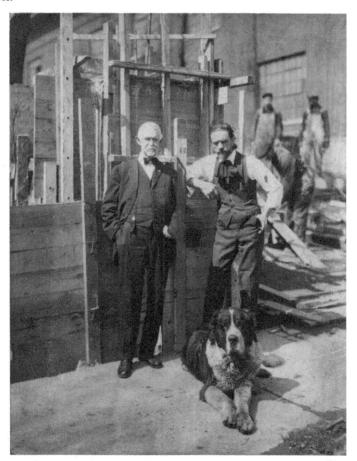

James Leroy Nixon, B.J. Palmer, and Big Ben, Vol. 14 (1920)

Nixon became a student at the PSC the year before the peak of enrollment, which occurred after the veterans returned from World War I. In 1916, there were 462 students, in 1919 there were more than 1,200, and in 1921, somewhere between 2,700 and 3,100 students. B.J. Palmer wrote that the 1919 Lyceum (homecoming) had 5,150 in attendance for the week. Lyceum was canceled in 1920 because the city was not equipped to house that many people. They were expecting more than 8,000 in 1921. Nixon's book captures the vibrant PSC culture.

Vol. 14 or *The Spirit of the PSC: Based on Facts Gleaned at the Chiropractic Fountain Head* is written from the student's perspective. The format is a story with dialogue. With a full-time faculty, large Lyceum parades, and a robust student body, Nixon decided to capture the culture in a fictional styled book.

Nixon's philosophical writings are socially-oriented and geared for any incoming student or alumni. It is a fascinating look at how the chiropractic worldview was emerging day-to-day in dialogue outside of the classroom. Students, who were training to bring chiropractic to the world, were also grappling with an entirely new way of viewing the world, the body, health, healing, and the universe. Nixon captured this. He writes:

> In writing the following story the author has been actuated solely by a strong desire to convey to the public a more intimate knowledge of actual conditions at The Palmer School of Chiropractic, the great Fountain Head of that new and wonderful science which seems destined to revolutionize the art of healing as applied to the human body and eventually bring to the inhabitants of the earth, it is not improbable, a return of that remarkable longevity which seemingly attached to our earlier forbears. So much of misrepresentation has been circulated through the direct or veiled activity of Medical professional jealousy, that it is only fair to those deluded ones who have believed the vaporings of selfish detractors, that they be given a true picture of the actual life of the school; the extent of its educational resources, the personal characteristics and charm of its capable faculty; the scope of its curriculum; the cosmopolitan character of its student body and the marvelous results which have attended the application of its art.

Nixon's style is colloquial, down to earth, and simple to understand. A few lengthy quotes will capture how he embodied the culture and philosophy through his prose. These quotes enact elements of chiropractic that no other Green Book captures. All of the topics are covered throughout B.J. Palmer's books but Nixon's ability to include the first-person and second-person perspectives is an important contribution to the PSC body of literature.

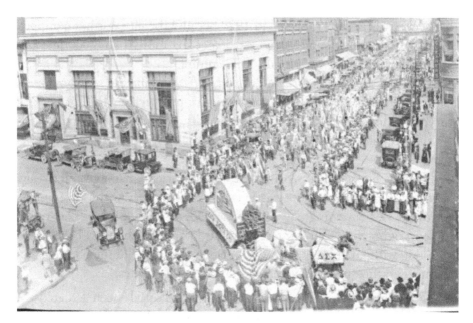

PSC Lyceum parade down Brady Street, Delta Sigma Chi Fraternity float
rounding the corner pulled by four horses (1921)

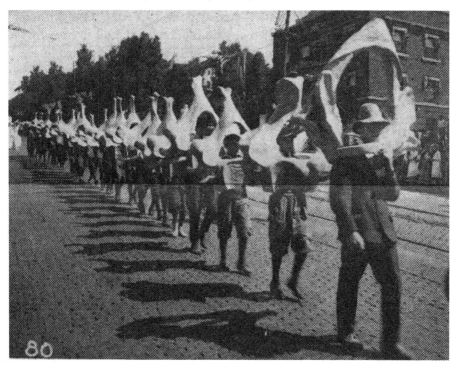

PSC 5th Annual Lyceum parade (1919)

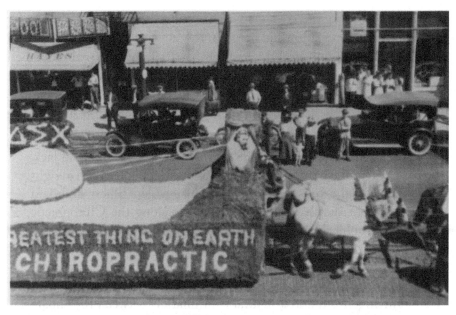

Delta Sigma Chi Fraternity float in the PSC Lyceum parade (1919)

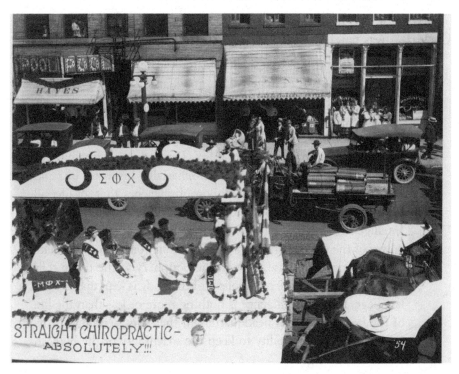

Sigma Phi Chi Chiropractic Sorority float in the PSC Lyceum parade (1919)

The following quote covers a very complex aspect of the philosophy of chiropractic, the relationship between the interior of the individual and the interior of the universal. It describes the type of personal embodied and intuitive action that B.J. Palmer had been advocating for more than a decade. Nixon even uses B.J.'s mentor, Elbert Hubbard, as an example. Hubbard died on the Lusitania, which was a passenger ship sunk by the Germans at the start of WWI in 1915. The dialogue goes like this:

> "That of itself is evidence of greatness, Ah believe," said Jack.
>
> "Yes," Clawson returned, "and it was the courage born of right living and a broad perspective, that enabled Elbert Hubbard to die heroically as he did. Following along the Chiropractic philosophical idea, one might say that Innate found in him a most efficient vehicle of expression."
>
> "Well, partner, yeh're pretty deep for me, but Ah reckon Ah understand what yeh're driving at. Yeh mean that Universal Intelligence found a natural coordination between the Innate mind and the Educated mind of Elbert Hubbard, not usually possessed by the average individual."

Nixon jumps from there straight into B.J. Palmer's Normal Complete Cycle as it was taught by John Craven at PSC. He writes:

> "Something like that, Jack. Nearer to the creative idea. But to tell you the truth I'm getting somewhat into the fog of doubt as I study the normal cycle as explained by Doctor Craven."
>
> "What's bothering yeh ?" Jack asked with a smile. "Ah think the Professor is pretty clear in his analysis."
>
> "Well, what do you think of this?" Clawson asked, hitching his chair nearer to his companion and emphasizing his words by rapid gesture with his hands. "Our philosophy teaches that all life; all force in the body; all power to function proceeds from Universal Intelligence, as reflected in the brain by Innate Intelligence. That power of the various organs properly to function is sent by Innate over the line of impulse through the periphery to the tissue cells and in this manner the metabolism of the body is kept up. In plain language, Innate Intelligence is nothing more or less than the life of the body, having its headquarters in the brain, sending out its constant stream of vitality to keep the machinery of the body in motion. Am I right?"

"That's about as Ah understand it," Jack replied, hesitantly. He could not quite grasp the sudden philosophical turn the mind of Clawson had taken.

From there, Nixon explores one of the most profound aspects of the philosophy of chiropractic: what happens to Innate Intelligence after death. He writes it as though all students of the philosophy have these types of questions. Nixon writes:

"Now, then, if Universal Intelligence is the supreme force, God, the Supreme Being, the designer and creator of all things, and Innate is the reflection simply of Universal Intelligence, what becomes of a human life when it quits the body? From the viewpoint I have suggested, life is no more, no less than a reflection of Universal Intelligence first expressed in the embryo, gradually developed and sustained from the same source until final dissolution. When that occurs, what becomes of the reflection, the life? Does it wander like a vagrant gleam of light through eternity's space, or does it follow the more natural and reasonable course of returning to the fountain head to be again absorbed by Universal Intelligence, much as the sailor returns a bucket of sea water which has served its purpose in washing the decks, back to volume of the ocean?"

For a moment Jack made no answer. He had been watching Clawson with surprise, not unmixed with apprehension while he had been speaking. Now he arose and going over to the elder man's side, placed his hand inquiringly upon his gray hair.

"What's the matter, partner? Don't yeh feel well? They say the flu is getting a strong hold for the season's campaign. Ah do hope yeh ain't going to be ill!"

"Oh, quit your fooling, Jack!" Clawson protested. "I'm entirely serious. This, you understand, is a conjectural hypothesis. It's not an attempt to refute the idea of the immortality of the soul, but an argument in its support. Wouldn't it be immortal if it returned after performing its mission here in some human frame, to be taken up and reabsorbed by the great Universal Intelligence from which it had originally come? Wouldn't it now?"

He gave Jack a friendly slap on the back and turned his attention for the moment to refilling his pipe.

"Yehr getting hold of the subject from a new angle to me,"

Jack said, resuming his lounging attitude on the bed. "Why don't yeh ask Craven about that?"

"I'm going to," Clawson answered. "It's new ideas, they tell me, that pleases both B. J. and the instructor. You spoke of the fact that when B. J. talks to the students, he always says something that makes one think. He certainly proved the truth of that estimate when he wrote his philosophy. It certainly opens a broad road to conjecture and investigation which may lead into entirely new realms of reasoning. Now as for this suggestion I have presented. Humanity in general bases its faith on the Scriptural writings. What do we find there? Something like this: 'For the body shall return to dust, and the spirit to God who gave it.' To continue the argument, what does that mean? What is the spirit? Life; the soul; the immortal part of man! If when it leaves the body it goes back to its source, then it must return to Universal Intelligence, to be absorbed into the great source of all things as the bucket of water is absorbed by mother ocean; losing its individual identity, but remaining an atom of that supreme something. Such an idea might be accepted by the profound thinker with consistency. We have long since abandoned the idea of a literal hell of fire and brimstone, such as the clergy of my boyhood used to some advantage in their revival efforts; why may we not with equal reason question the supposition of a literal Heaven with streets of gold and gates of pearl? What do you think? Understand, Jack, I'm not trying to destroy any images, simply talking for argument's sake. Is the idea altogether at variance with the teaching of Chiro philosophy?"

"Well, partner, Ah don't know sometimes what to think! Just when Ah begin to believe Ah've got the idea down pat, along comes some suggestion which sort of upsets my former analysis of the subject. Ah'd really like to have yeh take it up with Craven and see what deduction he'll make. He's a shrewd reasoner, no doubt about that."

"Oh, I shall, never fear," Clawson answered. "He has shown a willingness to explain all questions that are presented. You have noticed that sometimes the entire period has been occupied in answering inquiries handed up by the students. He meets my idea of a capable teacher."

Nixon's writings capture the practical and integral way that people lived the chiropractic paradigm, which was never just a health care profession

SPECIAL Reduction

IN THE PRICE OF

Two Famous Books of the CHIROPRACTIC LIBRARY

Now $3.00 POSTPAID

VOLUME I

PHILOSOPHY

By B. J. PALMER

Going beyond the mere "back-punching" for money. During the time that this book was written (and subsequently revised with each issue), The Palmer School was going through its hardest struggle for recognition. Contains articles on Orthopedy, Innate Intelligence, Suggestive Therapeutics, and many other subjects of interest. Last pages have dictionary of common terms used by practitioners. Three hundred and thirty-two pages.

Regular Price $3.50.

VOLUME XIV

THE SPIRIT OF THE P. S. C.

By LEROY M. NIXON

Without the history of The Palmer School the story of Chiropractic would be incomplete and lacking in interest. Much of the philosophy of Chiropractic is given in easily readible form in this book for the practitioner to present to his patients and prospects. No chiropractor's office equipment is complete without this book. Two hundred pages.

Regular Price $2.00.

In ordering specify NO. VX-56—Chiropractic Library
(Two Books) $3.00, Postage Paid

The PALMER SCHOOL of CHIROPRACTIC
Davenport, Iowa, U.S.A.

Advertisement for Vol. 1 & Vol. 14 (1921)

but a new way to live and be in the world. The chiropractic perspective included a viewpoint from within outward, ideally, a view from the nervous system free of subluxation.

Nixon's novel also explores the transformation of consciousness that many patients have always associated with the chiropractic adjustment. Often such states of consciousness are related to a more attuned and coherent sense of being. Sometimes these first-person experiences relate to somatic memories of physical, emotional, or psychological trauma, what B.J. Palmer called retracing. This was closely aligned to D.D. Palmer's idea of overcoming the abnormal habit of a vertebra. It also relates to what B.J. referred to years later as illumination. Nixon writes:

"Ah hope yeh have not been disappointed," said Jack, regarding Clawson with earnest inquiry.

"Disappointed?" said Ralph. "Far from that! After the first three adjustments, my conscious self began to assert its restored sovereignty. It was as if memory's hand went back into the obscurity of the past and dragged out and posted up for my inspection one by one, those connecting incidents which have already served partially to bridge the gloomy gulf of my forgetfulness. Daily I can feel my hold upon that past becoming more and more tangible. Daily my mental vision appears to grow stronger. There are still many things I would know that have not yet been revealed, but I sincerely believe that Innate Intelligence is urging on the educated brain to increased effort at more clear interpretation. I feel absolutely certain now, that eventually I shall be able to clear up all the doubts and uncertainties, and come into full possession of that clear retrospect which will answer all questions and remove all doubts. I already feel like a new man. It has been much like being put away in a tomb under a mistaken impression of death, only to be rescued at the eleventh hour and restored to life and action. But for all the great benefit I am deriving from the art of Chiropractic, I feel confident I should never have considered the matter of adjustments as a relief from this strange incoordination, had it not been for the appearance of what I, at the time, believed to be a spiritual visitation of the one woman who had blessed my life. Is it not wonderfully strange that the inspiration should have come immediately on my entering the school and on the day that I began my regular course of study of the science through which I was to find the road to recovery?"

"Why, the whole story sounds like a fairy tale," said Jack. "If it ever becomes known publicly, it will be a clincher for those wooden-heads who maintain that the science is a dream of ignorance. Have you ever said anything to B. J. about this?"

"Not a word; to no one except what I have just told you. Even my adjuster does not know why I urged him to take the atlas and other cervicals. To tell you the truth, I expected that were I to tell them why, they would shake their heads, in doubt of my sanity! I wanted to be sure, and once I am fully restored, as I have every reason to believe I shall be, I shall be quite willing to tell it to the world."

"Well, yeh certainly have my best wishes that the time may come speedily," said Jack. "Ah realized up there in Uncle Jerry's room that yeh were hard hit, but Ah hadn't any idea it was Innate giving yeh a lift into the right road. Reckon Universal Intelligence had something to do with it, after all."

"I am not prepared to dispute that," Clawson returned, "but it is taking the real Chiropractic course—retracing. Is it not remarkable that the first thing I accurately remembered was the explosion in which I was hurt, and after that the incidents leading up to the accident, in recessional."

Capturing the culture even further, Nixon includes a graduation scene. Since there were no videos back then, this is as close as we will ever get to understanding what it was like for the students at PSC during that era. He writes:

Exercises were brief but impressive. After a short but forceful address by B. J., in which he congratulated the members of the class upon their success and praised them for their diligence, as well as giving them practical advice to guide them in the great work for humanity upon which they were about entering, the graduates formed in single column, marching before the assembled faculty, each being handed his or her diploma by Dr. Palmer; each receiving from their former instructors, the men whom from long and intimate association they had come to love and esteem, hearty congratulations and best wishes for successful, profitable and pleasant field experience.

Then the chimes again rang out their silvery toned notes of a gladsome welcome to the full-fledged Chiros, and student friends crowded forward to add their good wishes to all that had gone before.

Advertisement for Vol. 14 (1921)

One last element of Nixon's philosophical approach is his writings about the future. The culture of chiropractic always held a promise that the world would be changed, one person at a time, which will lead to a better and healthier world. Nixon's inclusion of this vision is congruent with the view of the Palmers. Furthermore, this passage captures the vision and engages the reader who just might be a prospective student. He writes,

> "Then in time we should have an entirely new type of citizenship, providing all children were given Chiropractic attention as they developed?" Margaret asked.
>
> "That should be the result," Ralph answered, "though it might take several generations to accomplish the full reformation. There would be incoordinations of heredity to overcome, which no doubt would prove the strongest obstacle to speedy readjustment of conditions. Really, the future possibilities of Chiropractic are more remarkable even than the secret wrung by chance from nature by Dr. Palmer's father. I think that B. J. himself believes that his remarkable art is still in its infancy. Even his building plans indicate that. Today there is no student in his school who is studying as hard or as conscientiously as the president of the institution."

"I have found it a most absorbing subject," Margaret said. "Walter and Beatrice have both been enthusiasts, and even before coming here I had become impressed with the idea that in giving his new art to the world, Dr. Palmer had conferred an inestimable blessing upon suffering humanity. I have been almost tempted to myself enroll as a student." Ralph laughed.

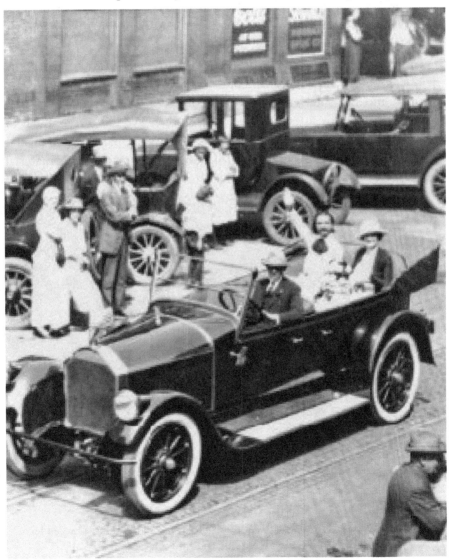

B.J. and Mabel Palmer in the PSC Lyceum Parade (1919)

Vedder's Chiropractic Advertising: Vol. 16 (1924)

Harry Vedder, DC, PhC, was not only the head of the Department of Physiology at PSC, he also oversaw the printing and advertising for the school. He edited the *Chiropractic Educator*, which was a magazine for laypeople that grew to a distribution of three million. Vedder also wrote a column in *The Chiropractor* called, "Get This," along with some other essays. Prior to publishing his third book, Vol. 16 or *Chiropractic Advertising*, he published at least two articles on related topics.

In 1920, Vedder wrote an article called *Compensation*. He considers the law of compensation, which B.J. Palmer wrote about years later, as always operative and not solely related to material gain. Vedder concludes that this was the law of cause and effect. He writes, "We fail to see much of the compensation because we see only the material." Character, honor, and real friends lead to the beaming smile of old age, no matter one's material success.

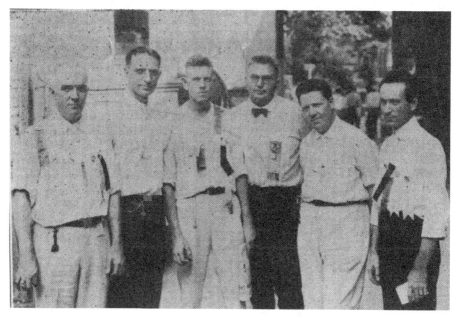

PSC Faculty at the 5th Annual Lyceum:
From left to right Drs. James C. Wishart, Henri L. Gaddis, Harry E. Vedder,
Fank W. Elliott, Otis E. Cronk, and John H. Craven (1919)

Vedder's 1922 article on *Selling* became Chapter 7 of his new book. The article emphasizes advertising psychology as a way to create interest and desire in the prospective buyer. Since the average person only views health as "a means to an end," and because focusing on sick patients in advertising is a limited market, Vedder proposes that chiropractors educate the public on preventative care, maintenance care, and any signs that the body's function is becoming deficient. He gives the example of the new ways in which the auto industry was teaching the public to take care of the rattles and loose bolts. He also suggests chiropractors increase their scope by including care for a wide spectrum of non-acute ailments. He writes:

> Why not apply this same fundamental advertising principle to Chiropractic? Why not convince the public through education that the little rattles, the little attacks of indigestion, the passing spells of headache, etc., are danger signals which precede a coming collapse. They are merely nature's way of acquainting us with the fact that something is becoming deficient in our physical make up.

Vol. 16 was written as a guide for chiropractors based on a survey of 150 chiropractors in the field with an average of 6.4 years of practice. Vedder mailed out a questionnaire to successful practices in a wide variety of urban and rural locations. It contained 24 questions. Some of the results were as follows: 71% used newspaper advertising, 44% contracted for advertising space with average use of 1475 inches of newspaper columns per year, 65% tried to get newspaper articles about their business published, 56% used more than one newspaper, 65% used pictures, 54% did not write their own ad copy, 92% focused their ads entirely on chiropractic and did not compare it to other methods. The book is mostly comprised of practical applications of daily advertising practices based on the results of the survey.

Vedder acknowledges that the chiropractic profession was the first health profession to use advertising "on an extensive scale." He writes, "Unquestionably, the Chiropractic profession uses more printers ink per year than all other professions combined." This is why he was concerned that the science of chiropractic would be influenced by the business, which could be detrimental to viewing chiropractic as a profession.

In considering the difference between duty and ethics, Vedder makes a plea for chiropractors to ethically fulfill their duty. This viewpoint is reminiscent of D.D. Palmer's writings on the topic. Vedder writes:

Some chiropractors seem to feel that they are going beyond the limits of propriety when they presume that patients, who have received benefits from them, should be expected to concern themselves further in the welfare of the chiropractor. Some of these practitioners call it unethical to push themselves and their ability or to seek publicity about these important facts. Nothing, however, could be further from the facts. Every chiropractor has spent a world of concentrated effort and considerable time in obtaining a knowledge which fits him to bring to the people of his community a service, and any thing which will effectively apprise that community of his ability to render that service is not only a privilege which he possesses, but a duty under which he is obligated.

The privilege of being a chiropractor comes with an obligation to increase "the circle of his beneficent influence," by telling everyone about the benefits of chiropractic.

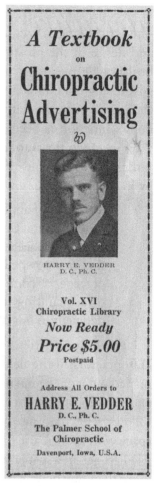

A Textbook on Chiropractic Advertising

HARRY E. VEDDER
D. C., Ph. C.

Vol. XVI
Chiropractic Library
Now Ready
Price $5.00
Postpaid

Address All Orders to
HARRY E. VEDDER
D. C., Ph. C.
The Palmer School of
Chiropractic
Davenport, Iowa, U.S.A.

Advertisement for Vol. 16

Vedder implores his readers to garner confidence by being sincere, truthful, professional, dependable, and not exaggerating claims. He also recommends the cultivation of a genuine interest in others as a way to increase one's natural friendliness.

Finally, Vedder criticized the profession for the infighting, and suggests that the court of public opinion should be paramount. He concludes the book like this:

I refer to the spectacle on our stage of striving to gain laws calculated to protect the chiropractors rather than the public. I refer to the petty squabbling which is indulged in for personal reasons and which sets at naught the interests of our audience. I refer to the kind of advertising which attracts the public to our stage only to find that the advertising was far-fetched or wholly untrue. I refer to the wearing of beautiful masks turned to the footlights while behind those masks are faces showing the ugliness of deception and the glint of greed. I refer to everything that is not open and above board and which is calculated to deceive the public. This we must learn, and I grant that the best element in the profession is rapidly learning that the only justification for our existence lies in public service and that in the last analysis, whether it be in one country or another, the only final law is the law made by public opinion for the benefit of the public.

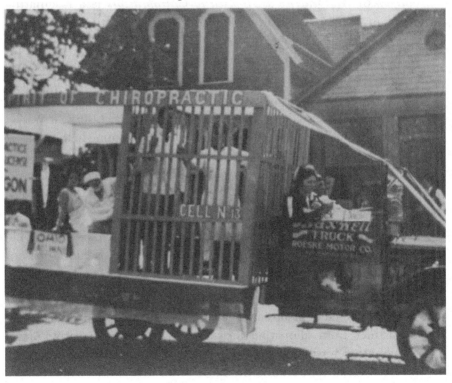

Ohio Alumni float PSC Lyceum parade (1920)
"Spirit of Chiropractic/Cell N13"

Malpractice as Applied to Chiropractors: Vol. 17 (1924)

Arthur T. Holmes, Esq., was born in 1887 in LaCrosse, Wisconsin. He earned his law degree from Wisconsin State University. Holmes joined Morris and Hartwell's law firm in Lacrosse in 1915. He was assigned to the legal defense of chiropractors charged with the various forms of illegal practice all across the country. Some years, Holmes spent 300 days on the road defending chiropractors in court. He became chief legal counsel to the Universal Chiropractors Association in 1925 when Tom Morris resigned. By 1932, Holmes became the legal counsel for the National Chiropractic Association. He kept that post until his death in August 1966.

Vol. 17 or *Malpractice as Applied to Chiropractors* is a fascinating document in the annals of the philosophy of chiropractic. It provides a perspective on the legal question.

Of Holmes, Tom Morris writes:

> Mr. Holmes of the firm of Morris, Winter, Esch and Holmes, has been associated with me for some years past. With the increasing activity in the form of malpractice suits, it was thought well to write a book which could be of some help to the Chiropractor and devoid of many legal problems which are only interesting to attorneys. Several questions and problems not yet settled, are not discussed, and as soon as settled by the courts, information concerning them will be given.

The book explains the legal practicalities as to how philosophy should be used in practice. Philosophy was, after all, one of the core legal reasons why chiropractic was viewed as separate and distinct from medicine.

Holmes defines chiropractic as a distinct science. He writes:

> Chiropractic is now a science unto itself. It is separate and distinct from allopathic medicine and from osteopathy, or any other form or system of healing. It has its own particular methods of ascertaining the cause of disease, and its own particular means of eliminating the cause and allowing innate to restore the patient to health. Its strides in the past twenty-five years have been marvelous and it has overcome the opposition and hatred of several other health sciences, some of which still persist in their efforts to belittle Chiropractic. However, the results count and there are now in the United States millions of satisfied Chiropractic patients who recognize Chiropractic as

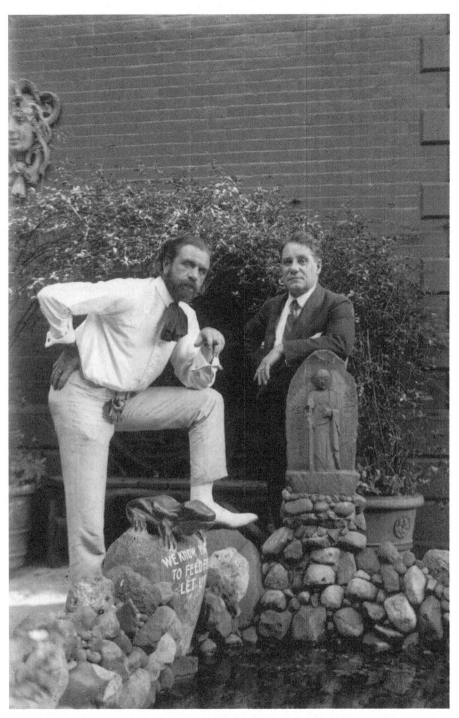

B.J. Palmer with and Tom Morris (1925)

the most simple and still the most efficient system in the science of health which exists today. Many Chiropractors realize the wonderful thing which they have in the form of a science. They realize that so far as the health science is concerned, it is the best of any so far devised or thought out.

Holmes proposed that the "real good Chiropractor" is the one who sells the patient the philosophy of chiropractic. The chiropractor should emphasize how nature cures and how the chiropractor eliminates the cause. This takes away the "promise to cure." He writes:

> The last warning advice to all Chiropractors should be, "No matter how much you believe in your science or how confident that you can benefit your patient, do not make the mistake of promising your patient something which you may not be able to fulfill, probably because of causes beyond your control." The only excuse for such a promise is that the Chiropractor wishes to procure the patient, feeling confident he can benefit the patient. However, that should not be considered. You don't need patients that bad and if you explain the Art, Science and Philosophy of Chiropractic clearly enough to your patient he will sell himself, and upon his recovery, you as a Chiropractor and Chiropractic as a science, will get the credit.

Holmes emphasizes that the best approach, especially in terms of winning court cases, is for chiropractors to use "Chiropractic adjustments solely." Chiropractors should not mix chiropractic with other allopathic modalities. Advertising for these increases legal risk.

Also, Holmes felt that the chiropractor that "mixes" allopathic medicine into chiropractic cannot conscientiously practice chiropractic because the two are "diametrically opposed." Chiropractic's theory of disease is distinct. In this regard, he suggests great care be used in making a diagnosis and recommends that chiropractors "always use the words 'Chiropractic Analysis' instead of diagnosis." This is not only a legal maneuver but "in reality different." The chiropractor's analysis is distinctly different from the medical doctor's diagnosis.

Finally, some of Holmes' advice is still applicable today, almost 100 years later. He writes:

> There is the Chiropractor who does not particularly love Chiropractic, who doesn't know its philosophy, who never did

make a rattling good success of Chiropractic and who buys an electric vibrator because he thinks it will give him something more to sell. This fellow Mr. Straight Chiropractor, you and I can't reach. He doesn't care about Chiropractic and he hasn't got sense enough to know that the patient who gives the credit for his cure from pneumonia to violet rays instead of Chiropractic adjustments it not a particularly good advertisement for Chiropractic. I suspect the straight Chiropractor must fight this kind of mixer to avoid twenty-five cent adjustments...

Which do you want, Mr. Chiropractor? Do you want to be regarded as a professional man with a wonderful science which gets marvelous results or do you want to be known as a man who gives very good baths which tone you up and gets results, or further be known as a good "rubbin" doctor.

Well, the Chiropractor who loves Chiropractic wouldn't do a thing outside of Chiropractic for anything because he wants Chiropractic to get the credit for the recovery. He wants to place Chiropractic on the plane of a science.

But the fellow who doesn't love Chiropractic, doesn't care.

Holmes recommends referrals for cases that may require prescriptions of diet or medicine. Chiropractors should limit their liability by explaining to the patient that diet and drugs are not part of the chiropractic profession and that "Chiropractic adjustments allow a normal flow of innate intelligence to the different organs which will make them function normally."

On liability, he concludes:

If you want to test a Chiropractor ask yourself these questions:

Are you striving to perpetuate and raise the standard of Chiropractic science?

Do you care whether the Chiropractor is known as a professional man or as a masseur?

The question has often been asked, "Would I be mixing from a malpractice standpoint if I advised foods, exercise, etc." The only answer the writer can make is to give the rule:

First—The Chiropractic system contains its theory of what is the cause of the patient's disease.

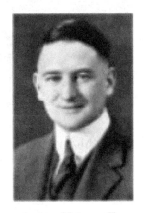

Arthur Holmes, Esq.

Second—A method of determining what is the cause of the patient's disease.

Third—A method of eliminating the cause of that disease.

A more complete discussion of that theory is contained elsewhere.

The rule is this: If the act is contained within the purview of the system as defined, and is incident to and in harmony with that system then for the purposes of malpractice it would come under that system.

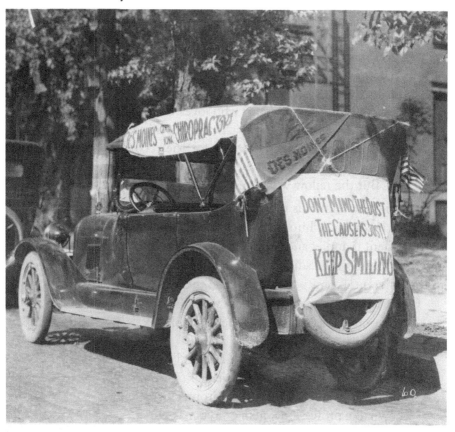

Des Moines Central Iowa Chiropractor's float, PSC Lyceum parade (1919)
"Don't Mind the Dust/The Cause is Just! Keep Smiling"

FOUNTAIN HEAD NEWS   Page 13

MALPRACTICE
as applied to
Chiropractors

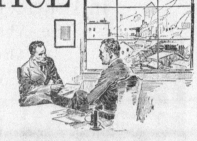

Volume 17
THE SCIENCE OF CHIROPRACTIC LIBRARY
By ARTHUR T. HOLMES
Endorsed by TOM MORRIS, both being members of
The U.C.A Counsel of the firm of Morris,
Winter, Esch and Holmes

MORE than that ought not to be necessary. That such a firm should write such a book on such a timely subject should be sufficient to place a copy in the hands of EVERY Chiropractor who wants to know what to do, what not to do, how to advertise, how to protect his interests against malpractice suits, what to avoid saying or doing to protect himself; what to do in the event suit is started—all of this is more wonderfully covered in this book.

Just to give you a more specific knowledge of this book, there are separate chapters each on the following general subjects:

Chapter 1—Malpractice In General.
Chapter 2—Relationship Between Chiropractor and Patient.
Chapter 3—Specialists.
Chapter 4—Contracts to Cure.
Chapter 5—Liability for Diagnosis.
Chapter 6—Liability for Mixing Other Sciences with Chiropractic.
Chapter 7—Chiropractic Theory.
Chapter 8—Negligence.
Chapter 9—Note On Contributory Negligence.
Chapter 10—Speed vs. Tomlinson.
Chapter 11—Nelson vs. Harrington.
Chapter 12—Ennis vs. Banks.
Chapter 13—State vs. Smith.
Chapter 14—Wilkins vs. Brock.
Chapter 15—Damages.
Chapter 16—Services Rendered Gratuitously and First Aid.
Chapter 17—X-Ray.
Chapter 18—Defective Appliances.
Chapter 19—Practice Without Consent.
Chapter 20—Fees—Liability of Third Party for Services.
Chapter 21—General Advice.

The book consists of 250 pages. Cases are constantly cited bearing upon the questions in view. Bits of evidence are quoted from actual cases tried, showing how witnesses are trapped, etc.

The book sells for $5.00 and can be purchased ONLY through The Palmer School of Chiropractic, who are acting as the exclusive agent for Mr. Holmes.

Enclosed find a separate order blank, which fill out and remit for immediate shipment. The book is in stock and will be shipped the day order is received.

Hundreds of orders were sold at Lyceum this year, this being the first announcement of its coming.

THE PALMER SCHOOL OF CHIROPRACTIC
Chiropractic Fountain Head   DAVENPORT, IOWA, U.S.A.

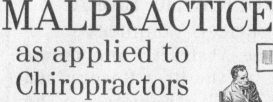

Advertisement for Vol. 17

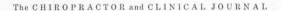
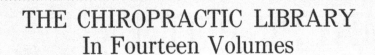
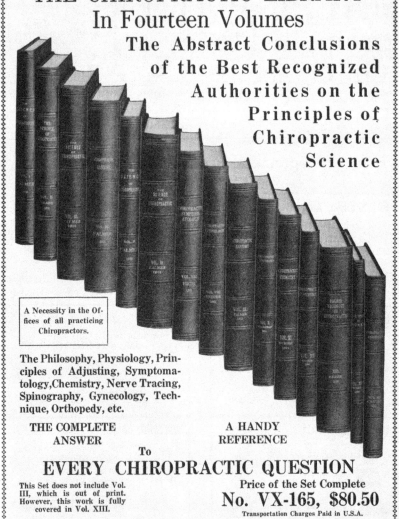
The Chiropractor, Volume 19, Number 1 (1919)

Chapter 8
The Legacy of John H. Craven

John H. Craven, DC, PhC, was born in 1880 in Kansas. He graduated from PSC in 1912 and joined the faculty in 1913. Craven was the head of the Department of Philosophy and also the Department of Orthopedy. He left PSC on July 1, 1926, and taught for Logan Chiropractic College in the 1930s.

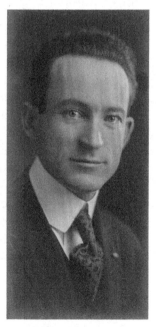

John Craven (1924)

Rolf Peters notes that prior to enrolling at PSC, Craven went to Kansas Wesleyan University and was ordained in the Methodist Church, where he was a pastor for 11 years. He officiated at the weddings of many PSC students. Peters also reported that Craven contributed more than 20 articles to *The Chiropractor* about philosophy, NCM research, and also, hygiene and public health.

Craven left a philosophical legacy in chiropractic through the impact of his students, his role as B.J. Palmer's collaborator and revisionist, and his own writings like *Chiropractic Orthopedy* and *Chiropractic Pediatrics and Hygiene*. Craven's student, R.W. Stephenson, wrote one of the most well recognized and influential texts of the entire Green Book series. Craven's collaboration with B.J. Palmer on new editions of Vol. 1, Vol. 2, and Vol. 5, helped to craft those books into their final printed forms.

Between 1916 and 1919, Craven saw to the revision and republication of B.J. Palmer's core philosophy texts. In 1916, he collaborated with B.J.

on the second edition of Vol. 5. In 1917, he helped B.J. to revise the third edition of Vol. 1, and in 1919, the revision of Vol. 2. He is listed as a collaborator on Vol. 5 and Vol. 2, but not Vol. 1. However, in 1917, B.J. Palmer writes:

> On the whole, we are frank with you in admitting, that Vol. 1 is largely what it is in the 2nd edition. It has, however undergone many revisions at the hands of our Doctor Craven who spent many an hour mauling over its pages.

Most of the first edition of Vol. 1 was written by D.D. Palmer, so, we know that Craven studied the Founder's writings even though B.J. removed his father's name when he published the second edition in 1910.

Craven's ability to teach the chiropractic philosophy is evident in his 1919 address to 4,200 people at Lyceum, where he sums up his understanding of chiropractic. Craven's words were captured as follows:

> Man is a living being, therefore there must be life. We cannot define life, although we recognize its presence. It is the quality or character which distinguishes animal and vegetable life from inorganic or dead bodies. No definition is great enough to define life. They tell us about it, but do not tell what it is. It is impossible to define the best things in life, and how helpless we are when we endeavor to define life itself.
>
> We are not so much concerned about the definition of life as we are concerned in the expression of life. The difference between the dead body and the living body is that in the living body there is this elusive, evanescent something that proves the negative material and makes it living material. This force we have been told is the result of the working of the laws of chemistry and physics, but Chiropractic teaches it is the producer of this physical action.
>
> The nervous system neutralizes this force, but does not produce it. This force is the life that is innate to the body. Chiropractic maintains that life is the same wherever found and that life is intelligent. The object and function of Chiropractic is to get sick people well... If there is function when the life is present and no function when the life is absent, then the presence of the life must be responsible for the function. If there is no function in a part of the body, we reason that it is because of the absence of life in that part.

It is, then, the object of Chiropractic to get the life to that part of the body. Now, no man can manufacture life... And since we cannot produce life we must look for the cause of the absence of the life in the affected part and try to get the life that is already in the body to flow to this part.

The nerves are the conveyors of this innate life, and Chiropractic removes the rheostat that is stepping the current down, by its increased resistance to the current of impulses that are sent out from the brain and circulated through the nervous system to every tissue cell in the body. You cannot improve upon nature. You cannot add life to the body. Therefore, the only thing necessary to restore incoordination to coordination is to remove the pressure from the impinged nerve, that this innate life which is already in the body, may get to every part of the body and produce its proper function.

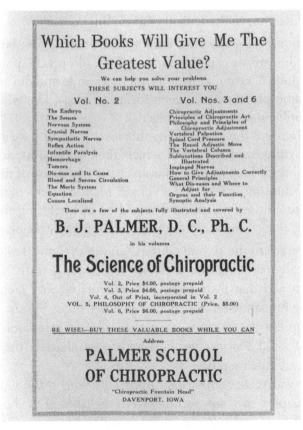

Advertisement for Vols. 1-6 (1917)

Craven's Philosophy of Chiropractic: Vol. 5 (1916)

In 1914, Craven published his first articles elucidating the steps of B.J. Palmer's NCC. The articles were published with Craven listed as author, along with several others essays, in the second edition of B.J. Palmer's Vol. 5, in 1916. The title page includes, "Collaboration by J.H. Craven, DC, PhC, Professor of Philosophy in the Palmer School of Chiropractic."

Craven's personal copy of the first edition of Vol. 5 is preserved in the archives of the Western States Chiropractic College Library. The edition contains Craven's signature along with dates and edits throughout the text in purple ink. An advertisement for the book from 1916 reads:

> This edition of Vol 5 is the same as the original edition with the exception that 5 lectures have been omitted and the entire book rearranged by our Dr. Craven to make it more practical as a text-book.

In the dedication to the second edition, B.J. Palmer writes:

> Among those close and friendly helpers, none have been more true, diligent or conscientious to the Chiropractic philosophy than John Craven. Having formerly been a studious minister, he came prepared to accept advanced ideas. His willingness was only exceeded by his sincerity.
>
> Many are the happy hours this teacher and I have analyzed and synthesized the detail which then became a part of his teachings; which now become an elaborated phase of this book.
>
> To him must be given all credit for the production of this second edition, therefore, it would be but befitting that unto him, belongs the honor of the dedication of this book.

In the Preface to the second edition, Craven explains that the impetus to systematically rearrange the book was to develop a textbook for use in the classroom and that instructors and students wanted such a text. He notes that the fundamental principles were unchanged but the science was updated. They cut the sections on specific disease processes in order to make room for B.J.'s newer writings and to emphasize "the philosophy applicable to all" disease processes.

The goal was to develop a logical introduction to the topic. For this reason, the chapter on *Power* was moved to the front of the book followed by the chapter on *Cycles*. Power is expressed as life transmitted through the cycles. The book then takes the reader through the application of the philosophy in terms of the various ways life can be expressed both normally and abnormally. Craven writes:

> There is no question but this book stands alone, it is in a class by itself so far as Chiropractic Philosophy is concerned. It contains the very latest and most recent conclusions, and will be found invaluable to every Chiropractor, as well as interesting and instructive reading for the laity. The science of Chiropractic is in its formative period, and the past few years have seen great progress along every line of Chiropractic. As nothing is permanent except change, we must expect men's minds to keep abreast the times. Dr. Palmer has more than kept pace with his contemporaries, he has lived and is living many years in advance of his time. In the years to come this work will be more appreciated than it is now.
>
> This volume does not by any means exhaust the subject, but sets forth the fundamental principles covering every phase of the Philosophy of Chiropractic.

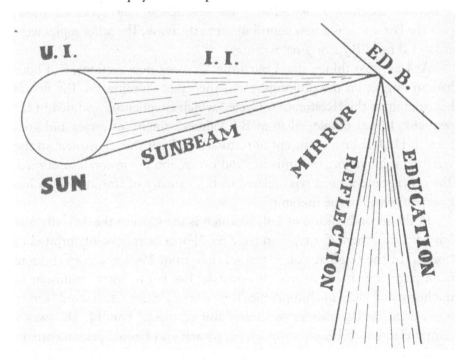

Diagram added to the second edition of Vol. 5 to depict B.J. Palmer's metaphor of U.I as sun, I.I. as sunbeam, Ed. B as mirror, and Education as a reflection

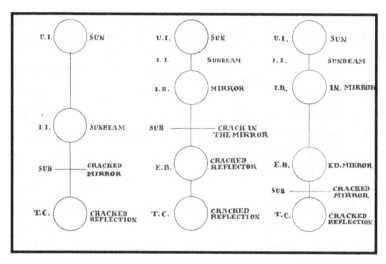

Diagram added to the 2nd edition of Vol. 5 to depict the metaphor with subluxation

The new sections written by Craven were mainly about the NCC. They include: *Universal, Innate Intelligence, Mental, Innate Mind—Educated Mind, Creation, Brain Cell, Transformation, Mental Impulse, Propulsion, Sensation—Ideation, Habit—Poison Formed, Restoration Cycle.* Of these, only the last one was a new contribution to the book. The other topics were expanded from B.J.'s original writings.

At least two things stand out from Craven's new sections, and both had an impact on the philosophy and theory of chiropractic. The first is his coining of the "Restoration Cycle," which Stephenson codified in his textbook. It was developed from B.J. Palmer's theory of cycles and goes back to D.D. Palmer's concept of restoration. After the adjustment of the vertebral subluxation, transmission and expression are restored to normal. The other standout is a typo related to B.J.'s theory of "forun," which has gone unnoticed in the literature.

In the second edition of Vol. 5 (which is identical to the 3rd, 4th, and 5th editions), there is a typo on page 65. "Form" is mistakenly printed as "forun." In the original Vol. 5, first edition, from 1909, the correct quote is on page 361. It is possible this mistake has led to some confusion in the history of ideas in chiropractic. This is because the actual word "forun" was coined by B.J. Palmer to mean "unit of force." For B.J., this was a central element of his philosophical approach and figured prominently in his theory of cycles. The typo itself is within a quotation from Vol. 8 of the *Encyclopedia Britannica*, from the section titled "Energy." The quote is referring to the conservation of energy, which is a law of physics. The law certainly does not include B.J.'s term "forun." Hence, the added confusion makes it seem like forun may be a term from physics rather than coined by B.J. in 1909.

Craven also wrote a *Preface* to the third edition in 1919. In the preface he acknowledged the success of the second edition as a textbook in the classroom. He writes:

> More and more the Chiropractor is realizing the value of Philosophy and that "Vol. 5" contains the foundation principles of this philosophy. As a matter of fact the expressions "Chiropractic Philosophy" and "Vol. 5" have practically become synonymous.

The third edition included slight edits and a hope that it would become embraced by the profession.

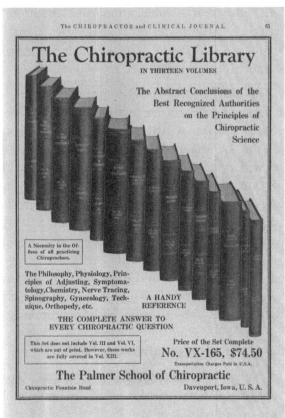

Advertisement for Vols. 1-14 except Vols. 3 and 6 (1923)

Craven's Chiropractic Orthopedy: Vol. 15 (1921)

Craven's book, *A Textbook on Chiropractic Orthopedy*, Vol. 15, was the first detailed textbook on the spine written from the perspective of the chiropractic paradigm. In the acknowledgments, Craven thanks Dr. M. Bell Larson, philosophy professor at PSC; R.W. Stephenson, PSC faculty member, for drawing all of the illustrations in the text; P.A. Remier, technician from the PSC Spinograph Department; and also Mabel and B.J. Palmer. Mabel counseled him on anatomical illustrations and he used her textbook as a reference along with Cunningham, Gray, Piersol, Lovett, and others. He also thanked the students, who asked for the book to be written. Finally, he gives tribute to the PSC Osteological Studio as his primary source for research.

In the book, Craven makes the case for the vertebral subluxation model developed at the PSC based on anatomical and physiological evidence. He proposed the idea that a subluxation could interfere with its own holding elements, an early model of Degenerative Joint Disease, and a precursor to Stephenson's Vertemere Cycle, which opened the door to later proprioception models of subluxation. Craven writes:

> The subluxation of a vertebra producing pressure upon a spinal nerve and interfering with the transmission of motor impulses to the spinal structures, such as the ligaments and muscles, that are attached to the vertebrae, these ligaments and muscles will lose their tonicity. If the interference be the same on both sides of the spine, then the lack of tonicity in the spinal structures will allow the spine to bend abnormally with the convexity of the bend toward the Posterior.
>
> The subluxation which is producing the pressure on the spinal nerve may be interfering with the transmission of nutrient mental impulses to the body of the vertebra or to the bodies of several vertebrae in the same locality. If this is the case, then there is likely to be an NCR condition in the bodies of these vertebrae, producing a molecular decay and resulting in caries of the spine, spondylitis, or Pott's disease.

NCR refers to Nutrition minus, Calorific plus, and Reparation minus, which was a type of equation system to assess symptomatology originally developed in the second edition of Vol. 2.

Craven developed the cord pressure model originally proposed in B.J. Palmer's chapter, *Spinal Cord Impingements*, in his 1911 edition of Vol. 3. In Craven's chapter, *Cord Pressure*, he hypothesized that cord pressures depend on the degree of subluxation and could exert pressure on only a few nerve fibers. This occurs mainly in the middle cervical and could cause pressure on any area of the spine. He writes:

> There are three ways in which cord pressure may be produced:
>
> (a) Traumatic.
> (b) Pathological conditions in the cord.
> (c) A pulling upon the cord from a subluxation of the sacrum or coccyx.
> (d) A subluxation may be produced which will, because of its exaggeration, produce pressure upon the cord as shown in Fig. 10.
>
> The number of fibers involved would depend upon the degree to which the vertebra was subluxated. Clinical observation has revealed the fact that in the majority of cases the location of cord pressure is in the middle cervical place.

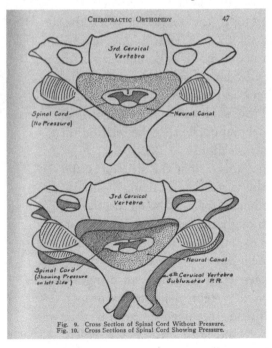

From Vol. 15 demonstrating a vertebral subluxation of C3 and C4 causing cord pressure on left side. Illustrated by R.W. Stephenson (1922)

Craven also includes chiropractic philosophy in his orthopedy text. Innate was discussed mostly in terms of intellectual adaptation. This term was originally coined by B.J. Palmer in Vol. 5 in 1909, as a way to merge intelligence with evolutionary adaptation. Craven emphasizes equalization of weight-bearing to take pressure off intervertebral discs. This could lead to changes in vertebral shape and prevent pressure on spinal nerves. It might also lead to a buildup of exostotic growths to support weakened postures. This perspective was congruent with D.D. Palmer's original definition of Innate from 1902. Craven extends this view to the restoration process as well, after the correction of vertebral subluxation, which could lead to "readaptation for the purpose of removing the exostosis." He also includes Innate's attempts to compensate for decreased muscle tonicity related to subluxations in other areas. Craven described the philosophy of the adjustment as follows:

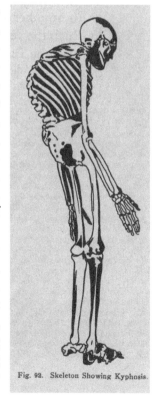

Fig. 92. Skeleton Showing Kyphosis.

From Vol. 15 (1922)

If a vertebra is subluxated very slightly to the posterior with very great laterality and the adjustment is given as though there was more posteriority than laterality, the results will not be as good as if the adjustment is given according to the degree in which the vertebra is subluxated. This is one reason why we get better results in some cases than in others. One adjuster may get better results than another because he has a better mental picture of the subluxation and having a better mental picture, he sees the relation of the different directions.

Let us not forget that the structures attached to the vertebrae are living tissue in which intelligent force is being expressed and even though the adjustic force is not applied in exactly the proper direction, Innate Intelligence is capable of using the vibrations to an advantage in bringing the subluxated vertebra back to its proper position. Innate Intelligence can do this much quicker and with greater ease when the adjustic force is applied in exactly the proper direction.

Craven's Hygiene and Pediatrics: Vol. 3 (1924)

Craven's second book, *A Textbook on Hygiene and Pediatrics From a Chiropractic Standpoint*, was designated the new Vol. 3 in the series. Craven helped to revise new editions for Volumes 1, 2, and 5, so, he was aware that the second edition of Vol. 3, from 1911, was not being reprinted or revised. It was replaced in 1920 by Vol. 13. Also "Vol. 4" was now being reused for the new edited compilation of D.D. Palmer's writings published in 1921. The original Vol. 4 was integrated into the second edition of Vol. 2 in 1913. Thus, "Vol. 3" was open and Craven grabbed it. This probably made the marketing of the *Chiropractic Library* less confusing.

Craven wrote the book because there were no texts on hygiene that were congruent with the philosophy of chiropractic. He proposes that the chiropractic standpoint adds to the discipline of hygiene by taking the perspective that cleaning also comes from the inside out. He writes:

> The body is capable of great possibilities in intellectual adaptation. It is possible for Innate Intelligence to maintain a degree of health in widely different conditions. Even where the environment is extremely adverse and objectionable Innate will adapt herself to the abnormal condition and maintain the normal processes of life in the body. However, it must be remembered that a greater amount of internal force is required to bring about an intellectual adaptation to an adverse environment than to a normal, natural or more perfect environment.
>
> There must be a constant process of adaptation to the environment even though that environment be a most desirable one. All internal processes must of necessity be adaptative to external conditions.

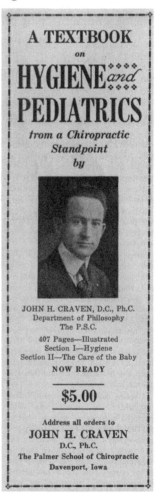

A TEXTBOOK
on
HYGIENE *and*
PEDIATRICS
from a Chiropractic Standpoint
by

JOHN H. CRAVEN, D.C., Ph.C.
Department of Philosophy
The P.S.C.

407 Pages—Illustrated
Section I—Hygiene
Section II—The Care of the Baby
NOW READY

$5.00

Address all orders to
JOHN H. CRAVEN
D.C., Ph.C.
The Palmer School of Chiropractic
Davenport, Iowa

Ad for Vol. 3 (1924)

Craven refers the student to Vol. 5 to learn more about the poison cycle and the causative relationship between poisons and subluxation.

Craven wrote in general on what we might refer to today as the chiropractic lifestyle. For example, he advocated that the individual should live in the proper dwelling, in the right location, both chosen to enhance health and the expression of life in the body. Craven also wrote about Innate eating, where a person should eat what agrees with them. "Innate is the best judge." This perspective was echoed years later in the writings of Ratledge who was a student of Carver and a colleague of D.D. Palmer.

Craven considered immunity as an adaptive process. He writes:

> If the public could read what the hygienists have to say on the subject of immunology and could read it in the light of chiropractic philosophy they would realize that chiropractic adjustments will not only restore health to the sick, but will prevent the well from getting sick.

Section 2 of the book is the first systematic writings on Chiropractic Pediatrics. It covers early child development and unique factors to watch for in pediatric anatomy and physiology that apply to chiropractic analysis. Craven also covers adjusting during dentition as well as analyzing and adjusting infants, which should emphasize the birth history. The book goes through myriad types of incoordinations associated with children and the various major adjustments required to achieve results.

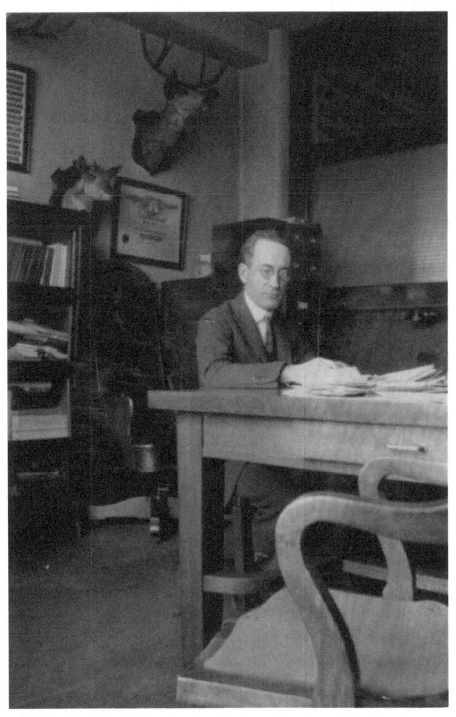

John H. Craven (1924)

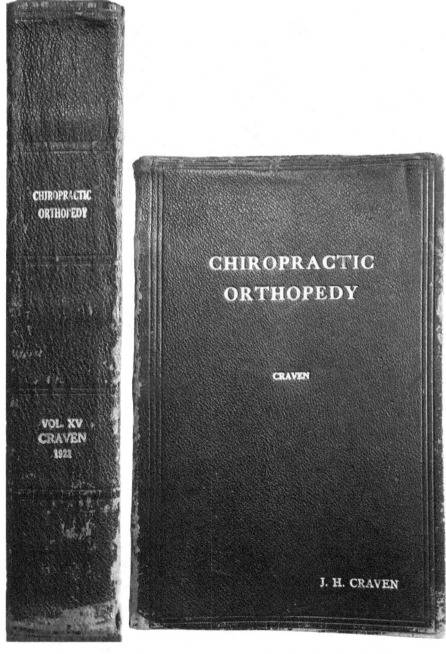

Chiropractic Orthopedy, brown leather first edition.
Author's mock up, double thickness. Craven's personal copy (1921)

Chapter 9
The Life and Work of R.W. Stephenson

Ralph W. Stephenson, DC, PhC, wrote Vol. 14 or *Chiropractic Text Book*. The book had a significant impact on chiropractic theory and practice. In the first 75 years of the chiropractic profession, 75% of chiropractors graduated from the PSC, and Stephenson's text was required reading for 43 of those years. The book was used by three generations of chiropractors, not only at the PSC, but also in schools founded by PSC alumnus like Life University, Life Chiropractic College West, and Sherman College, and also in schools founded by their graduates including the New Zealand College of Chiropractic. R.W. Stephenson's second book, *The Art of Chiropractic*, was also published in 1927.

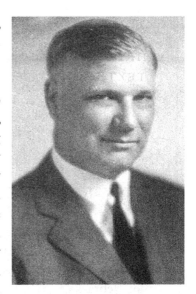

R.W. Stephenson

A Brief Look at R.W. Stephenson's Life

R.W. Stephenson was born on December 6, 1879, in Lincoln, Illinois. He lived in McLean, Illinois, as of 1900. Rolf Peters notes that Stephenson went to elementary school in Seward, Nebraska and attended Highland Park College at Des Moines, and Iowa State College at Ames, Iowa. In 1910, he was working as a farmer in Nebraska and was married to Nina Stephenson, who was from Alberta, Canada. They moved to Alberta, where Stephenson taught school.

According to Stephenson's World War I draft registration card from Seward, Nebraska, dated October 18, 1918, he was listed as tall, of medium build, with brown hair and hazel eyes, and teaching school in Gadsby, Alberta. Considering that Alberta set new standards for its 1,200 rural one-room schoolhouses starting in 1910, he could have taught as many as one hundred students.

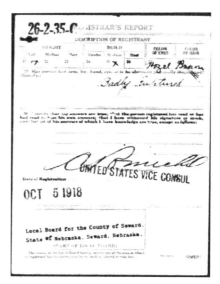

R.W. Stephenson's Voter Registration Card, Seward, Nebraska (1918)

After he and Nina divorced, Ralph moved back to Iowa and entered the PSC in 1920 at age 40. After graduation he became a faculty member in July 1921. He married Gladys Tilden on October 9, 1922. Gladys was also from Nebraska.

Stephenson started teaching in the Department of Orthopedy in 1923 and the Department of Philosophy in 1924. In November, 1925, Henry Gaddis resigned and Stephenson became the head of the Department of Technic and Director of Clinics. He resigned from the PSC in 1929, announcing a planned 2 year rest in southern California. The limited historical record shows he resided in Redondo Beach, California, initially and was a violin maker before returning to the PSC in 1935.

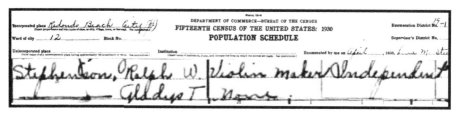

Excerpt from *Fifteenth Census of the United States* (1930)

In 1936, it was reported by Davenport newspapers and the PSC that Stephenson had practiced for six years in Boulder, Colorado, during his absence from the PSC. There is no historical evidence to support that Stephenson was indeed in Boulder as reported. It is unknown why he was reported to have been in Boulder for six years. Peters, whose material was based on the PSC archives, writes:

> After practicing in Colorado for some 6 years, Stephenson returned to the PSC in 1935 to study HIO Technique, and was again attached to the faculty. He planned to prepare a second edition of his *Chiropractic Text Book*, by replacing old applications with the new, while keeping the neverchanging principles of chiropractic. Unfortunately he was not able to conclude this project, as in March 1936 he was hit by a bus, which tore loose his right kidney, and he passed away on 5 April 1936, less than 2 weeks after the accident, at the young age of 56.

Tributes to Stephenson from Students

In 1922, one student wrote that Stephenson's teaching of science and philosophy emphasized cause and effect. He taught the science of the theory of Innate Intelligence in such a way, "that even those outside the school who fail to grasp it would understand."

After he died in 1936, there were tributes to him from students and faculty alike. The 1936 class referred to themselves as the Stephenson Class. He was their class adviser. They wrote, "The highest verbal tribute we can pay him is to say that he was a Chiropractor and a man." The Alpha chapters of the Sigma Phi Chi Sorority and the Delta Sigma Chi Fraternity also wrote tributes. The sorority wrote:

> Dr. Stephenson was even more than a teacher and a bene-factor to mankind's problems and health; he sought to perfect in the musical instrument, the violin, the all perfect reception and interpretation of sound vibrations, the ear. His instruments are masterpieces in their field...
>
> They needed a philosopher in Heaven, so God took "Daddy" Stephenson away.

During his hiatus from teaching, Stephenson took up violin making in Redondo Beach. He was listed in the 1930 U.S. Census as violin maker, not chiropractor. The fraternity wrote:

He always answered to the best of his ability the numerous questions with which he was constantly besieged by the student body. Although he was always working, he was never too busy to lend a helping hand or to give good advice whenever requested. He was the one to whom we all went when perplexed by some question or problem. It was in this manner that he acquired the name "Daddy" Stephenson.

Even though painfully handicapped physically as a result of several ruthless bits of experimental surgery practices upon him when he was a child, he never permitted this to interfere with his work until it finally claimed his life.

He was admired, revered, and respected by all with whom he came in contact, not only for what he did, but also for what he was.

Stephenson's death certificate notes that cardiovascular and renal disease were other contributory causes of death, unrelated to the principle cause.

Stephenson's Illustrations

In 1921, Stephenson drew the illustrations in Craven's Vol. 15. These were pen line drawings from freehand sketches. In 1926, he drew *The Chiropractic Chart*, which was reproduced recently by The Institute Chiropractic. It is the first detailed nerve chart for chiropractors, which included a philosophical perspective and tips for NCM analysis.

Stephenson also sketched all of the illustrations in his *The Art of Chiropractic* and *Chiropractic Textbook*. He used sketches as slides in the classroom. Many of the images from his textbook have become iconic in the profession. Titles of the most well-known illustrations are as follows: *Safety Pin Cycle, Rotated Subluxations, Universal Diagram, The Normal Complete Cycle, Innate Body, Interbrain Cycle, Momentum* and *Re-tracing Chart*, as well as the *Schemes of Cord Pressures*.

Stephenson brought a new level of depth to teaching the philosophy of chiropractic through his detailed illustrations. His art embodied the philosophy.

From *Stephenson's Text*
(1927)

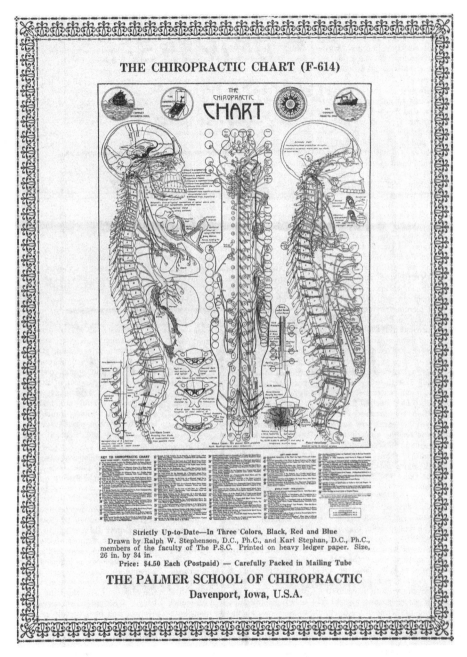

From *The Chiropractor* (1926)

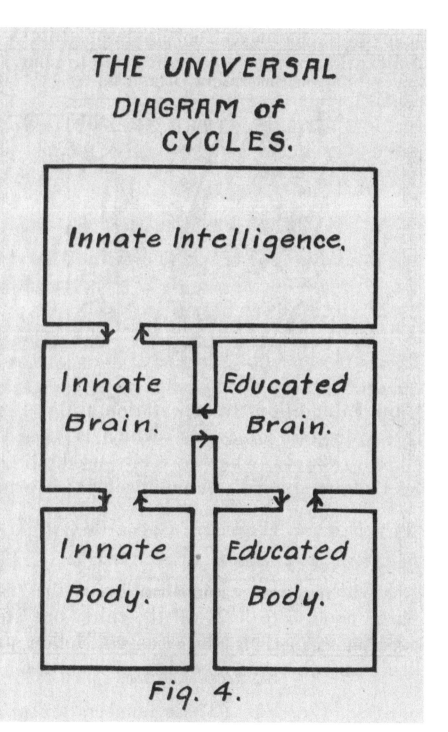

From *The Chiropractic Textbook* (1927)

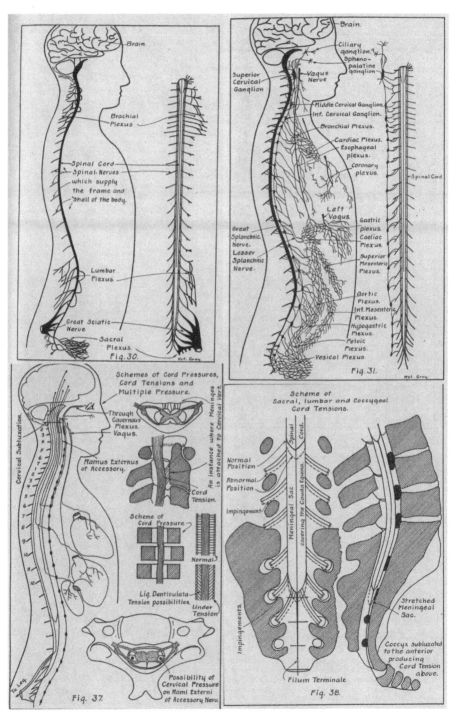

From *The Chiropractic Textbook* (1927)

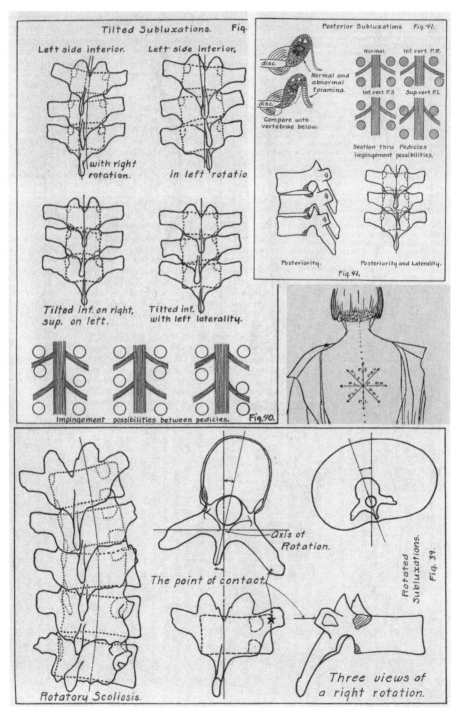

From *The Art of Chiropractic* (1927)

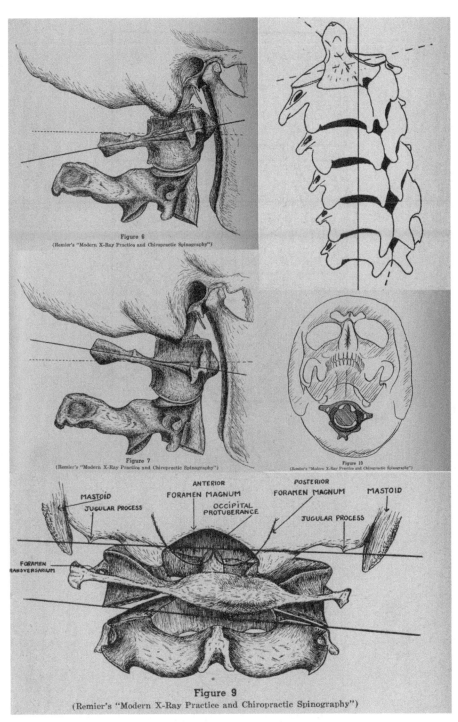

Figure 6
(Remier's "Modern X-Ray Practice and Chiropractic Spinography")

Figure 7
(Remier's "Modern X-Ray Practice and Chiropractic Spinography")

Figure 10
(Remier's "Modern X-Ray Practice and Chiropractic Spinography")

Figure 9
(Remier's "Modern X-Ray Practice and Chiropractic Spinography")

From *The Art of Chiropractic* (1927)

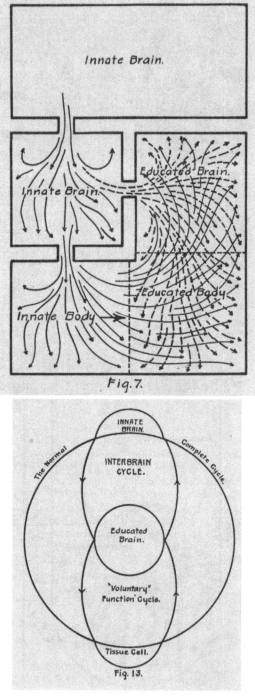

From *The Chiropractic Textbook* (1927)

Stephenson's Writings Prior to 1927: PhC Thesis

On February 26, 1923, Stephenson earned his postgraduate degree, the Doctor of Chiropractic Philosophy (PhC). His thesis titled *Chiropractic* was accepted by Craven, the head of the Department of Philosophy.

In the thesis Stephenson gives "a brief explanation of its principles," and lays out much of the argument for his future text. The emphasis is on the insight that "Chiropractic is based upon axioms," which are "basic principles." He writes:

> This premise might be stated: Life is intelligent and governs all matter.

He emphasized that the intelligent forces behind tissue growth, healing, and repair are different from the forces of physics and chemistry. Later in his 1927 book, he uses a similar distinction to define Innate Intelligence as a Law of Life.

Other precursors to his textbook are found in the PhC thesis, such as his deductive approach and his reference to chiropractic as a radical and deductive science. He noted that geometry teachers were trying to "revolutionize Euclid's Geometry (a good example of pure deduction) by changing to inductive reasoning." Perhaps geometry was one of the topics he taught in a one-room schoolhouse in Alberta before attending PSC. In the thesis, he complains about that type of education because, some things, like Chiropractic, are "for deduction only." In 1927, in the Preface to Vol. 14 he writes:

> The entire work is tied together by references, article to article, where it was deemed necessary; and proof given, by use of the fundamental principles, in the manner of deductive geometry.

In the PhC thesis, we learn his initial reasoning for this approach.

From this deductive perspective, Innate Intelligence is viewed as a hypothesis that is proved through logic. He writes:

> Chiropractic is based upon the hypothesis that man has an Innate Intelligence residing within his body and this intelligence sends intelligence from its headquarters over the nerves to the various parts of the body. From the inside to the outside. It is the only power with intelligence enuf to heal any tissue... Therefore if there is anything interfering with the

forces of nature coming from within, he strives to remove this interference, knowing that it is the cause and knows that it is useless to try to remove the effect.

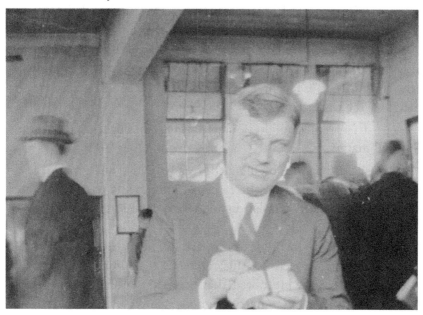

R.W. Stephenson (1924)

Stephenson's overall approach to Universal Intelligence (source) and Innate Intelligence (subsource) is generally the same as in his textbook. However, the way he describes them is sometimes different, especially in terms of the oneness of all energy and the radiation of energy. He writes:

> The infinite Intelligence is everywhere, it is Universal, common to every locality, and does not deny attention to the smallest molecule or atom. Our study of physics show us that there is energy everywhere, throughout the Universe. It also shows us that energy is in many forms but is after all one energy. What does that signify? Any of these forms of energy can be transformed into another, and every moment we see it being done all around us. In its radiant forms there is no corner of the Universe it does not reach, and consequently every bit of matter receives some energy.

Other analogies he uses for Universal and Innate are the sun and its rays, the ocean and a dipper of ocean water, and a tiny spark or thunderbolt, surrounded and governed by the Universal Life, which ignites the bolt by induction.

According to Stephenson, the energy that scientists have overlooked is Life Force. He writes:

> This form of energy is the Life Force, which Chiropractors call Mental Impulse. Its purpose is to cause vibration in the cells of organic matter. It too, can cause matter to move. It can be transformed into any of the lesser energies.

The Mental Impulse is described as a more highly organized form of energy and is conducted over the nerves as an intelligent current. He even states that the Life Force can "get hold of matter and move it." By 1927, he uses the metaphor of a magnetic field to describe how Intelligence "gets a grip on matter." He reasons that a field is a better physical analogy than something that is not tangible like "hope or charity."

Several of his core axioms from 1927 are also in the PhC thesis such as: nerves conduct mental forces, there are limitations of matter, the intelligent force comes from the brain, the function of matter is to express force, the five signs of life mean the matter is alive, and Mental Impulses will never harm the tissues; they are physical forces that are not evident until expressed. Also, that the afferent nerves carry mental forces containing intelligent messages to the brain just like the efferent nerves carry mental impulses away from the brain.

There are also interesting points in the thesis that are not in the textbook. For example, he refers to the Cerebrum as the Educated Brain and the Cerebellum as the Innate Brain, although he emphasizes that those are really functional designations not anatomical. D.D. Palmer made a similar proposal in response to B.J.'s early writings.

In the PhC, instead of naming the Normal Complete Cycle, which is the cornerstone of his textbook, Stephenson writes about the Material Cycle (how forces move through the body) and the Immaterial Cycle or "the life which operates the equipment." Innate Intelligence is defined as the power that creates force. Transmission is defined as the missing link leading to Expression, which is the union of matter and force. He writes:

> Thus Intelligent forces come from the inside to the outside - that is, ex-pressed. Hence Chiropractors name the steps of the cycle of mentality to and from the tissue cells.

He also writes that all living things have Innate Intelligence. Plants have an intelligent force and the plant "knows how" because it has sensibility. This approach foreshadowed late twentieth-century theoretical biology, especially the theory of autopoiesis and cognition, that living cells create their own parts from their own parts and "know." Autopoietic theory was also developed by contemplating the sensation of nerve cells.

Stephenson arrives at transmission, subluxation, impingement, and interference toward the end of the thesis. He uses a similar approach in his famous 33 principles. In the PhC, he writes:

> Innate is hindered by subluxations.
>
> Subluxations are the physical representations of incoor-dinations. A subluxated vertebrae is one that has lost its proper juxtaposition with the vertebra above and the one, below, to an extent less than a dislocation, and which impinges nerves and causes incoordination at the periphery of those nerves.

He also describes the different kinds of forces including adjustive forces, resistive forces, and the concussive forces that cause the subluxation.

Stephenson emphasizes that adjusting the vertebra is very different from mechanically "setting" a vertebra. He writes that an audible sound upon adjustment is meaningless, and:

> There is a clean cut feeling of "response" and consequent movement that always tells an adjustor whether, he has made a successful adjustment or not. You may "crunch" a vertebra into place by sheer strength and technique, but unless you call forth from your patient "the adjustic concussion of forces" you cannot give a successful adjustment — the kind that Innate accepts.

At the conclusion of the PhC thesis, Stephenson briefly explains the art and analysis of chiropractic. He also goes through the nine functions, and the ways in which the functions may be incoordinated due to increased or decreased action. Incoordination is used instead of "disease." He concludes:

> The writer believes that a pretty fair exposition of the philosophy of Chiropractic has been given wherein the funda-mental principles have been introduced... The fact that Life is intelligent, that the expression of that life depends upon a triunity of perfection, the combining of that intelligence with matter, the manner of its combination, the interference with that combination, and what happens when there is such interference, and how it may be remedied by man has been the theme of this thesis.

Stephenson's Articles: 1920s

Stephenson expands on the ideas in his thesis in five articles published in *The Chiropractor* between 1923 and 1926. The articles are important to the history of ideas in chiropractic because they offer a glimpse into the topics that Stephenson was most passionate about during this time. After all, in the *Introduction* to Vol. 14 in 1927, he writes:

> Art. 1. REMARKS.
>
> This book is written for use in the class room. It may, however, be studied just as easily by the field practitioner, and is not too technical in most of its parts to be readily grasped by the layman. It has grown, rather than having been written; it is the expansion of the notes which were tested in the class room for six years, and the writer believes that, with the constant arrangement and betterment to suit the requirements of the students of Chiropractic, this has created a real textbook, rendering easily understood a subject that students have always said was difficult.

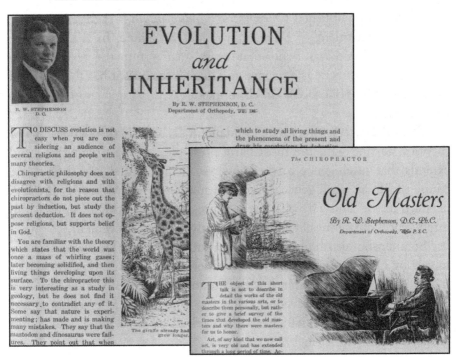

From *The Chiropractor* (1923 & 1925)

It was during these six years that he was also testing his ability to write down his thoughts in an understandable fashion as articles.

In October 1923, he published a short article called *Evolution and Inheritance*, which emphasized that all movement of living things is "actuated by intelligence," each action of life is an act of creation, and an adaptation. Successful adaptation may also result from the removal of subluxations.

Successful adaptation "can be inherited." Dis-ease is not inherited because it is a failure to adapt. In his textbook he would repeat this dictum but also suggest that diathesis, which he learned from Firth, may be inherited. This distinguishes dis-ease from diathesis, the predisposition to disease.

Stephenson proposes that modern man is more subject to subluxation than natural creatures because of Educated mind's influence over Innate and civilization in general. He writes:

> There is a continual battle between his normal Innate Mind and his abnormal educated mind. Chiropractic restores to him what civilization takes away.

In 1924, he published *Chiropractic Fundamentals*. It is the only article that lists Department of Philosophy under his name. In the article he develops the basic arguments that would evolve into the textbook. He states that chiropractic is a science and like all sciences it has fundamental principles. The philosophy of chiropractic is the explanation of these principles.

From there, in Chiropractic Fundamentals, he goes through the major theories starting with the most basic principle, "Life is Intelligent," and extends that intelligence to the universe and all matter. He defines the triune of life as intelligence, force, and matter, whereby force is the link between cause and effect. Matter expresses force, which comes from intelligence. He defines life as "Intelligently directed movement."

Stephenson also builds on his ideas about energy. He suggests force travels by radiation and conduction, which leads to the supposition that transmission can be interfered with. The interference of Mental Impulses leads to immediate detectable evidence. One example is radiant heat detected by the NCM, which was first tested by B.J. Palmer and Dossa Evins, one year earlier in 1923.

One of the most interesting analogies in this article that does not make it into the textbook, which is reminiscent of D.D. Palmer, is that Intelligence branches into things. This embodied metaphor is a useful way to approach this difficult topic. He writes:

> The intelligence of man recognizes in the living thing an intelligence that is localized or branching into and looking after the welfare of the thing in which it resides. This is called Innate Intelligence. Being an intelligence it is a power. Being a power it performs its function—that of creating force. This force assembles molecules and atoms into what we call organized matter. As long as this thing is alive, these forces keep it organized by using or dodging or overcoming its environmental conditions. This is called adaptation. If it fails to make adaptation to the other forces of nature it cannot keep up its proper organization and disintegration into the elements of which it is made.

The failure to adapt is also a result of the pressure on nerves due to subluxated segments. This reduces the nerves' capacity to carry the force and intelligence. Adjusting the spine can lead to restoration of transmission and coordination because the pressure on nerves is removed.

In February 1925, he published an article called *Old Masters*, on the evolution of art and music in civilization. He concluded that there is an evolution of culture, which he viewed as a "slow unfolding of destiny." In his textbook, he includes a section on B.J.'s Utopia, which builds on those arguments.

In December 1925, Stephenson published *Moves*. The article built on his main point at the end of the thesis that a true adjustment is when it is given scientifically and in such a way that Innate can accept it and make the change internally. This was central to his *Art of Chiropractic* and also an important part of Vol. 14.

In November 1926, he published *Transmission*, which expanded on his theories of radiant energy, mental energy, and universal energies permeating every point of the universe and all cells. Transference of energies and interference to Mental Impulse transmission were the main focus. He concludes the article with a 1920s rationale for the use of NCM in relation to the emanation of heat from nerves of the spine.

Stephenson's Art of Chiropractic (1927)

In November 1925, Stephenson was named head of the Department of Technique and Director of Clinics. It is unclear exactly what courses he taught but upon studying an advertisement for a postgraduate course, reviewing the rationale and methods for using the NCM, we may understand some of the topics Stephenson taught in his classes. The course was offered throughout 1925 and 1926. In August 1926, Stephenson gave daily lectures from 1:30-2:30 p.m. His topics were: *Visualization in Adjusting, The Patient's Posture, The Adjuster's Posture, The Mechanics of Adjusting, The Palmer Toggle-Recoil, Innate Contraction of Forces, Rotations and Their Mechanics, Definition and Study of Moves, The Value of Fundamental Drills, The Art of Relaxation and Speed*, and *The Philosophy and Art of Palpation.*

In August 1927, Stephenson's book, *The Art of Chiropractic* was advertised in *The Chiropractor.* The book was revised and republished by W. Heath Quigley and other faculty of the Technic Department in 1948. The new edition included new sections on the upper cervical technique. Perhaps this was related to the revisions Stephenson was planning before he died. In the original *Foreword* to the book, B.J. Palmer writes:

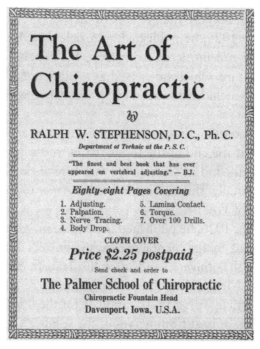

From *The Chiropractor* (1927)

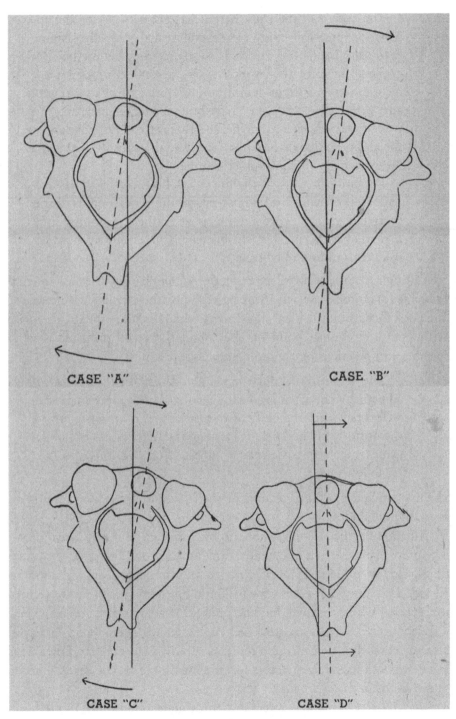

From *The Art of Chiropractic* (1927)

The author of the work herein has given this scientific application practical study for several years, gradually shaping his ideas, assembling his facts, systematizing his methods of explanation until this work is now, beyond all question the most exacting work of description upon the art of adjusting of any work I have ever seen. I have only one regret, in seeing this work appearing over his name, and that is that I did not possess the ability to do what he has done; but, that it is done is cause for extreme joy in Chiropractic ranks.

I regard this work as the finest and best work that has ever appeared on vertebral adjusting, giving us essentials alone, every fact strictly proven, minus goat-feathers, confining itself to demonstrated mechanistic principles which any scientist can read, try and find to be true.

The object of the book was to bring the student back to the fundamental principles of chiropractic, which are based "upon the intelligence of nature." The book focuses on the ideal adjustment, which includes the toggle-recoil at the simplest contact point on the spine. The recoil principle is what specific chiropractic is based upon. Stephenson writes:

The technic of adjusting is art. The Palmer method of adjusting is the art of producing recoil or the Innate contraction of forces within the body of the patient. It is an art requiring the utmost skill and belongs among the highest arts of human achievements because man's noblest efforts are those to help his fellow man.

The book includes detailed technic instructions and breaks new ground on several seminal ideas.

The first detailed definition of chronic subluxation in any Green Book is printed on page 5. Chronic subluxations are long standing, with abnormal tissues due to prolonged interference to transmission. Longer treatment periods are required. It takes time to "build up the tissues of the vertemere to the point where they will hold before lasting adjustments can be given." This abnormality leads to stretched or hardened ligaments, a distorted intervertebral disc, contractured muscles, all of which make it difficult for Innate to use the adjustor's forces for placement. He also discusses chronic subluxations in the *Chiropractic Textbook*.

The Art of Chiropractic integrates the Innate philosophy throughout. Stephenson writes:

INNATE INTELLIGENCE IS THE ADJUSTOR

Innate Intelligence always strives to replace a misplaced vertebra. If it is a subluxated vertebra, it is so because Innate's replacing forces are cut off from the region of the misplaced vertebra. This subluxation, which is interfering with the transmission of mental Impulses to some organ, remains in that position because it also is interfering with the transmission of Impulses to its supporting tissue. Sometimes this is to such an extent as to make the vertebra, or the tissues holding it in situ, pathological.

He learned this model of subluxation from Craven and integrated it with the Innate adjusting and recoil theory of B.J. Palmer. Stephenson continues:

Innate can replace a vertebra if the adjustor produces concussion in those tissues. This concussion is called the recoil. Recoils are brought about by concussions; concussions may be accidental or scientific — Dr. Palmer prefers the latter. Concussions may be the result of mechanical forces, or intangible physical forces, chemical forces or mental shocks. Both subluxations and adjustments are produced by recoil to concussions. Unbalanced resistance subluxates; balanced resistance adjusts. A spontaneous adjustment is one accomplished by Innate without the intervention of outside forces. Accidental adjustments are brought about by accidental recoils, which happen to be just right. The adjustor should try to produce recoils scientifically, so they will not "just happen," but so he can bring that "phenomenon" about at will.

As soon as a subluxation exists, the body combats it. Stephenson describes this interior perspective in terms of the internal corrective force resisting the external invasive force. The corrective force is the natural response of the body to reduce the nerve pressure and restore "normal energy conduction." This "Innate Activity" follows the fundamental principles of mechanics.

When the external invading force overcomes the internal resisting force, the forces within body takes a new direction, through the segments. Stephenson writes:

In an effort to dissipate, it travels through the osseous structure of the body and finally it will move the weaker segment from its normal position. The procedure of adjusting is simply that of determining the resultant of the forces that are trying to move the segment to its normal position and manually applying a force to act with this resultant of the internal reparatory forces to produce a perfect and complete resultant which will move the segment to its normal position and reduce interference. The internal reparatory forces begin to correct a pressure at the instant that it appears in the body these same corrective forces synchronize the energy which we apply with its established force resultant in an effort to re-position the segments.

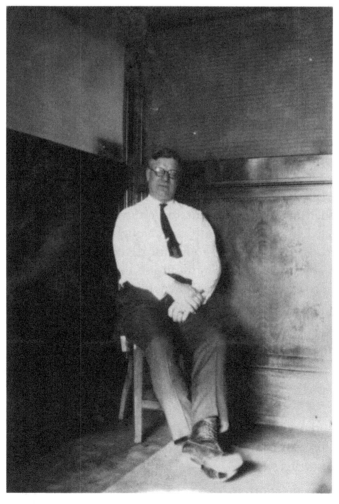

R.W. Stephenson (1924)

This explanation included a dissipative approach to the body's Innate response and an energetic and synchronistic description of correction. Theories like "dissipative structures" in relation to the self-organization of biology and "synchrony" within the body, would not enter the language of theoretical biology until the end of the twentieth century. Stephenson and his mentors were decades ahead in their understanding of how the organism maintained its holistic organization.

Stephenson provided over 100 drills to train chiropractors in the art of chiropractic. Some of these included first-person viewpoints and practices for palpation. He taught how to get into the proper frame of mind and body for delivering the ideal adjustment. He included ways to "develop the art of relaxation" and "build certain brain patterns which will Innately guide the procedure." Relaxation of the body while setting up and delivering the adjustic thrust was very important. Mental drills included concentration, listening to the fingers, and even projecting "educated mind into finger tips."

Stephenson presents the most comprehensive explanation of palpation in any of the Green Books. D.D. Palmer wrote of the distinction between palpation and sense of touch. Stephenson takes this to a new level of careful and precise explanation. He also includes sections on Nerve Tracing as a form of palpation and suggests that students study Vol. 6 to learn more about it. When Quigley republished *The Art of Chiropractic* in 1948, B.J. Palmer was no longer advocating Nerve Tracing or full spine adjusting.

Stephenson's Chiropractic Textbook: Vol. 14 (1927)

The Chiropractic Textbook by Ralph W. Stephenson, was designated Vol. 14. This was an odd numbering choice considering that Nixon's *Spirit of the PSC* in 1920 was also Vol. 14. If it followed the series, Stephenson's text should have been designated Vol. 18. A second edition of Stephenson's Vol. 14 was published in 1940, by PSC. Price was a 1936 graduate, Stephenson's student, and became head of the Department of Philosophy. Like Quigley's addition of an upper cervical section to the 1947 edition of Stephenson's *Art of Chiropractic*, Price added a new chapter to the book, *Occipito-Atlanto-Axial Region*.

Stephenson's *Chiropractic Textbook* is comprehensive. He codified the philosophy of chiropractic and subluxation theory with precise definitions. It includes his classic 33 principles and 411 articles offered as proof for his deductive approach. In a letter from B.J. Palmer printed at the front of the book, B.J. writes:

> Of ALL the books written and compiled on Chiropractic Philosophy, this is by far the best, not excepting my own. The one great, grand and glorious thing you HAVE done has been to compile the many principles which are in my writings, into a systematic, organized manner, building them up from simple to the higher forms, so that any layman inclined could investigate and find out what CHIROPRACTIC IS, IS NOT; WHAT IT DOES AND DOES NOT; HOW AND WHY IT DOES WHAT IT DOES. YOU have clearly, carefully and consistently compiled the many PRINCIPLES of Chiropractic into a readable, understandable book, simple enuf for the layman, deep enuf for the savant.

B.J. concluded that students should consult his volumes for more "complete information on a specific subject," but for those looking for "the working approximate principle," *Stevie's* book was the best choice. He also wrote that the book fills a niche.

The book itself is built upon the previous volumes. Stephenson writes:

> I have quoted freely from Dr. Palmer's books, and from Dr. Mabel Palmer and Dr. Craven; viz., Vol. V; Vol. IX; Vol. XV; Majors and Minors, (M&M).

Stephenson's text references Vol. 5, with page numbers at least 50 times, Vol. 15, 13 times, Vol. 9, eight times, Vol. 2, five times; and Craven's Vol. 3, one time. He thanks Craven for "intimate instruction in Chiropractic and its Philosophy." Stephenson sought to create a book that faithfully contains B.J. Palmer's teachings and chiropractic's fundamental principles.

Because of the book's straightforward approach, definitive explanations, its logical progression of ideas, and its presentation of the core principles of chiropractic in a deductive geometry, it has become known in the profession simply as *Stephenson's Textbook*.

Even though Stephenson's text is so well known in many corners of the profession, there is very little critical literature about the book. The majority of references to the book through 90 years of chiropractic literature reference his classic 33 principles. That literature usually takes either a dismissive approach or views the text as the ultimate authority.

For brevity's sake, and since many of his major concepts in the book have already been discussed, the remainder of this chapter will explore how Stephenson integrated the 33 principles with the 31 steps of B.J. Palmer's NCC. This is followed by an exploration of some of Stephenson's innovations to theory. Finally, we point out a few important areas that future critical analyses might pursue.

Stephenson's Integration of 33 Principles with 31 Steps

Stephenson builds upon his previous writings by establishing the core principles of chiropractic. The principles may be traced back to D.D. Palmer's original ideas and B.J. Palmer's development of those ideas. Central to the book is B.J. Palmer's theory of creation, transmission, expression, from Vol. 2 and Vol. 3, and the 31 steps of his Normal Complete Cycle, from Vol. 5. Throughout the text, Stephenson goes into those steps, defines every element, and continually refers the student back to whichever of the 33 principles applies in each instance.

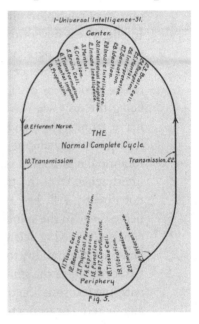

From *The Chiropractic Textbook* (1927)

The following lengthy quote sums up how Stephenson integrated the way human biology uses neurologically mediated intelligent organization to adapt. On page one, Stephenson writes:

Article 25. CHIROPRACTIC.

The Science of Chiropractic holds that a Universal Intelligence created and is maintaining everything in the universe. This is manifested by movement and is called Life. A specific, definite portion of this intelligence, localized in a definite portion of matter and keeping it actively organized, is called by Chiropractic, Innate Intelligence. The function of an inborn, localized intelligence is to adapt some of the forces and matter of the universe in a constructive manner. Organization points to centralization, or having a point of control. In animals, this point of control is in the brain. From this organ, Innate Intelligence sends its controlling forces via the spinal cord through the spinal column, thence through the nerve trunks emitting from the spinal cord and passing through the intervertebral foramina to nerve branches ramifying to all parts of the body. Perfect adaptation of universal elements for this body, depends upon perfect control by Innate Intelligence. Perfect adaptation results in health, and imperfect control results in dis-ease. Defective control by Innate Intelligence is never from any imperfection of Innate Intelligence, which is always perfect, and assembles perfect forces in the brain, but from interference with the transmission of those Innate forces through or over the nerves. Owing to the spinal column being the only segmented structure of bone through which the nerve trunks pass, and the possibility of the displacement of its segments, changing the size and shape of the intervertebral foramina, it is possible for subluxations to occur there and offer interference with the transmission of Innate forces indirectly, if not directly. All dis-ease is thus traceable to impingements of nerve tissue in the spinal column. Chiropractic is a science which consists in having scientific knowledge of this cause of dis-ease and the artistic ability to adjust and correct these displacements of the segments of the spinal column, thereby removing interference with the transmission of Innate forces. Adjustment does not add any material or forces to the body but allows Innate to restore to normal what it would have had, had there been no interference. In this manner, health is restored. Chiropractic includes the study of all life, but that of the human body in particular. At the present time adjustments are almost entirely confined to the human spine and restoring health to the human body. Therefore, our studies, with the exception of the fundamentals, will be in regard to the human Innate Intelligence, chiefly; the human body and the functioning of its parts; and incoordinations of the same in order to arrive at proficiency in ascertaining and removing the cause of dis-ease.

Stephenson's real genius was an ability to explain all of B.J. Palmer's core philosophical and theoretical models understandably and practically.

Stephenson's Contributions to Chiropractic Theory

There are several areas where Stephenson not only explains the latest understanding of chiropractic theory but also contributes some new innovative approaches. These include: the *Vertemere Cycle*, *Cord Pressure and Cord Tension*, *Universal Forces*, *Innate Forces*, *Momentum of Dis-ease Processes*, and *Transformation* as a field-effect.

He coined the term *Vertemere Cycle*, which was developed by Craven and may represent the first proprioceptive model of vertebral subluxation. It also explains why Innate can't correct subluxations that have reached this point. It is defined as follows:

Art. 375. THE NORMAL VERTEMERE CYCLE.

The Vertemere Cycle is the cycle from innate brain to the tissues holding in situ the vertebra in question.

A subluxation impinging a nerve from brain to organ, also impinges the nerve supplying its own tissues; that is why it exists as a subluxation.

Stephenson also expanded on the cord pressure models of B.J. Palmer and John Craven when he hypothesized, there are multiple causes of cord pressure such as sacral impingements, cervical subluxations, and pathologies like tumors of the meninges, the cord, or the canal. He referred to cord pressures as distortion of the meninges and cord tension. He developed several illustrations to clarify these points.

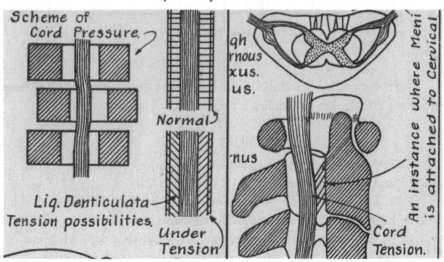

From *The Chiropractic Textbook* (1927)

The Chiropractic Textbook elaborated on the role of forces in chiropractic theory. He coined the terms Universal Forces and Innate Forces. Stephenson writes that "Invasive Forces are Universal Forces" and "Resistive Forces are Innate Forces." These terms were developed from earlier theories of B.J. Palmer and D.D. Palmer.

Stephenson also innovated on B.J. Palmer's 1913 theory of momentum, which was developed from D.D. Palmer. Stephenson developed a time and momentum chart for practitioners to determine the patient's location on the spectrum between health and death.

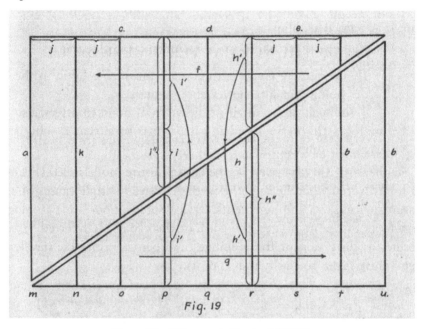

Fig. 19

From *The Chiropractic Textbook* (1927)

The more embedded and chronic the subluxation patterns and disease processes are, the longer it takes for restoration. He writes:

Art. 135. MOMENTUM.

Momentum is the possession of motion; requiring effort and time to stop it.

Chiropractically, Momentum is the progress of dis-ease or health, requiring time and effort to stop it.

The Momentum of either health or dis-ease depends upon the survival values; which are material values requiring time to change. There is no process that does not require time. (Prin. 6)

He also added the terminology for the theory of survival values, which B.J. Palmer adopted in Vol. 18 and thereafter.

As noted above, Stephenson added a novel contribution to B.J.'s 1907 theory of transformation. He suggests that the act of transformation begins when the thought is created from a stepping down process. The process begins with Universal Intelligence, then Innate Intelligence and then the Mental Realm. According to B.J., the newly created thought then merges with the raw force, and becomes a mental impulse. Stephenson proposes that transformation is much like a magnetic field. He referred to this as the way in which intelligence "gets a grip on matter." This field-like approach to the mental impulse points to areas where the mental impulse might be researched with modern technology.

Critically Analyzing Stephenson's Text

It is important for chiropractic's advancement that all of the Green Books be subjected to critical analysis. These texts are the foundation for modern theory and practice. This is especially important for influential books like Stephenson's text. Without examining a text's flaws, the circumstances of its creation, the references it rests upon, along with its contributions, a book could run the risk of being reified on a pedestal. To avoid such freezing of theory, ideas, and innovation; critical analysis using contemporary scientific and philosophical sources are crucial.

While critical analysis is not one of the objectives of this book, since Stephenson's text has had such an impact, it is important to at least point out some areas of inquiry to examine the text. Perhaps future works could take these up systematically. Two areas for example are the forun theory and Stephenson's use of logic.

B.J. Palmer's original theory was explicit that foruns or units of force entered the body from the environment and were eventually transformed into mental impulses. The transformation included the newly created thought and the unit of energy. Craven said that the forun itself was created in the brain and Stephenson reflects that. Stephenson writes:

> When Innate assembles universal forces in the brain cell they are in the form of thoughts. In this non-specific state they are called foruns.

This is not how B.J. Palmer explained the theory in 1909. The thoughts and the foruns were distinct until merged during the transformation process. In fact, Stephenson captures all of the other steps of B.J.'s NCC, but he does not include the original idea that the brain absorbs energy in an osmotic fashion from the environment and then transforms it into usable power to express intelligence as action and function.

Stephenson's approach to the "forun" is a break from B.J. Palmer's original theory from 1909. It is more congruent with the writings of Craven in the 1916 edition of Vol. 5. This is an interesting distinction, especially because in 1934, B.J.'s only reference to Stephenson's text is about this newer idea and B.J. seems to agree. Therefore, it is difficult to say whether this was a modification of the original. However, the new approach is not as logical as the idea proposed in 1909.

Since B.J. published Craven's writings on the topic in the second edition of Vol. 5 and also referenced these newer ideas that the brain creates the energy *and* the thoughts, we can only surmise that the idea was changed and Stephenson captured that change.

Other areas of the text that rely on the use of logic and reason have yet to be analyzed by philosophers trained in logic. It would be useful for the profession to subject the book to scrutiny at the highest levels of academia, learn from the analysis, and develop new theoretical frameworks from there.

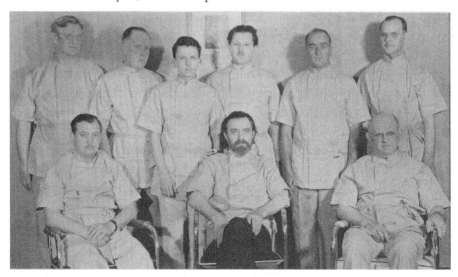

Seated from left to right is WL Heath, BJP, AB Hender, standing in background RW Stephenson, PA Riemer, K Cronk, HC Hender, Evans and HC Chance (1935)

Early Systems Thinking in Stephenson's Text

Stephenson's text offers three levels of theory: the expert mastery of facts with its logical progression of ideas, the scientific viewpoint relying on anatomical and physiological models in clinical practice, and the early systems approach to viewing life and science. The third level is the most complex. For example, biology was viewed in terms of the interior organizational logic of the biological system and how that related to the environmental forces impacting the organism.

Stephenson's approach was a pioneering integration of a body/mind viewpoint. For example, he describes increasing levels of complexity in terms of biological and mental development. Living systems could be classified in terms of gradations. Each new level of complexity in evolution contains intelligence "exactly proportionate to their state of organization." Also, Stephenson links the increasing complexity of the nervous system to the ability of organisms to adapt more readily and reason more completely. Because of this he writes, "Man gives himself the highest rank, this rank being based upon his superior powers of adaptability." He also writes:

> Man has the most powerful organ of Intellectual Adaptation, the Educated Brain, hence a greater adaptability. He rates himself higher in the scale of life because of his higher powers of sensibility and reasoning.

The increasing complexity of the organism's organization is correlated not only to the greater ability to adapt but also to the development of reasoning faculties. This viewpoint has roots in the writings of D.D. Palmer and foreshadowed later theories like Piaget's genetic epistemology and Maturana and Varela's autopoietic theory.

Another important holistic viewpoint that Stephenson expands upon was a distinction that can be traced to B.J. Palmer's 1916 pamphlet called *Laboratorical Findings and Inductions vs. Clinical Findings and Deductions.* Stephenson contrasts the overly rational approach utilized in the laboratory, whereby living systems are viewed as parts that could be analyzed, versus what he called "the clinic" or the "clinical" approach, where the Innate perspective is always considered. This could be viewed as a transition to an early-systems way of thinking that was found in many of the Green Books. He writes:

> The Chiropractor's reasoning upon laboratory material, in which the physicist sees nothing but matter, is recognizing the

intelligence that governs the matter in question and is therefore clinical. Also, the chiropractor does not treat matter with matter, in order to cure dis-ease; but calls upon the only power that can cure it—the inborn intelligence within the matter.

Therefore the true meaning of clinic in Chiropractic is the recognition of the intelligent guiding force in all "living things."

Distinctions between interior and exterior, laboratory and clinic, normal and abnormal, were central to the chiropractic paradigm and would not enter philosophical discourse in academia until the second half of the twentieth century. In many respects, the chiropractic paradigm was leading the culture.

The CHIROPRACTOR   37

Chiropractic
Fundamentals

By R. W. STEPHENSON, D.C.
Department of Philosophy, THE PSC

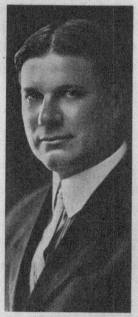

R. W. STEPHENSON, D.C.

EVERY science has its principles, theories and hypotheses. Every science has a number of principles which are established, upon which that science is based. According to the exactness of its fundamental principles, is a science exact. The science of mathematics is made up of a countless number of exact principles. Chemistry and physics are studied according to a number of established facts; music, art, drawing, designing have their principles, and even medicine is practiced according to established procedures.

Chiropractic, no less a science than any of these, also has many principles. Those principles which every chiropractor uses in his science, whether he knows it or not, whether he believes it or not, are the fundamental principles of Chiropractic. The explanation of these principles is Chiropractic philosophy.

In the limited scope of this talk we can only name and explain a few of the main ones. Perhaps one of the most basic of these principles, is one which is universal and states that life is intelligent. The reason that Chiropractic looks to gence. Therefore, we must admit that some power is most almighty intelligent, in order to know that much.

To Chiropractic this fact is universally true; not limited to mere animals and other creatures but to every movement in the universe. As we recognize the intelligence directing every natural law with a precision not to be denied, whether it is a molecule or a planet, do we recognize life.

We state the Chiropractic idea of life by saying that life is a triunity; the combination of three important factors; intelligence, force and matter. Matter moves — it gives us evidence of force. Can you conceive a force unless matter shows it to you? Where does this force come from? By its precision, we know it must come from some power intelligent enough to make it precise in its movements. This is usually called Law or Natural Law. Then Law must be Intelligence itself.

Scientists have studied matter for many years, but did not look back to the cause. Some scientists studied intelligence but did not look forward to the effect. Chiropractic studied both and recognized the link between them, i.e., force. In-have discovered some of the ways in which it travels. For instance, they speak of radiation, and conduction; they speak of forms of energy and that these forms are interchangeable; hence, there is possibly one form which we see manifest in many other forms.

Energy radiates at a very high rate of speed. In spite of that fact it seems to prefer to travel at a slower rate in or through matter. Heat, a form of energy, prefers

From The Chiropractor (1924)

Stephenson's Utopian Vision

Stephenson ends his 1927 textbook with a vision for the future world, where culture and society are transformed by chiropractic's philosophical influence and its scientific application. The ultimate vision is a world where subluxations are regularly corrected and where Innate flows more freely through all humans. He writes:

Article 399. B.J. Palmer's Utopia

In accordance with the hopeful idea given by the Universal Cycle, Dr. Palmer's love for the human race and solicitude for the suffering, lead him to hold that chiropractors have a great mission to perform. "Not to improve the basic law—this is impossible—but to remove any negative obstructions brought about by perversions of that law, to the further end of a greater and freer expression of what the law of cycles demands in every phase and attribute." If Chiropractic would be allowed to do this, an ideal state of affairs could be brought nearer. This state of affairs, which is not impossible for chiropractors to bring about, if they had the chance, would approach the ideal. An ideal state of sociology is a utopia.

An ideal sociological state would be a country or a world without sickness, insanity, blindness, feeble-minded people, deaf and dumb, backward children; social evils, criminality, drunkenness and its attendant evils, abnormal reproduction, etc. If Chiropractic were given a chance to do its miracles and reasonable time allowed for the results to be brought about, it could do much; more than any other human agency has done or can do, in reducing the above named abnormalities to a minimum. This would be a great economic saving, because there could be fewer public and charitable institutions and penal institutions.

This type of vision was expressed by many early chiropractors such as D.D. Palmer, B.J. Palmer, J.N. Drain, Willard Carver, T.F. Ratledge, and other Green Book authors.

Stephenson's Final Article: The Ubiquitous Mixer

Stephenson wrote a final essay in *The Chiropractor* in May 1935, the year before he died. The article is titled *The Ubiquitous Mixer*. We include this final writing not because of its philosophical merits but because there is something familiar to it for modern chiropractors. There will always be those who are unscrupulous and use a good profession like chiropractic for their own benefit. And yet, some of the specifics he writes of in 1935 are still with us today.

Stephenson writes of a parasitic type of "mixer," or a chiropractor who preys on other chiropractors by opening an office in their town and using their good reputation to lure in prospective patients. He writes that there are two kinds of this peculiar person:

> First, the chiropractoid who may be sincere in his solicitude for mankind, but does not know what Chiropractic is. He distrusts it and seeks to bolster up what he thinks is a weak modality, by using old fashioned medical modes. Second, the chiroquactor who well knows that he is cheating sick people and does not care. He distrusts everything, even himself.

According to Stephenson, the "chiroquactor" knows the chiropractic princi-ples but does not care and is often a moral pervert, a dope, a criminal, and always unscrupulous. The goal of this type of mixer is business, not profession, where money is more important than getting the sick patient well. Stephenson continues:

> It is impossible to name or describe all of the apparatus which may be found in a mixer's office, but suffice it to say that in mixer exactly answers the idea that medical doctors universally have about chiropractors—that they are practicing illegally and incompetently an offshoot of medicine...
>
> The mixer, in his publications, always discredits the brand of Chiropractic taught at the Fountain Head and refers to D. D. Palmer as proof of this discredit. If these mixer writers and publishers really knew the principles that D. D. Palmer laid down they would know that they are the same that B. J. Palmer upholds. The Fountain Head is not opposing D. D. Palmer's findings, and conclusions: but is carrying on the work that D. D. Palmer started, in the direct line

of evolution. The mixers' propaganda in trying to oppose the Palmers is clearly the act of the parasite in trying to destroy its host...

Someone, and I suspect the mixer, among others, has taught the general public that Chiropractic is all right for some things but perfectly helpless in other directions. The idea is, that Chiropractic is the only thing for "sore backs" but under no circumstances should a chiropractor take a case that is a disease. Sore backs for chiropractors, and all other troubles to the M.D.

Of these last two points, only education of historical facts, ethical development training, and good scientific research on the correction of vertebral subluxation will remedy problems that have been with the profession for far too long.

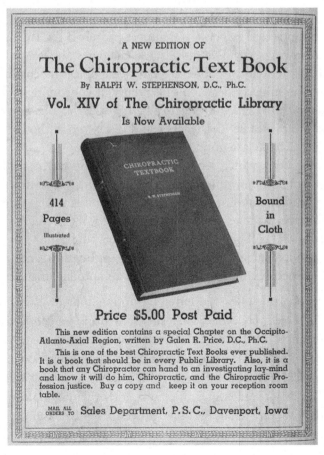

Advertisement for the second edition of Vol. 14 (1940)

Stephenson's Final Thoughts on Chiropractic's Advance

In March 1935, a letter from R.W. Stephenson was published in *The Chiropractor* as a reply to other letters. In Stephenson's letter, several important statements stand out. For example, he notes that in writing his textbook, he "had no thought of being considered as an authority in Chiropraictc." His central aim of the book "was to help students of Chiropractic the world over." Since chiropractic was so new, he sought to organize the literature in a concise way. He writes:

> My aim was to save the students the trouble and delay in reading extensively and laboriously in the library of Chiropractic to obtain their classwork. Therefore I arranged the material which I had learned at the P.S.C. from 1920 to 1927 and the material from "After Tomorrow What," from "Majors and Minors" and from "Volume V." The material used in the "Chiropractic Textbook" was almost entirely B.J.'s. The theories, the drawings, the illustrations, the analogies, the examples, the explanations in my book are but pedagogical mechanisms to "put the subject over" and give plenty of concomitants. While always thinking Chiropractically, I worked at this book with the mind of a school teacher and not as an authority—I do claim to be a darn good teacher.
>
> The book which I prepared is still useful to the student— most of it is not obsolete, for throughout, it lays stress upon the fundamentals of Chiropractic. The fundamental principles will never change. If the reader or user of the "Chiropractic Textbook" will remember the date of publication, omit the outmoded subjects which deal with **application**, and study it for **principles**, he will be using it in an uptodate manner.

Stephenson concludes the letter by noting that in 1927, he viewed himself as "a stage in its evolution; a stepping-stone—a cog in the gears of scientific advance." In that regard, he felt that by staying up-to-date on the latest chiropractic science, he was able to be a "sound cog," and continue to "mesh with science in a useful manner." His intent was to update the book with new illustrations, analogies, diagrams, and explanations by questioning all prior theories and retaining only "proven FACTS." On continuing to evolve and grow, Stephenson writes:

I believe a competent scientist does not become mentally static—he does not become wedded to his own or any one else's pet theories and "set" in his beliefs. He does not believe that his thoughts are super-human and immortal just because they are his own. The competent scientist knows that, appearances to the contrary, he might be wrong. Such a scientist advances as he learns and does not shut himself away from learning. He never "arrives." The one who is successful is the one who IS succeeding, and he is no longer successful if he HAS succeeded. The successful one is an is-er and not a was-er. He is kinetic, not static.

If in my own experience the most astounding thing should happen; namely, that what we now believe to be the Fundamentals of Chiropractic should prove to be not the fundamentals at all, I would scrap them without protest. An astounding thing in Chiropractic has happened, and Chiropractic is no longer the thing it was in 1920 or 1924 or 1927. Therefore I am declaring that those parts of the Chiropractic Textbook not in line with HIO principles are now obsolete. My reasons for saying so are not politic.

I am not "yessing" B.J. for a job. I have not asked him for one, but I am immeasurably gratified to have the chance to become an up-to-the-minute Chiropractor and try to be of more value to myself, to Chiropractic and to the P.S.C.

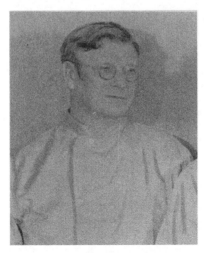

R.W. Stephenson (1935)

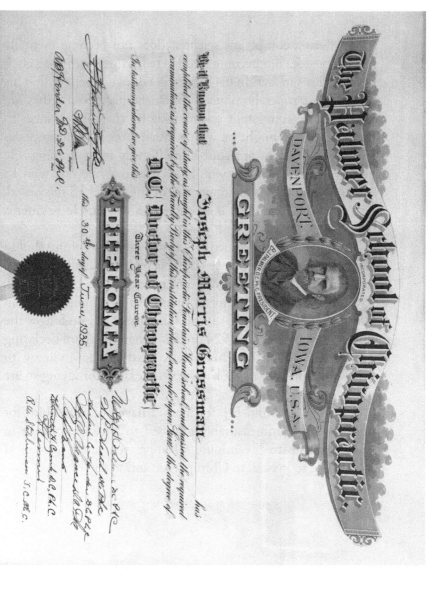

PSC diploma signed by
R.W. Stephenson
(June 30, 1935)

Chapter 10
The Research Pamphlets: 1924-1933

To understand the Green Books that came after Stephenson's text, it is important to examine B.J. Palmer's pamphlets published between 1924 and 1934. The pamphlets were basically B.J.'s lectures transcribed as short books. The pamphlets were designed to update the profession on the latest research. B.J. may not have published any Green Books during this decade, but many of these pamphlets were eventually published in later volumes.

B.J. Palmer began testing the NCM in 1923 and announced it to the profession at Lyceum in 1924. He researched the NCM, tabulated his statistics with his faculty, and presented the findings every year at Lyceum. These talks were published as pamphlets for sale at each Lyceum.

At the beginning of Vol. 18, which was published in 1934, B.J. writes:

> During 11 years since introduction of NCM, we have been gradually climbing the scale of understanding of much that before was mystery. We have left behind much theory and taken on much science. As developments occurred, we have written them into our publications. The past few years we have issued an annual of research work of year previous. To bring this book to its fullest value, would mean to reprint most of those into this. As those productions ARE in print, and can be had as separate units, we do not feel the necessity of reprinting and incorporating them into this.

He lists eight pamphlets that contain the research leading up to Vol 18. They are: *The Hour has Struck* (1924), *Why Did B.J.?* (1925), *Reasons for my Faith* (1928), *A Hole in One* (1930), *The Hour Has Arrived* (1931), *Manual of Instruction in Gliding Technique for Use of NCM No. 2* (1931), *Crowding the Hour (1932), and Disciplining The Hour* (1933). Not only did the pamphlets form the basis for discussions and new theories in all future Green Books but they became part of the books.

B.J. reprinted at least four of the pamphlets in other textbooks. *The Hour Has Arrived* was included in Vol. 24 on page 610. *Crowding the Hour* and *Disciplining the Hour* were included as chapters 2 and 4 of Vol. 25. Also, a ninth pamphlet was published in the fall of 1933 titled *Torqued Subluxation Torque Adjustment*. It was integrated into several chapters of Vol. 18 in 1934 and published as chapter 5 of Vol. 25 in 1951.

One theme of these pamphlets was "the hour." This metaphor was a way for B.J. to impress upon his students and colleagues that the new innovations were crucial to chiropractic's future. The significance of thermography, HIO, the Specific, and the upper cervical chiropractic analysis model was stressed through the course of these eleven years of lectures.

The research during this time led to new models of subluxation and new theories and practices of chiropractic. This led to new research and philosophical insights, and eventually, 16 more books from B.J. Palmer over the next two decades. By his late 70s, B.J. mostly wrote about how the research and the history of innovations inspired his evolving philosophical insights.

The Hour Has Struck (1924)

The Hour Has Struck was delivered on a Sunday evening on August 24, 1924, at the Eighth Annual PSC Lyceum. The lecture was published as a 19-page pamphlet introducing the NCM to the profession. It laid out the science and the rationale, as well as the leasing options for chiropractors.

At the start of the talk, B.J. acknowledges that "chiropracTIC" is based on a principle and yet "chiropracTORs" have a problem. Many chiropractors are seeking more patients for financial gain. They are in a "little rut and groove," scraping by each day and they are used to the comforts of modern life. He classifies the profession in terms of fifty percent who should not be chiropractors because they have no ability, twenty-five percent are commercially successful, fifteen percent who are involved

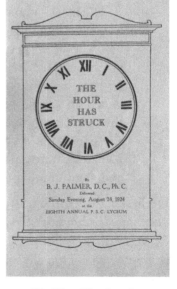

The Hour Has Struck
cover (1924)

in chiropractic politics locally, five percent who are aware of chiropractic problems at the level of their state, and only 50 people in the profession who understand the national problems chiropractic faces. Of that, there are only about 25 people who understand "the problems facing the International Chiropractic movement." The vision and scope of those 25 people are regulated, governed, and controlled by the ninety-five percent through legislation, education of the public, and practices of chiropractic boards and associations. The "group mind" of the profession is destructive towards pure chiropractic.

This talk was given two years after B.J.'s 1922 talk, *Cleaning House*, which described the UCA Model Bill, which was a legislative agenda designed to introduce pure chiropractic laws in every state. That talk also proposed that competing state organizations should "clean house" and get rid of boards and associations that were not in-line with a strictly chiropracTIC agenda, meaning no alternative methods, practices, or theories to be used alongside chiropractic practice.

B.J. claims that public confidence in chiropractors is at a 28-year low. This is mainly due to chiropractors who claim the right to "do anything he pleases." He proposes the new NCM is the way to save the profession. He writes:

> Chiropractic is a natural right which men cannot destroy. Chiropractors, though, can through a destructive majority group mind destroy the rights of chiropractors. If chiropractors who are, will get squarely and unswervingly behind this BACK-TO-CHIROPRACTIC-NEUROCALOMETER-MOVEMENT, we will yet save you chiropractors.

For B.J., the NCM was a scientific and financial solution to the problem chiropractors were facing.

In the talk, he describes the early history of the NCM. Dossa Evins, a young chiropractor and engineer, introduced the idea to one of B.J.'s inner circle, Frank Elliot, who convinced B.J. to test it out. The PSC hired Evins and together they completed ten months of tests with 500 cases. They had yet to explain the new device to anyone in the profession. Patents were applied for in 17 countries. After the tests were complete, B.J. writes:

> When finally realized that we had in our profession the most valuable idea that has ever been given by man for man in

the history of the world, the appalling immensity of the thing grew upon us, and then we figured out that we had three ways of giving it to the world.

The first plan was to keep the NCM only in the clinic, the second plan was to sell it, the third plan, which was enacted, was to lease the device to chiropractors.

This third option was controversial because of its financial benefits to B.J., especially because the price was $1,500, even though that included ten years of instrument servicing, and training twice per year, which included reviews of technique and palpation, even if it took several days. Considering that in 2018 dollars, the lease would cost $22,106, it is no wonder that B.J. got a great deal of push-back from the profession. He also made a small fortune.

He explained that the collections from leases would go toward a staff of ten men to travel the country doing servicing and training, a national publicity campaign, lawyers for patents, as well as royalties, taxes, and development and repairs. Also, he was planning to increase the wattage and output of the WOC radio in order to advertise nationwide.

In defense of this pricing strategy and a rationale for why B.J. made the analogy that the majority of chiropractors had been "milking the cow," that a minority of chiropractors had been feeding for many years, he writes:

> Whose cow is Chiropractic anyway? Is it more my cow or your cow? Must I always stand at that feeding end? Can't I get a glass of milk once in a while? Who is that man that speaks to me about the rights of the sick to get well? Who is that man that dares say I am the downfall of this profession? Do you know of any chiropractor adjusting for fifty cents when he could collect five dollars, just for the love of the rights of the sick to get well? Do you know of any reducing their price on the theory of their love for the rights of the sick to get well if he could get it?

He viewed the NCM as a way to ensure that he, and the PSC, and the wider international chiropracTIC movement would stay financially viable so that they could continue to bring TIC into the future. He even described the monthly payments as an insurance policy for the profession.

B.J. Palmer emphasized that he was not only in it for the money. If that were the case, he would offer a contract to any chiropractor who asked. Instead, there were hundreds of contracts that were marked "hold," pending

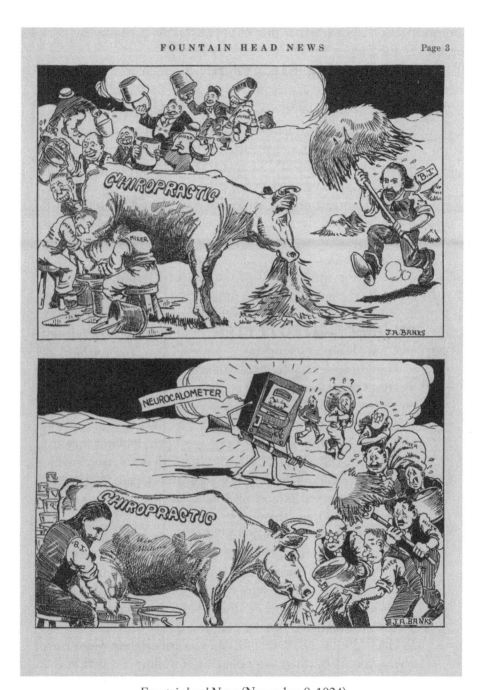

Fountainhead News (November 8, 1924)

an investigation as to whether that chiropractor has been feeding the cow or milking the cow.

A lengthy quote from the talk will explain his further defense of the new leasing structure and criticisms he had already received. He writes:

> You know, folks, Chiropractic is my birthright. It is my heirloom. I could no more do anything different than I am doing, because I am not the master of my own destiny. I am in the hands of an All-Wise Creator that carries me on and on. Everything I have or everything I ever have had, is bounded by Eighth Street on the south, Eleventh Street on the north, Brady Street on the east, and the alley on the west—centered on Chiropractic and nothing else. I own no stocks, nor bonds, nor dry oil holes. I have specialized all my life on Chiropractic, and I have centralized all of my life on Chiropractic. Every dollar I ever made-it is here and in you. You know that just as well as I do. I have given everything I ever made back into Chiropractic—and that is more than the most of you can say who have been criticizing me.
>
> I have risked forty-four years of my life, and my reputation—whatever that is worth—and all that I have got in the world in putting over this Neurocalometer campaign, the hardest, the safest and the best way for Chiropractic.
>
> I went into this fight with my eyes open, looking forward and upward, believing that there was enough of you worthwhile people that would help me carry on my message—the right of the sick to get well tomorrow. I believed there was enough of you to help do that. There were easier ways that I could have made money, Money, MONEY! There were easier ways that I could have made mine. There were smoother paths that I could have trodden; there were richer incomes at my command.
>
> Now, what would you have done, if you had placed into your hands today the monopoly of the greatest thing in the world in seventeen countries? What would you do? I challenge you—WHAT WOULD YOU DO? Yet you criticize me when I am saving you. Why, there isn't one out of a thousand within the speaking range of my voice that would have taken the hard way through, every inch of the way and all of the way back again. There isn't one out of a thousand that would have done it. Why for years, I have been endeavoring to save Chiropractic. I have

thought and taught, written and printed, analyzed, traveled and lectured; I have struggled with every means at my command to be worthy of your confidence in all things Chiropractic, and while ChiropracTIC has been getting better and better, chiropracTORs have been getting worse and worse.

Why, in July of this year we ran short of jail fund money, but I hadn't the courage to ask you for more. With your great misunderstanding of me, I couldn't ask you for more. I couldn't have stood any more insults like what I had been getting—I couldn't have stood it. I just took the necessary amount from other funds. I would rather pay in cash than heartaches. Why? Was it because I was always so far behind that none believed me worthy of leading you on? Or was I so far ahead that you couldn't see me?

For years I have been compelled to do many things I did not want to do to keep this school on a financial balance. Why, you haven't any conception of the worries that go with an institution of our magnitude, where our overhead is exactly $3,000.00 a day—THREE THOUSAND DOLLARS A DAY to keep this institution alive. Why, that is beyond your average understanding. Why, I am compelled to keep down costs and to keep on rendering service and build, if you please, on a declining income. That was my problem for years.

Then came the great solution—the Neurocalometer. Oh, I have been in some very unpleasant situations before, but none anywhere near equaling those of the past eighteen months.

B.J. concludes that the first ten months involved him convincing himself that the NCM was right. Then he realized the PSC needed more resources to bring the NCM to the world, even though it would be risky to rely on the profession to embrace it and his followers to sign up. Nine months were spent developing the program followed by the backlash from the profession including his followers. He acknowledged in the talk that the criticism was so fierce it drove him "to the ragged edge of insanity and a breakdown." The criticisms and daily letters were so intense that B.J. eventually spent some time in a sanitarium to rest and recover. Of the criticism he writes:

Why, thousands of these chiropractors got together in groups, in districts, and in conventions, and they heaped maledictions upon me from all sides. Most of them were induced to keep on with that sort of thing because of the vehement expressions of one person to another, piling them up. That thing has kept on for three months, weekdays, and Sundays, day and night. Letters, telegrams, long distance phones—there was no rest for the weary.

Nobody will ever know—nobody but Mabel can ever know—the sleepless, tossing and rolling nights, night after night, the hours spent, Sundays all day included, week in and week out! Why, the problems that we worried through when our friends were misunderstanding us, night after night, fighting to get a bit of respite, a bit of sleep, to appear smilingly the next morning in the classroom, because I knew I was right!

You know, from year to year, we look forward to these Lyceums. Months in advance we begin planning for the coming event. We begin planning, and we dream the day dreams for the homecoming of our Chiropractic kids; we look forward to the smiling, shaking hands and the "howdy-do"—BUT NOT THIS YEAR, NOT THIS YEAR. We dreaded this Lyceum. Every conscious hour has been a constant nightmare. We have dreaded this year. We have dreaded this Lyceum, and we have looked forward to the relief of the week after.

And yet, he mastered his self through knowing he was right and getting feedback from the field chiropractors that were having success with the new NCM.

He concludes that he is forgiving of his detractors and that "Chiropractic is greater than any man or any set of men in it." He drew inspiration from reading biographies about Abraham Lincoln and decided, in relation to the harsh critiques, "I will take anything from anybody, if the sick will be benefited by my taking it."

He concludes the talk with:

I place in your hands the most valuable invention of history, because it picks, proves and locates the CAUSE of all dis-eases of the human race.

The future of this Chiropractic profession is in your hands, for you to accept or reject. **The Hour Has Struck!** THE HOUR HAS STRUCK! Hold high the sacred trust! HOLD HIGH THAT SACRED TRUST THE HOUR HAS STRUCK!

B.J. Palmer's Reasons for My Faith (1928)

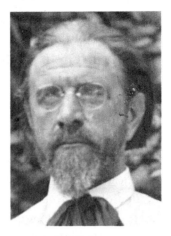

B.J. Palmer

In 1926, B.J. Palmer lectured in 37 states. One of his main talks was *Reasons for My Faith*, which he referred to as *Conclusions of Facts as they Applied to Chiropractic Principles and Practices*. It was published in 1928 as a pamphlet.

The pamphlet described a survey of the field chiropractors conducted in 1918. They found that only 35% of patients were "getting well." B.J. and his staff used these statistics to upgrade their "incomplete applied system" of chiropractic analysis. This led to the development of the NCM.

B.J. and his staff concluded that one reason for the 65% of failures was that chiropractors were finding acute subluxations but they were not detecting and correcting chronic subluxations. This was because one clinical finding for acute subluxations was the emanation of heat or "the hot box." Such heat is detectable by the human hand.

This type of chiropractic analysis dates to 1902. In the early days, the location of subluxation was found by running the back of the hand over the spine to find the hottest spot. In a private letter from D.D. to B.J. on April 27, 1902, which includes D.D.'s first known use of the term "sub-luxation," D.D. writes:

> Observe the difference in temperature of your patients along the spine, of those having fever, by placing your hand at different points; where you find the greatest heat, there you will find the sub-luxation causing the inflammation which produces the fever.

It was proposed that the NCM ended the need for heat detection by hand.

In the pamphlet, B.J. explains that the "rule of the hot box" was laid down in Vol. 3. It states that the interference caused some Mental Impulses to get sidetracked because they can't get through. He writes:

> Being energy, they create abnormal action at point of interference, generate extra heat, which is dissipated to the surface at that point. This is an ACUTE subluxation.

When the subluxation becomes chronic, then a "chronic hot box" develops, which has reduced intensity "outside the range of human sensitivity." This claim was based on six months of research. He writes:

> The minimum and maximum temperature range of the CHRONIC subluxation was within 1-100th of a degree centigrade.

The research study using the NCM, or what B.J. refers to in the pamphlet as the Mechanical Chronic Hot-Box Heat Finder, examined 486 failed chiropractic cases. For each case they collected information as follows: name, address, former history, names of diagnosticians, diagnosis, classification of conditions, previous adjustments, results of adjustments, method of adjustments, how many places were adjusted, how often these had been changed, length of time each was given, and results of each. Cases were then brought to the new PSC clinic. Conditions were determined. Spinographs were taken and analyzed. NCM readings were taken. The Major vertebral subluxations were located and adjusted. Frequency of adjustments were noted along with any changes. Daily pre and post checks were made. Cases were followed through to dismissal.

According to the pamphlet, conclusions from this first cohort study of the NCM on a population of poor-responding chiropractic patients was a success. B.J. concludes from the research that the classic meric system was only accurate 35% of the time. The NCM located the chronic subluxation in the other 65% of cases.

Several new theoretical and physiological models were introduced into subluxation theory. According to B.J., it was now possible to detect the location of interference to the nervous system caused by subluxation using thermographic instrumentation. Also, a vertebra could be manually moved without it being an adjustment. He hypothesized that if the misaligned vertebra was not causing interference, then there was no restoration

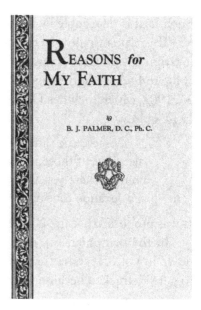

Reasons for my Faith
cover (1928)

to the transmission of impulses required. Thus, it was possible to move a vertebra and increase the pressure on the neural structures. This new approach challenged the clinical protocols of the entire profession.

B.J. includes a simple diagram of the brain-cord system with five anatomical and physiological types of interference: 1. Superficial Visceral Nervous System Interference, 2. Cord Pressures, 3. Spinal Nerve Pressure, 4. Cord Tensions, and 5. Inflammatory Pressures. This was the first time B.J. wrote about Cord Tension and Cord Pressure in 30 years. He found that the majority of missed cases were due to this type of interference.

In the pamphlet, B.J. references Crile's *Bi-Polar Theory of Living Processes* for the first time. Crile's book was published in 1926. For B.J., Crile's research on living processes confirmed his energetic theories of life. He would continue to cite Crile's work throughout his books from this point forward. B.J. even advertised copies of Crile's book, which could be purchased at PSC with reproductions of his own underlining from his private copy.

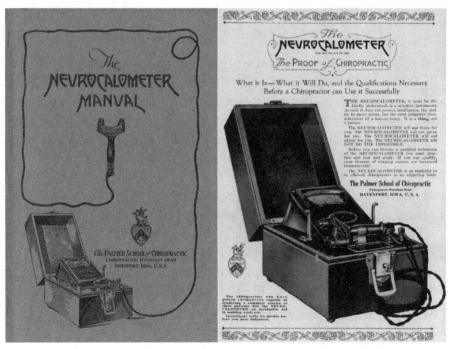

Neurocalometer manual and promotion (1924)

B.J. Palmer's A Hole in One (1930)

In October 1929, B.J. Palmer delivered his talk, *A Hole in One* (HIO), for the first time. It was an invited lecture presented to the Minnesota Convention of the first American Chiropractor's Association. B.J. writes that even though they were "composed of mixers," they invited him anyway. He writes:

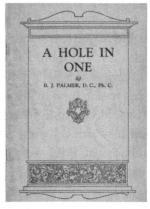

> They knew in advance that my subject would be Chiropractic and they knew that what I might say was not favorably or kindly inclined towards chiropractoids. In spite of this, I was still invited.
>
> Sunday, Oct. 20th was the day. I spoke 2 hours in the morning on The Backwash, 2 hours in the afternoon on my latest, A Hole in One. They seemed tremendously pleased. Enthusiasm ran high.

A Hole In One cover (1930)

He hoped the talks would help them "get back to the back." A few years later, HIO would become synonymous with B.J.'s upper cervical chiropractic analysis. Initially, the theory emphasized the importance of locating the optimal one or two specific vertebral subluxations in the spine.

B.J. delivered the talk throughout 1930. His largest audience was at the Chiropractic Health Bureau Convention in New York City on February 21, 1930, to 7,000 people. *A Hole in One* was published as a pamphlet in July of that year. In October 1930, he gave the talk to 2,500 people in New Zealand, and in November, to 650 at King's Hall in Sydney, Australia.

Considering the talk was first delivered only two years after *Stephenson's Text* was published, it is notable that in the talk he mentions principles that are different from Stephenson's classic 33 principles. However, B.J.'s principles are congruent with Stephenson's principles. B.J. writes, "Chiropractic gradually grew. It is now premised upon certain principles." Here are some of the principles he proposed:

> Fifth: The fixed physics fact that matter cannot move without force or energy.
>
> Sixth: Human matter is in motion as human energy gets to the human matter.

Seventh: Human matter moves in exact ratio as human energy is delivered to the human matter.

Eighth: More mind in more matter equals more motion.

Ninth: The quantity flow of mental energy, between brain and body, predetermines the quality of function at the periphery.

Overall, *A Hole In One* is an overview of the chiropractic perspective and consistent with prior chiropractic theory. It does offer some new philosophical perspectives. B.J. Palmer writes:

Man, to the chiropractor, is a spiritual, electrical, mechanical, chemical being-spiritual as to his intellectuality; electrical as to the internal thot-energy flowing thru nerves; mechanical in its every active functional movement: chemical as to the by-product of the mechanical.

The chemical is a by-product of the mechanical. The mechanical is a by-product of the electrical. The electrical is a by-product of the spiritual. The spiritual, being source within itself, is a by-product of none other than itself.

We approach man, then, according to that basis. We approach man first as to his being a spiritual being; second, as to his being an electrical being; third, as a mechanical being, and fourth as a chemical by-product of the other three, in that order of study and evaluation.

In regards to the research, B.J. sends the reader to *Reasons For My Faith*. He proposed that the NCM brought the abstract theory of mental impulse into the realm of science.

The subluxation model is consistent with his earlier theories. There are few updates to the theory, mainly in terms of finding the one adjustment that will make the biggest impact. *The Hole In One* is described towards the end of the talk. He writes:

If a "chiropractor" **plays at his** adjustment with shotgun things, which are **not** Chiropractic, he proves in exact reverse ratio that he doesn't **know** Chiropractic and can't deliver it. As he **knows** it, he does it. As he **does not** do it, he does not know it. **A competent chiropractor knows his Chiropractic** and will see **how little** he can do to see **how much** he can accomplish. More than likely, he will adjust **no more** than two places in one back in one day. This is because he **has** located the specific subluxation and adjusted **that** to the exclusion of fol-de-rols.

B.J. Palmer's The Hour Has Arrived (1931)

At the 1931 Lyceum, B.J. Palmer presented *The Hour Has Arrived*. It was in this talk that he unveiled the upper cervical model of chiropractic. The talk was published as a pamphlet and sold at the Lyceum.

In the pamphlet he explains how this new model was developed. In the spring of 1930, B.J. and his staff started testing the NCM 2, which was introduced at Lyceum in 1929. The NCM 2 was smaller and could be held with one hand using a gliding motion. The instrument was less sensitive and picked up half of the points of the NCM 1. According to B.J.,

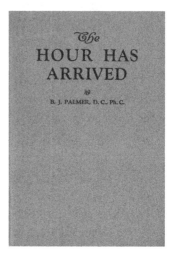

The Hour Has Arrived
cover (1931)

this gliding technique led to the new focus of HIO because it located the interference. He was, however, referring to the new modified theory of HIO, or the "HOLE IN ONE major superior cervical subluxation."

They found that by adjusting the upper cervical spine, NCM readings were not only reduced at that vertebral level but also in other regions of the spine. Majors were "usually found close to the skull line as in the atlas or axis." B.J. hypothesized that the upper cervical adjustment may release cord pressure and release "congestion superior to itself." By clearing the Innate Brain of "damming back" impulses, even more positive changes below were likely.

In *The Hour Has Arrived*, B.J. writes:

> In 1924 THE HOUR HAD STRUCK. In 1931 THE HOUR HAS ARRIVED when the NCM is established and no one has successfully challenged its scientific service; whereas thousands have successfully proven it IS a Chiropractic necessity in Chiropractic service by a chiropractor.

The new model was worked out by B.J. and his staff. New definitions for old terms were developed. Also, new terminology was proposed. However, the fundamental elements of the chiropractic paradigm were unchanged. New definitions included misalignment, alignment, realignment, and subluxation. Of subluxation he writes:

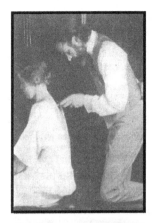

B.J. Palmer using NCM2

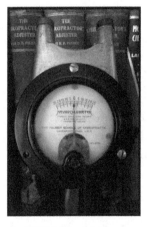

NCM Model No. 2

1st. It must be out of relationship to its correspondents above and below.

2nd. There must be an occlusion of a foramen or spinal canal.

3rd. There must exist a pressure or tension upon spinal nerves or spinal cord.

4th. There must be present an interference to transmission of mental impulse supply.

5th. Resistance of that transmission is always present.

6th. An increased abnormal local resistance heat is present in adjacent immediate tissues. To which there may or may not be present any, all, or none of the following:

7th. Taut fibres.

8th. Tender nerves.

9th. Contractured or prolapsed muscles.

10th. Under palpation, an irregularity of position may be ascertained.

11th. The Spinograph may illustrate a misalignment of correspondent position.

A subluxation could only be confirmed with NCM and spinograph, and an adjustment is only complete if the interference has been removed, which is confirmed with a post-check. He writes:

> An ADJUSTMENT can be given ONLY upon a SUBLUXATION. An ADJUSTMENT can be given only to a living body.
>
> "THE ADJUSTMENT WITH THAT EXTRA SOMETHING" is the SUBLUXATION that is ADJUSTED which remains in normal situ for an extended period of days or weeks; which makes possible A CONTINUED open foramen, which permits a long CONTINUED flow of mental impulse supply; which gets Cases well quicker and reduces the number of places necessary to "adjust"; proves that each ADJUSTMENT

is such in fact, and makes possible a definite knowledge of WHERE, WHEN, and HOW to ADJUST. "The adjustment with that extra something" releases interference at one place without creating more at others; thus making it THE HOLE IN ONE ADJUSTMENT.

He builds on this statement and then integrates the new model of HIO, with Stephenson's new terminology "accumulative constructive survival value," and the 1907 theory of Innate Recoil. He continues:

> The adjustment with that "extra something" is the net result of the additional accumulative constructive survival value that accrues as a result of an exclusive Innate recoil ADJUSTMENT upon a SUBLUXATION which was the major in each case. It is the marked brevity of time and rapidity with which cases get well in contrast to the long time and slowness with which cases formerly got well, even tho by accident, wherein the case is "adjusted" upon many "subluxations" none of which were ADJUSTMENTS upon THE SUBLUXATION which was THE cause of that case's sickness.

HIO took on a new interpretation because B.J. felt it was now understood that one subluxation, usually found in a superior location, in the upper cervical spine, was the cause for multiple readings throughout the spine.

This new approach of relying on thermography to detect neurological and hence, mental impulse interference coupled to spinography, did away with the older chiropractic models for B.J. and the PSC. Thus, history taking, tracking symptoms, and nerve tracing were no longer necessary to locate the vertebral subluxation. He writes:

> Now they arrive the first day; no history is taken; none is needed. We use our NCM to LOCATE the nerve pressure interference; the Spinograph to gain knowledge of POSITION of the subluxated vertebra at that place. We ADJUST and check to see what effect THAT subluxation has had upon EVERY OTHER reading up and down the entire spinal column. If it changes the evaluation, either by increasing or decreasing; and it does this consistently day after day, week after week, then it is proof that ONE subluxation is creating MANY readings and the ADJUSTMENT of ONE vertebra releases MANY readings, rather than ONE "subluxation" for every reading for every disease in every organ or symptom that the patient complained about.

B.J. proposed that chiropractic completely move away from patient reports of symptoms and only utilize objective measurements to detect vertebral subluxation. Patients might come in with symptoms but without a subluxation, and so, no adjustment is required. He writes:

> And in that lies one REAL secret, "the ADJUSTMENT with that extra something", for the additional step upward and forward, WHEN THERE IS NO INTERFERENCE THEN THERE IS NO NECESSITY FOR AN ADJUSTMENT. We must learn to rely upon the NCM as the truth teller, rather than the patient's telling of his or her ills, symptoms, and feelings. WHERE is determined BY THE NCM. WHEN is determined BY THE NCM. So far as reliable information from the patient is concerned, it can he discounted out of the picture completely and entirely. Follow the patient's lead and he will get worse; or, if he gets well, it will be in spite of him rather than because of what he tells you.

This led to the new dictum, "ALL SUBLUXATIONS ARE MIS-ALIGNMENTS. BUT NOT ALL MISALIGNMENTS ARE SUBLUXATIONS." This was yet another challenge to a profession that relied on palpation as a distinctive chiropractic methodology. According to B.J., as of 1931, it was established that palpation could not determine the difference between misalignment and subluxation.

In the remainder of the 70-page pamphlet, B.J. presents dozens of cases and NCM readings, and then describes his reasoning as to why the major subluxation is usually upper cervical. He writes:

> Adjustment of the one vertebral subluxated realigns the occiput, atlas and axis into correct alignment, and this in turn releases pressures and interferences and restores transmission between the Innate and Educated brains, which in its turn also releases the congesting above and interference below in a multiple interference commonly known as a cord pressure. We thus do TWO things: 1st, restore normal function to the thinking brain above; 2nd, restore function to the working body below—two VERY important things in the proper working health of the body, both mentally and physically.

B.J. Palmer's Crowding the Hour (1932)

At the 1932 Lyceum, B.J. Palmer presented *Crowding the Hour*. It was advertised as follows:

CROWDING	189 Pages of Printed Matter
THE HOUR	Issued during Lyceum, 1932
	$2 per copy—1c per page
B. J.'s LATEST BOOK	Limited First Edition. 600 sold at Lyceum upon presentation. Ready for immediate delivery

Crowding The Hour advertisement

The book was reprinted as Chapter 2 in *Chiropractic Clinical Controlled Research*, Vol. 25, which was published in 1951. B.J. writes:

> CROWDING THE HOUR is a continuation of scientific research work which took place during 1931-32. It was presented at Lyceum, 1932. It enlightens us on demonstrated proof of correctness of SPECIFIC work as applied in Chiropractic adjusting.

> To CROWD the hour is to make time valuable — to concentrate each minute in greater human service.

B.J. writes that between 1923 and 1930, he and his staff demanded scientific facts. They were no longer satisfied with developing chiropractic by relying on successful cases. He writes:

> Let some of us buckle into hard thinking, researching, and developing the scientific side of practice and improving adjusting art of chiropractic to where it reached high value of principle of chiropractic.

He then expands on the move away from relying on symptoms to detect vertebral subluxation. After 1930, they did not rely on case histories in the analysis. The new method was to "completely ignore questionable methods of symptomatology, pathology, and diagnosis." All research was directed at the spinal column, location of the cause, and cure of all dis-ease.

By the fall of 1932, they modified subluxation theory based on their findings and found that subluxations would sometimes stay adjusted even after one adjustment. Prior to that, the theory was that patients needed to be continually adjusted until well.

According to B.J., any previous conflicts between principle and practice were now resolved. Adjustments were only administered when there was interference detected by NCM and a structural distortion traced on spinograph. The object was to make chiropractic reproducible and scientific while getting cases well.

Partway through the 1932 booklet, B.J. Palmer introduces Stephenson's 33 principles. This is the only time he quotes the 33 principles or refers to them in their entirety. In future works he uses various principles but this statement, five years after Vol. 14 was published, stands alone. He introduces the 33 principles by saying, "Inasmuch as it sets forth the fundamental method of difference, we shall enlarge upon its premises." Then he names the first 33 followed by another 42, totaling 75 principles.

It is refreshing to see a laundry list of chiropractic theories tacked onto the end of the cherished principles of Stephenson. It demonstrates that B.J. Palmer had flexibility of ideas. He did not reify the deductive structure. Instead, he explored decades of theoretical and technical innovations. The new principles begin with the introduction of Cycles in 1909. The last ten principles include: the development of NCM, the history of adjusting techniques, a definition of toggle-recoil adjustment, the theory of the "hot box," the role of momentum in the restoration of health after the adjustment, the perfection of the adjustment with that something, the importance of understanding destructive survival values and constructive survival values, and the specific. Of this last point, principle 75, he writes:

Now we reach the last step— THE SPECIFIC. Because this is thoroly explained in another story, we will not go into detail here. We find ONE subluxation from which ALL symptoms and pathologies are caused. It EXCLUSIVELY is adjusted ONLY at such times and places WHEN and WHERE interference exists, to see how FEW times it can be adjusted to get case well.

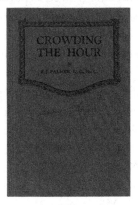

Crowding the Hour cover (1932)

He also gave details about how to practice SPECIFIC. These instructions included a list titled CONCENTRATION. He writes:

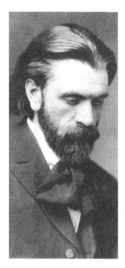

B.J. Palmer (1925)

In setting down various factors for successful practice of "SPECIFIC," we start when patient first enters office.

The procedure would be divided into four main divisions, from which numerous subdivisions could be deduced:

(a) Selling Chiropractic.

(b) Knowing and staying with your philosophy.

(c) Correct and scientific analysis.

(d) Complete case history for permanent record only, not letting it influence you in any other way.

(e) Careful visual observation of spine for objective defects, such as curvatures, that may enter into analyses or efficiency of adjustments or results.

(f) Scientific and accurate adjustment of cause.

(g) Checking, pre-checking, as well as post-checking.

Hovering over and intermingling between all features of SPECIFIC work, one factor predetermines success or failure—CONCENTRATION.

In the pamphlet, B.J. also describes important objective measures apart from NCM and spinography. He writes that the new standard, after 1923, was that the major subluxation would cause contractures of back muscles, which he viewed as pathology. This is followed by misalignments, abnormal curves, tipped pelvis, and leg-length inequality. Chiropractors who know how to read these changes may use them as a road map to discover the location, position, and number of subluxations. Upon successful adjustment, that chiropractor may note changes such as straighter spine, relaxation of the muscles, leveled pelvis, and even legs. He contrasted this with the older mechanical methods that focused on adjusting everything without a verifiable and repeatable methodology and practice.

Other new theories in *Crowding the Hour* include the concept of "Once a Major Always a Major," toggle-recoil as the evolution of adjusting practices, and to make sure that each case comes in at the same hour every day. He proposed that this final practice improves consistency, and, as he explains the following year, relates to subluxation periodicity.

B.J. Palmer's Disciplining the Hour (1933)

At the 1933 Lyceum, B.J. Palmer delivered *Disciplining the Hour*. It was, in part, a summation of the latest research study. He and his staff tracked the changes of 5,000 patients using the new HIO methods. The majority of major subluxations were found in the upper cervical spine.

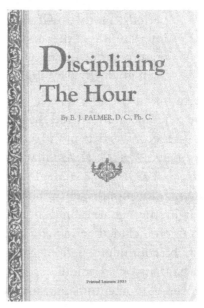

Two parts of the talk are worth exploring. He proposed that subluxations have frequency and periodicity. The two parts were called *Is there an Ebb and Tide to Subluxation Frequency* and *When is a Vertebral Subluxation?* Both articles were published in *The Chiropractor* in spring 1934. This topic was updated and reproduced as Chapter 4 of Vol. 25 in 1951.

Discipling the Hour
cover (1933)

In the April 1934 article, B.J. writes:

> It is interesting to study the conditions of frequency of vertebral subluxations, proven by frequency and locations of interferences; when such are most liable to occur and what reason seems apparent for them.

In the clinic, they observed that sudden changes in temperature, which were usually associated with a change of season, led to recurring subluxations. The body's natural resistance is then overcome by the external forces. A rapid change ensues, which is too quick for the body to adapt to. B.J. writes:

> Hence an old and long existing subluxation with interferences returns to the picture in a certain percentage

According to B.J., this type of observation of subluxation pattern frequency, is only possible with good case records. He referred to cases recorded over a three-year period, which demonstrated that this recurrence of vertebral subluxation happened with the major subluxation 50% of the time. Over time, after the individual gets used to the new season, regular graph readings appear again. He writes:

> We do find that regular cases will show more interferences at seasonal transitional periods than at regular inter-seasonal periods; or they will show up more frequent and increased interferences at the dropped or rising sudden changes in temperature periods than at regular seasonal weather that spreads itself gradually over the calendar.

He surmised that the muscle contracture or relaxation depended on the type of temperature change, heat or cold.

The second article in the series was published in May 1934. It includes the essay, *When is a Vertebral Subluxation?* In the article, B.J. explains that prior to 1930, it was thought that daily and regular adjustments were required "for months, until the patient was well." By the fall of 1932, they thought the subluxation was there constantly until adjusted. The new definition included periodicity and frequency. He writes that subluxations "may be continuous periods or they may be broken up into fluctuating, intermittent or spasmodic spaces of time." B.J. also relates this to the theories of momentum and survival values. He writes:

> This much is certain: if the damaging effect of a continuous multiple and accumulative interference is present more of the time than Innate Intelligence is able to adapt normally to or is able to rebuild and correct, then there is an accumulative destructive survival value and dis-ease is on the growth. If adjustment is given and the vertebral subluxation remains absent to where the effect is a continuous multiple and accumulative restoration of Innate Intelligence mental impulse supply and is able to adapt and rebuild, then there is an accumulative constructive survival value. In either case, whether the case is growing better or worse, depends upon how much of the time the vertebral subluxation is present or absent, whether it be a minority or majority of the time, and whether the bad works faster per hour than the good can repair or balance per the same time involved.

This model of periodicity of dis-ease was a new way to integrate the latest subluxation models with the process of pathophysiology. "Subluxations rise and fall, in periodicity, in degrees, as regularly as do observed symptoms which are their effect." According to B.J., NCM makes it possible to track the irregularity of subluxation periodicity, which offered new insight into dis-ease periodicity. B.J. explained this in terms of the tone of tissue structure. He writes:

> Idea that ONCE A VERTEBRAL SUBLUXATION it exists 24 hours a day must now give way to newer observation that all which is necessary to reduce health of an individual is that it be more or less present more or less of time, which gradually decreases distance of time between, which decreases health time periods and increases disease time periods, effects of which increase in severity or in periods of time and reduce resistance of tone of tissue structure and thus introduce its opposite or dis-ease of tissue function.

Additionally, B.J. described the dual perspectives of the chiropractic paradigm, a focus on internal and external experiences. He says there are two laws of demand and supply, one internal and one external. As an example he writes:

> A man walks along the street. He slips, internally. He meets the sidewalk, externally. Here is an external and internal law of demand and supply. As a result, a concussion of forces, a shock; a demand internally which he cannot meet externally; or a demand externally which he cannot supply internally. The net result—a vertebral subluxation. As a result, we now get squarely into the question of the law of internal demand and supply, for existing between is the vertebral subluxation which forecloses the impossibility of the internal demand meeting the internal supply.

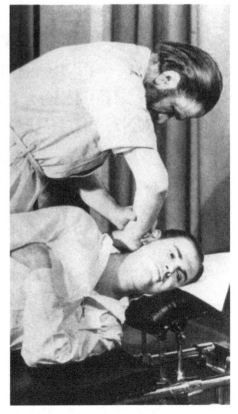

B.J. Palmer demonstrating toggle (1930s)

B.J.'s Palmer's Torqued Subluxation & Adjustment (1933)

In the August-September issue of the *Fountainhead News* in 1933, an ad reads:

Advertisement for *The Torqued Subluxation, The Torqued Adjustment* (1933)

B.J. Palmer's 30-page pamphlet published in 1933 was called *The Torqued Subluxation the Torque Adjustment.* At the start of the pamphlet, B.J. apologized for the promise of illustrations in the advertisement. He was just busy. In the time since that announcement he lectured in Colorado, California, Oklahoma, Missouri, Michigan, Indiana, and South Carolina. He crossed the continent twice in six weeks and planned, as of December, to complete the talk introduced at Lyceum in *Disciplining the Hour.*

The pamphlet was integrated into Vol. 18 in the following chapters: *The Exclusive Process of Deduction* (Chapter 5), *The Specific* (Chapter 6), *Locating the Specific* (Chapter 7), *Swanberg Denies Subluxation* (Chapter 8), *Why!* (Chapter 14), *Rules for Torqueing Adjustment* (Chapter 17), *The NCM More Important Now Than Before!* (Chapter 19), *"Uncanny" or Efficient* (Chapter 20), *A Miracle Happened During Pre-Lyceum Clinic Review Course* (Chapter 21), and *Axis Subluxations* (Chapter 29). The pamphlet was also reproduced as chapter 5 in Vol. 25, published in 1951, with some edits and commentary.

B.J. describes the growth of the HIO movement since 1930. By now, there were 5,000 successful documented cases in the field using "cervical major HIO adjustment alone." In this talk he explains why specific subluxations only occur in the upper three cervical vertebrae, with an emphasis on atlas and axis, and why a major is always a major.

The rationale for upper cervical involved vertebral structure, biomechanics, and spinal cord and spinal nerve distributions. The biomechanical emphasis focused on increased motion and torque found in the upper cervical spine. Torsion in three dimensions, twists the meninges and creates interference to the capacity of the spinal nerves and spinal cord to transmit mental impulses.

After the interference is determined with thermography, lateral and A-P spinographs were required. The x-ray analysis starts with the lateral view, and was designed to determine, which of the top three cervical vertebra were kinked, twisted, or torqued into a subluxation. A-P views are then taken to complete the interpretation. The vertebra causing the torque should be adjusted.

B.J. wrote that the dens was the reason why the upper three cervical vertebra were the cause of every dis-ease. He writes:

> Answer is simple: epistropheus, fovea dentalis or odontoid contains mystery as well as its solution. As many years as we have worked with, studied, adjusted spinal columns, we have

never realized mischief that is created in destruction of human health and life, as with this singular peculiarity that is not found connected with or between any other two vertebrae. As much as we have studied and researched spine, until recently none realized that this singular process on axis contained true solution to specific for restoration of all health to all organs of any human body.

After contemplating the completeness of the PSC osteological collection and the importance of malformations, he writes:

When it finally began to dawn into our consciousness that this odontoid process could be torqued in its position into and around in that spinal canal and that it was THE specific cause of ALL disease of the human body, we could hardly believe our conclusions.

The role of the odontoid process in spinal cord pressures was central to understanding the torqued subluxation and the torqued adjustment. Instructions for delivering the torqueing adjustments was included at the end of the pamphlet.

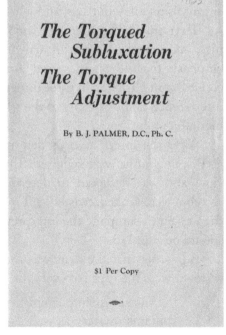

The Torqued Subluxation, The Torqued Adjustment cover (1933)

Chapter 11
The Research Textbooks: 1934-1938

Between 1934 and 1938, four new research-related Green Books were published as volumes 18-21 and the B.J. Palmer Chiropractic Research Clinic was opened. The books capture a unique moment in the history of chiropractic, when research and science were becoming integrated into the profession. There were many factors that pushed the profession to upgrade science teaching and research. The most significant forces were competition from other schools, economic leverage (such as advertising chiropractic as a science), the continual development of chiropractic technique and analysis, and confronting the medical lobby's new basic science laws, which were enacted in many states.

In 1935, B.J. Palmer published a pamphlet called *National Basic Science Data*. He writes:

> I have no quarrel with legitimate and honorable physicians and surgeons. They have their place and work to do. I do have a quarrel with the political physician and surgeon who, blames all professional failures on competitors and tries to cure that dis-ease by legislative elimination of competition; draws bills to operate on competitors, and if they die it was "the will of God."
>
> That's the set-up we are up against now.

Since the medical lobby was losing the battle against chiropractic in the courts and the legislatures, due to new licensing laws throughout the United States, basic science laws were crafted to keep chiropractors out of some states. In 1935, there were nine states with Basic Science laws. In those states, yearly chiropractic licenses dropped significantly. In some states licenses went to zero. The laws spread to dozens of states. All chiropractors seeking to be licensed in various states were required to take exams written by faculty at medical colleges. The last law was repealed in 1973. The profession dealt with this threat by upgrading basic science standards, conducting research, and working to overturn the laws.

The Green Books during this period mark a turning point for the PSC and the theory and research that it rested on. Previous books in the series up until this point were largely based on B.J. Palmer's first books, which were originally developed from his father's principles and practices. Vol. 18 and the research pamphlets are the foundation for all books in the series published after this period.

B.J.'s Subluxation Specific Adjustment Specific: Vol. 18 (1934)

Vol. 18 or *Subluxation Specific Adjustment Specific: An Exposition of the Cause of Dis-ease* was published in 1934. It was B.J. Palmer's first book in 14 years and it changed the course of chiropractic history. His last book was Vol. 13 (1920), the PSC technique manual, which was a collaboration with Vedder, Burich, and Firth. Prior to that, it had been more than 30 years since the publication of Vol. 6, in 1911, and the second edition of Vol. 2, in 1913. Vol. 18 was the first textbook update of B.J. Palmer's subluxation theories in 30 years. In the book, B.J. expands upon the new approach to upper cervical specific chiropractic.

In June 1934, B.J. ran the first advertisement for Vol 18. The advertisement noted that the cost of the book was ten dollars and it consisted of more than 1,000 pages, 480 illustrations, and 42 chapters. Delivery was set to begin at Lyceum. They already had 1,000 orders.

The 1934 Lyceum was expected to be the largest since the early 1920s. This was due to a drop in attendance after the Great Depression. In 1929 attendance was 1,200, in 1930 it was 1,956, in 1931 it was 3,035, in 1932 it was 2,776, and in 1933 it was 3,418. The growth of the PSC was fueled by B.J. Palmer. Now at age 52, he was

The Book You've Long Hoped For

The book you've hoped somebody would have the fearless courage to write.

The book that is full of intellectual surprises on every page.

The book that will make you mad—and glad.

A Chiropractic book written by the only Chiropractor who could write it.

A book you'll be proud to quote.

"The Subluxation Specific — The Adjustment Specific."

Now on the press. Ready for delivery Lyceum.

Almost 1,000 pages. 42 chapters. 480 pages, special drawings and fotos.

An author must write 49 books to write one. B.J. has written 49 others. This is his one!

Wm. P. Brownell, after reviewing the galleys, says: "This is the book of books."

This book presents and proves the existence of a SPECIFIC for the CAUSE of ALL dis-ease. It presents a SPECIFIC adjustment for the CAUSE of ALL dis-ease. Medical men have been seeking this for 5,000 years. It is revolutionary. It presents daring facts. It is going to be the most cussed and discussed, written about book in Chiropractic. Get it, read it first-hand and form your OWN conclusions. CHIROPRACTIC found THE SPECIFIC. It belongs TO Chiropractic. It is the prior art right OF CHIROPRACTORS.

Book sells for $10. First edition is limited. Over 1,000 orders already in and paid for.

Fountainhead News (June-July 1934)

entering another peak of his career. B.J. was determined to continually develop and grow chiropractic. The advertisement concludes:

> This book presents and proves the existence of a SPECIFIC for the CAUSE of ALL dis-ease. It presents a SPECIFIC adjustment for the CAUSE of ALL dis-ease. Medical men have been seeking this for 5,000 years. It is revolutionary. It presents daring fact. It is going to be the most cussed and discussed, written about book in Chiropractic. Get it, read it first-hand and form your OWN conclusions. CHIROPRACTIC found THE SPECIFIC. It belongs TO Chiropractic. It is the prior art right OF CHIROPRACTORS.

When the book came out in September 1934, it had 870 pages with 470 illustrations. An advertisement in May 1936 refers to it as "The Best Chiropractic Textbook Ever Written." The book was listed for $10.50, postage included.

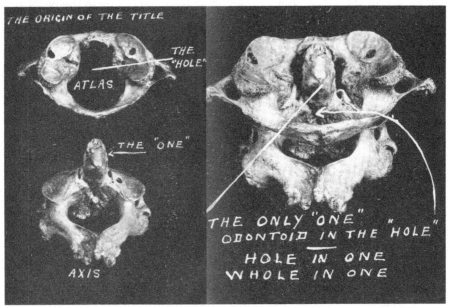

Illustrations from Vol. 18 (1934)

As a preface to the book, B.J. invites the reader to discard all previous "theories, beliefs, teachings, and practices." He also recommends that areas of the text that seem difficult to understand will become clear after first, letting it "lie passive in your mind," and then, reading the book two more times to allow for "mature reflection." He writes:

After you have given the book mature deliberation, if you wish to return to your old beliefs and ways of living, you are at perfect liberty to do so. But, for the time being, become as little children; for said the Master, "Except ye become as little children, ye can in no wise enter the kingdom of heaven."

The dedication in the book was written at Christmas of 1933. B.J. thanked Dossa Evins, inventor of the Neurocalometer in 1923. Evins died November 15, 1932. He also thanked his inner circle of faculty, the many loyal Palmer graduates, and lastly, his wife Mabel and son Dave. To the graduates he writes, "May Innate continue to bless their vision with understanding and encouragement to keep them keeping on."

The subluxation model developed in Vol. 18 was based on an expansion of the HIO technic being taught with the new emphasis on upper cervical. It also integrated some new findings by PSC graduate, A.A. Wernsing, who gave a monograph of his findings to B.J. on January 5, 1934, after Vol. 18 was already being laid out. B.J. acknowledged Wernsing in the book and told him personally that his ideas were being used. Years later Wernsing wrote that he did not feel his ideas were integrated correctly.

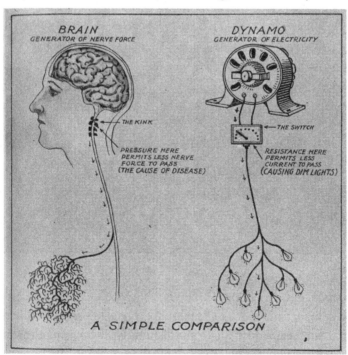

Illustrations from Vol. 18 (1934)

The method of analysis of Vol. 18 relied on spinographic evidence of Atlas laterality utilizing A-P open mouth views. Other instrumentation was developed alongside the NCM, to improve the detection of interference caused by vertebral subluxation.

Fountainhead News (May 1935)

B.J. Palmer referred to the "mental impulse supply" for the first time and also used a new phrase, "subtle mental impulse current." These additions to the terminology reflect a theoretical devel-opment fueled by B.J.'s research. This type of theory evolution would continue over the next two decades.

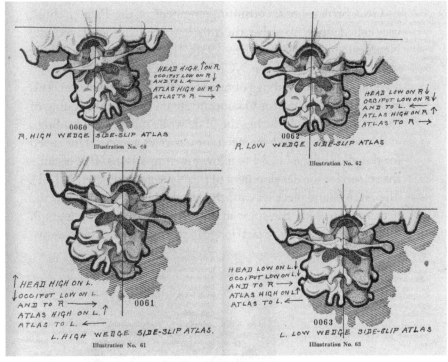

Illustrations from Vol. 18 (1934)

B.J. Palmer's The Known Man: Vol. 19 (1936)

Vol. 19 or *The Known Man or An Explanation of the "The Phenomena of Life" or Constants and Variables as Applied to Accuracy of The B.J. Palmer Chiropractic Clinical Procedure*, was the first official report from the new research being conducted at the B.J. Palmer Chiropractic Research Clinic. In his history of the PSC, Rolf Peters describes some of the technological innovations during the first years of the clinic's operation. Peters writes:

> B.J. Palmer established the B.J. Palmer Chiropractic Clinic on the ground floor of the classroom building on 15 August 1935. In trying to eliminate all variables, a new instrument needed to be developed, as using the Neurocalometer, watching the fluctuation of the needle, making a mental picture of it and then drawing by hand a graph introduced the element of human error.
>
> Otto Schiernbeck, consulting engineer of the Palmer clinic, was called upon to solve the problem, and he developed the Neurocalograph (NCGH) in 1936. The NCGH was a highly sensitive extension of the NCM, which recorded accurately on a graph sheet the readings obtained by the Neurocalometer. This allowed the chiropractor to concentrate on proper positioning of the NCM terminals during the glide while making the reading.
>
> He also recognized the need for a correct and constant speed for the glide of the NCM to allow for comparisons. This became the reason for the development of the Neurotempometer (NTM). The NCM hand piece was attached to the NTM, which drew the detectors up along the spine at a fixed speed, producing a graph reading of the same exact length in consecutive comparative readings.

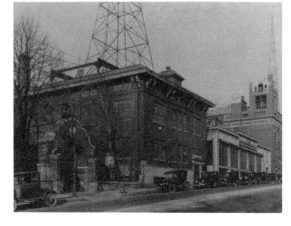

WOC radio towers
atop the PSC (1920s)

This equipment was used in a room that was completely screened with copper screening, while heavy iron plates surrounded the base of the room. This was designed to shut out all electrical and radio waves, as well as magnetic waves. A radio placed in this room would not pick up any transmissions, as all energy waves had been eliminated. The reason for this was that all known variables could be eliminated when taking a reading.

The research clinic was developed on the model of the Mayo Clinic. It was designed to help the worst cases. B.J. invited chiropractors to send their most difficult patients. The clinic staff completed a full analysis, cared for the patient for days or weeks at a time, and then sent them back to the referring office with a report. Many chiropractors sent their family members.

In an advertisement from April 1936, to pre-order Vol. 19, B.J. explains that the book was started just after the 1935 Lyceum. The B.J. Palmer Research Clinic officially opened two weeks before Lyceum. The advertisement reads:

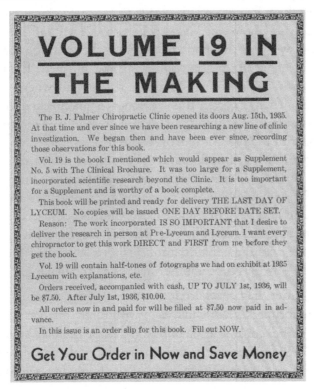

<figcaption>Fountainhead News (April 1935)</figcaption>

In the preface to Vol. 19, B.J. explains that the book was initially planned to be an article explaining why they built shielded and grounded booths to do NCM readings. The book expanded to explain why they were studying "by-products of mental impulse currents in the human body," and the importance of eliminating variables.

In concluding the preface he writes about his process of authoring books. These types of statements provide a first-person glimpse into the emergence of the final Green Books. B.J. writes:

> Books should be written only when something new need be said, or something old is stated in a new way; or some new and better service can be thus offered humanity. What is new or what can be better said must remain within the province of the thinking value of the one who writes the book. The interesting part about writing a book is that usually the author develops his methods or systems and then writes about them; or he writes about them as he develops those methods or systems. The aggravating part about developing methods and writing about them is that one idea leads to another as time enters his picture and he never knows when to cut off and print what he has written. This book has been in the writing over a year. The ideas we are writing about are not finished. The book is not ready to be printed. Shall we cut just anywhere, without rhyme or reason, even tho subjects are not finished, methods and systems are still in the making; or, shall we hold the book back until the present line of research is completed. Just about the time the neurocalograph was completed and in working order, we figured that the book was ready for press; but just then another new method or system was given birth and we started work on it. It of right should also be in this book because it was a clinical research problem we were solving. Before we get thru, we may hold the book up until this idea is finished, but—who knows—by that time another may be in the making.

The book itself had several references including an annotated bibliography in the form of 27 addenda, each with direct quotes. B.J. notes that while writing the book, Carrel published *Man the Unknown* and Crile published *The Phenomenon of Life*. Both books explored related topics so B.J. alluded to both titles with the title of the book. He quotes from both authors.

The Known Man includes twenty-one research tests and dozens of essays about the research. He writes, "We record human energies." To do this, they sought to eliminate all variables. Attempts were made to eliminate anything that might influence the energy of the human organism. It was reasoned that the NCM readings could be affected by various energy fields in the environment including radio waves, magnetic fields, and static electricity. For example, all wires connected to the instruments were grounded and patients were greeted by greeters wearing gloves and standing on rubber mats to ground the static electricity from the patient. He writes:

Book Volume 19 is Coming

This book will be out by Aug. 31st
Until July 1, 1936....Price $ 7.50
After July 1, 1936....Price $10.00

Containing new data, new information, new clinic facts. By many considered the best.

This is the booklet we mentioned in FHN of February. We intended then to bring it out as a Clinic Brochure Supplement. It is now coming out as A BOOK instead.

Many of you already have deposited your $7.50 for this book. Your orders will be filled first.

PLACE YOUR ORDER AT ONCE

Fountainhead News (April 1935)

> What matters it that instrument is grounded if patient and operator contain external variable and transfer them to instrument?

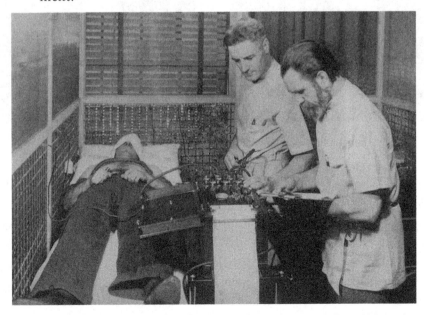

B.J. demonstrating Keeler polygraph in shielded grounded booth from Vol. 19 (1936)

B.J. and his staff were not only interested in pre and post checks for chiropractic care but the human energy system in general. For example, they conducted NCM readings inside and outside the shielded grounded booths on days when the atmosphere caused static. He writes, "We watched for 'radio static day... On static days, outside of booth, low average of number of break readings slightly increases." The radio speakers were mounted in the hallways. The powerful signal for WHO was broadcast from the radio tower on the roof. Of this phenomena B.J. writes:

> These are byproduct effects of external variables breaking thru skin insulation of atmospheric static electricity and backing into human receiving set, throwing NCM sensitive meter readings off usual constants established on regular days when static was absent.

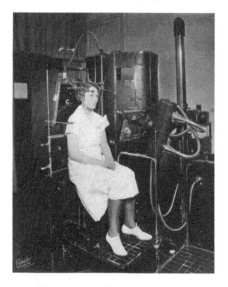 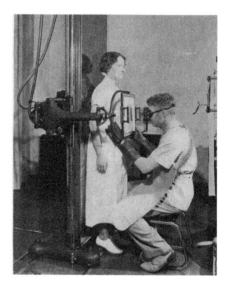

Illustrations demonstrating x-ray set up and procedure from Vol. 19 (1936)

B.J. developed a novel language describing the mental impulse based on his research in 1935 and 1936. For example, he wrote of "nerve impulse continuity," "mental impulse nerve-force flow," "nerve-force mental impulse supply," "mental impulse nerve-force constant," "intelligent human electrical current," "nerve current," "sensitive nerve force flow," "neuro-electrical mental impulse force," "health building mental impulse," "mental impulse health constant," and "mental impulse human electric nerve-force flow." From this new expansion of terminology, it is evident that B.J. Palmer was expanding his model of chiropractic.

B.J.'s Precise, Posture-Constant Spinograph: Vol. 20 (1938)

Vol. 20 was published in 1938. It was titled *Precise, Posture-Constant Spinograph, Comparative Graphs; An Exposition of Innate Natural Adaptation following HIO Adjustment Proving Measurement Correction of Vertebral Subluxations, Corrections of Abnormal Normal Adaptive Curves, as Well as Curvatures.* The book includes 100 cases with limited histories, images of spinographs, analysis of vertebral subluxation, and number of adjustments given. Most cases lasted two weeks because they were part of the "consultation service," which involved referrals from chiropractors in the field.

An advertisement for the book, published in March 1936, reads:

Announcing Volume 20

Contents of Vol. 20? That will be a REAL surprise. Take me on faith and believe me when I say it takes an entirely different angle on a new subject matter than any other book we have ever issued. It will contain about 800 two-color cuts produced at a cost of $5,400 alone. Book will cost around $8,000 to produce.

Vol. 20 is the type of book our profession has asked for for years. It will be THE FIRST of a new series. Upon ITS success depends whether others follow. Support THIS book and we will produce more covering different phases of vitally important evidence to prove CHIROPRACTIC DOES GET SICK PEOPLE WELL.

Every chiropractor has hoped, looked, longed for scientific, unimpeachable proof, that chiropractic does in practice what it claims in philosophy; that we practice what we preach and preach what we practice; we do what we advertise and advertise what we do. The advent of The B. J. Palmer Chiropractic Clinic, with its unequalled scientific laboratories and equipment, makes it possible to gather, assemble and disseminate just that. Vol. 20 will be THE FIRST book to answer those thousands of requests that have come to us for years. Its purpose is so gigantic that nobody else in our ranks would dare to attempt to produce it.

$7.50 until July 1, 1937. $10.00 AFTER July 1, 1937.

Rush checks pronto and we shall have the book ready for delivery BEFORE Lyceum, 1937.

Fountainhead News (March 1936)

Vol. 20 describes a cohort study designed to test the new procedures at the clinic to more fully understand the value of new protocols for the HIO system. The new protocols included new posture-constant patient placement for taking x-rays, as well as pre and post x-ray analysis, which included graphing any changes on the films. He writes:

One big objective, amongst others, attained in development of comparative graphs based on posture constant, is that it made it possible TO MEASURE subluxation distance and adjustment correction of malposition of a vertebra before and after adjustment; to measure curvature or adaptative curves distances and value of adjustment correction in correction of same as result of one adjustment, one place, as compared to another; which direction of adjustment corrected, which did not, etc. It was a research method of proving theories of "moves" which has worried our profession for many years. It permitted us to research scientific proof of long mooted medical prejudice that "chiropractors cannot move vertebrae by hand only", etc.

The book demonstrates the implementation of B.J. Palmer's new approach in practice. This included the emphasis on ensuring that all measures were as objective as possible.

The information collected at the clinic was comprehensive. Even though the intake included a history of symptoms and pathologies, these were not used in the analysis of vertebral subluxation. B.J. felt that vertebral subluxation could be located and corrected even without getting any information from the patient. He writes:

We could proceed along definite, positive, scientific lines, find information necessary to accurately and efficiently locate cause of his illness whatever or wherever it was, adjust it, observe and study his recovery, ascertain facts as to his progress and send him home well.

Many pages of the book include pre and post tracings of x-ray analysis. A running commentary across the footer of the text includes historical, philosophical, and theoretical prose. The commentary expands on the philosophy of chiropractic. B.J. concludes that the new objective approach to analysis was more scientific. He also ruminates on the similarities between scientific principles

Volume XX Shipped

On May 20, all orders on hand for Vol. XX were shipped. If anyone has placed an order with us and has not received his copy, communicate at once.

And this is a good time for those who have NOT ordered to do so. Order shipped day received. Price $10.50 prepaid, or $10.00 express collect.

Fountainhead News (June 1937)

and philosophical principles. He felt that by focusing on constancy in analysis, such as repeatable, verifiable procedures that would ensure the same outcome each time, then the practice of chiropractic would be congruent with a deeper level of constancy inherent to life itself. He viewed the life principle, the Innate Intelligence, as a constant force or pattern, which was inherent to the universe. A lengthy quote from the text captures this idea. He writes:

EACH human being is born into this world because of a consistent irresistible Intelligent Force, working according to a definite plan, designed to a definite pattern—all of which is constant.

Universal and Innate Intelligence are constants; the laws are constant, the purposes and designs are constants. They control earth, sea, sky, stars and planets, air, water, light and heat, by immutable constant control. The pattern from which man is made, the process of his make, his reproduction, is a constant. The life force in man, the by product of that force, such as skin, muscle, bone, is governed by a constant. Great and simple principles and practices are staid and sturdy and become monuments of lasting and permanent understanding which can never be destroyed—because they are constants. Why do we admire such men as Christ, Lincoln, Edison, Ford? Because of their constancy of thought and action.

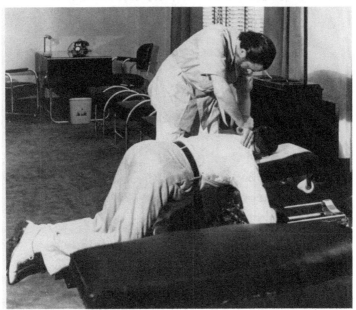

B.J. demonstrating Upper Cervical Toggle-Recoil Adjustment

Imagine what would happen to any of this if variables, with their ungovernable, irresponsible, and inconsistent ideas were to prevail. We don't admire or respect the wishy washy, undetermined, variable human beings who are gone with the North wind and come back with the South wind.

There is a constant underlying the Chiropractic principle and practice: subluxation, occlusion, pressure, and interference to mental impulse supply between brain and body; which slows down tissue cell activity; which, given time, creates disease; AND adjustment, opening occlusion, releasing pressure, restoring mental impulse supply between brain and body, which increases tissue cell activity; which, given time, recreates health. That constant is either right or wrong. If right, it is TOTALLY right. If wrong, it is TOTALLY wrong.

B.J. Palmer's either/or attitude towards the principles was amplified by his striving for objectivity through the use of scientific methods. Based on decades of clinical practice, he viewed the vertebral subluxation as incontrovertible fact. His research was designed to explore this phenomenon and perfect the techniques for practitioners to further master the principles and practice of chiropractic.

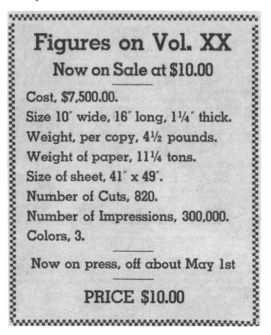

Figures on Vol. 20 *Fountainhead News*

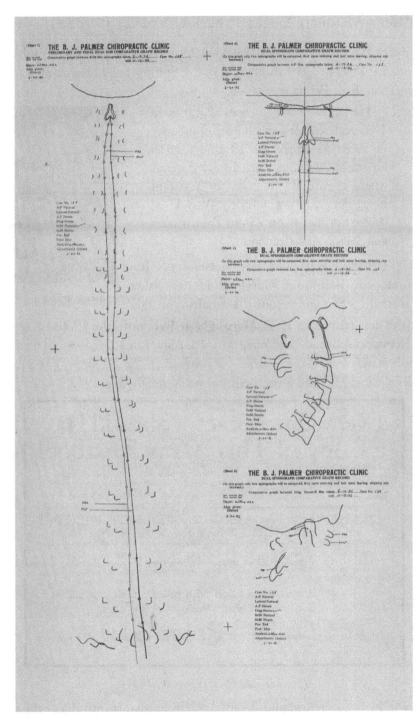

Illustration from Vol. 20 (1938)

Remier's Modern X-Ray Practice: Vol. 21 (1938)

Percy A. Remier was born on May 20, 1891 in Galesburg, Illinois. He enrolled at PSC in 1919 and taught in the Spinography Department upon graduation. Rolf Peters writes:

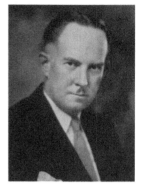

Percy Remier, DC

> He began his high school education in 1905 and became a machinist's apprentice in railroad shops in 1908. In 1910 he started work at Rock Island Arsenal, where eventually he rose to Assistant Foreman. During World War I he worked primarily on 75mm French guns and 3-inch American guns.

Remier left PSC in 1924 to start the Remier X-Ray Laboratory in Baltimore, Maryland. He was asked to return to PSC and rejoin the faculty and take over the department in 1932. He taught at PSC until the 1960s.

Remier published *The Chiropractic Stereoscope* in 1936. It was a 65-page pamphlet. *Modern X-ray Practice and Chiropractic Spinography*, Vol. 21, was published in 1938. The second edition was published in 1947.

Fountainhead News (February 1937)

Vol. 21 is a practical and detailed teaching text. It introduces the field of HIO to stereoscopic x-ray analysis. Remier writes:

Though this present volume carries the student of Chiropractic Spinography forward into the HIO Stereoscopic field it also dips back for clarity's sake into the old Meric period or regime so that this work will be found of value to all—no matter upon which step of Chiropractic progress they find themselves.

Vol. 21 includes begins with a history of x-ray and covers radiography theory and practice. The history includes the innovations initiated by B.J. Palmer in 1910 and the PSC x-ray lab in the 1930s.

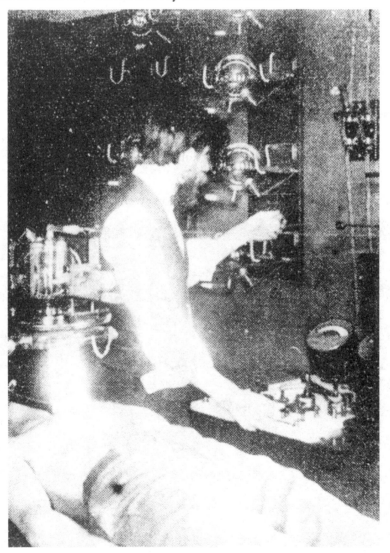

B.J. Palmer demonstrating X-ray technology (1910)

In his historical overview, Remier also wrote about the importance of HIO, which "became a working principle" in the fall 1930. He writes:

> With the advent of Hole-In-One came the demand made for Spinographic views taken before an adjustment with subluxation and after an adjustment without subluxation and then with the intermediate check sets of Spinographs so it became necessary to have a posture, as near constant as possible, which was fundamental and have all Spinographic sets of the same person taken exactly alike.

Stereoscopic views were developed in the spring of 1934, which led to 12-months of research to determine the best way of regarding atlas rotation. They determined three-dimensional images were necessary to visualize atlas. This led to increasing the x-ray facility in the new clinic. Remier writes:

> After many months of scientific research and experimental work... we did produce sufficient depth on our HIO pictures to bring out the third dimension.

He concluded that 65% of atlas subluxations were due to rotation.

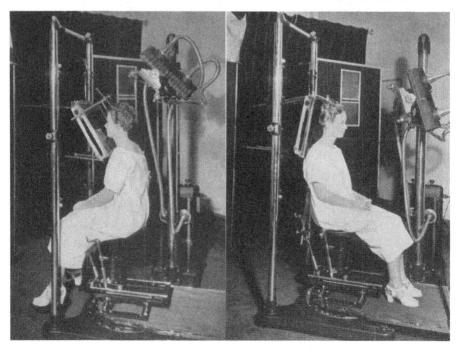

Vertex Stereo and Nasium—AP View from Vol. 21 (1938)

Remier designed much of the x-ray equipment so that the patient's posture would remain constant no matter which radiographers took the views. Rolf Peters includes a history of the PSC x-ray department in his *Early History of Chiropractic.* Of the Remier years Peters writes:

> His background as a machinist and tool-maker was of great benefit in the years to come, both for the commercial spinography department.

The clinic included x-ray equipment that he custom designed.

According to Remier, by 1935, atlas rotation was established. Base posterior views were developed in 1936. Also in 1936, the clinic took 18" by 36" stereo films, which required newly designed stereo-reading boxes to view the films. By 1937 the vertex x-ray procedures were in practice.

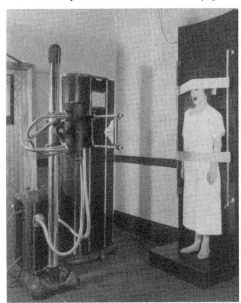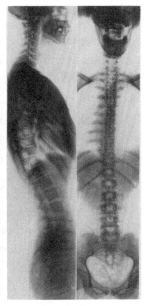

Full spine Anterior-Posterior X-ray set up & Lateral/AP films from Vol. 21 (1938)

Vertebral Subluxation was defined in the book from an "HIO point of view." Remier writes:

> Subluxation (Vertebral)—(HIO point of view) a misalign-ment of Atlas and Axis, Atlas relative to occiput, Axis relative to 3rd cervical. Therefore at least four directions are involved: Anteriority, Superiority or Inferiority, Laterality, and rotation of Atlas; Posterior-Inferiority, lateral tipping, laterality, and rotation of Axis.

Throughout the text, Remier implores chiropractors to use spinographs so that they might improve their service and become more thorough. This included no longer relying on palpation to determine misalignments.

In the conclusion, Remier describes the chiropractic perspective and Innate theory. He writes:

> Is it not definitely understood that Innate Intelligence always labors towards a normal position? Is it not true that one could work against Innate in the adjustment given by failing to pattern the adjustment to the misalignment even though the adjustment were given in accordance to the general listing which might be correct, but for lack of X-ray visualization would not contain the necessary quality of adjusting in just the opposite direction to the misalignment, considering all its directional values?

He concludes that the doctor's self-care is paramount with an emphasis on x-ray protective equipment. Keeping abreast of the latest science and research is vital. To adequately capture this sentiment, an extended quote is warranted. Remier writes:

> Health of the professional—How often do we observe that the very person who is caring for the patient's health is himself in a very poor physical state. No doubt this is due to neglect on his part to provide for himself that same service which he claims to be beneficial to others. Could there be anything more incongruous than the spectacle of an obviously sick man attending to the health needs of others? This is worth more than just a passing thought. Remarks have been made that such remedy was difficult because of unavailability of Chiropractic service, but difficult or not it can be and should be looked after.
>
> Perhaps one of the chief things that impairs the health of the X-ray technician today who is usually the Chiropractor, is the fact that he does not exercise the necessary care and precaution in securing full protection from the X-rays. It is not theory but fact that an overdose of such radiation leads to ill health of many kinds.
>
> It then behooves him to watch his own health and apply ample protection not only for himself but his assistants and any others who might be subjected to dangers from this insidious cause. The Chiropractor owes it to himself, to his patients, and

to Chiropractic to do all in his power to keep himself fit and in a healthy condition and to be himself a sound, walking, and living proponent of his profession.

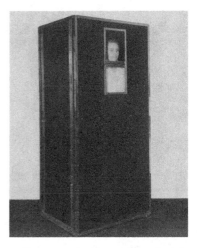

Chiropractic is always on trial. It seems to the author that it is the duty of everyone connected with this great science to make its continued presentation to the people of this and every other country where it is practiced, an example of efficiency, sound logical thought, justified claims, and established results. This can only be done by constant thought and experi-

Operators lead protection booth from Vol. 21 (1938)

mentation, by keeping abreast of the times in all channels of research, and making all the avenues of approach by the public, point to success in the art of Chiropractic in getting sick people well.

By your acceptance of this work which has been conscientiously aimed at establishing a keener perception of one of the essentials of the science; by reading it carefully with much study, and if possible, adopting the already tried principles which have been presented, you will be assisting in the march forward from the days when Chiropractic was a theory which worked rather, than a science which it is slowly but steadily proving itself to be.

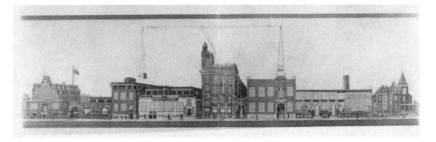

The Palmer School of Chiropractic (1920s)

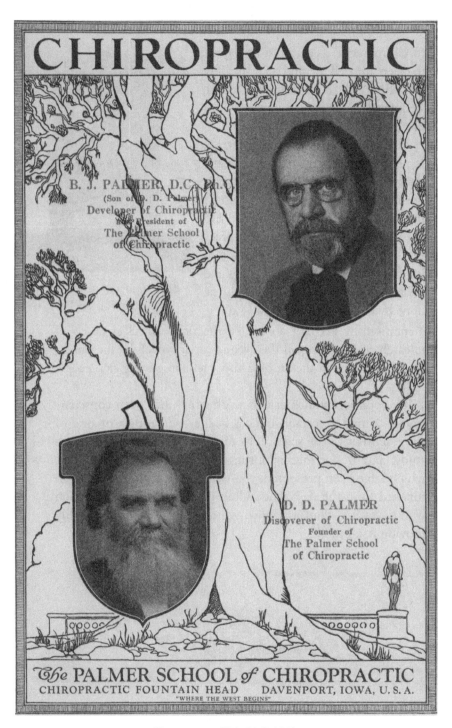

Frontispiece Vol. 20 (1938)

Chapter 12
B.J. Palmer's Tomes: Volumes 22-29

Between 1949 and 1953, B.J. Palmer completed eight large books, or tomes. The total page count of the books is 6,669. The smallest of the books was Vol. 24 with 715 pages. The tomes were written in the years after B.J. Palmer stopped running the Research Clinic full-time and his wife, Mabel, dying in 1949. He started spending winters in Sarasota, Florida, in 1950. He bought a home in Sarasota on Armand Key, an island on the Southwest coast of Florida, in 1951.

According to his nephew, W. Heath Quigley, B.J. confronted several health challenges in the early 1950s, including a sometimes painful ulcer and an enlarged prostate that required surgery due to a congenital anomaly blocking the ureter. B.J. also had a surgical intervention in the summer of 1953, whereby the pyloric opening was virtually "non-existent," due to scarring. This led to a disastrous attempt at a barium x-ray study. The barium did not make it to the stomach and heroic efforts were needed to dislodge it. After this traumatic event, B.J. would not consent to surgery until talking with two of his inner circle, Herbert Hender and Ralph Evans. Quigley writes:

> For the past two weeks Ralph and B.J. had been angry with each other and were not speaking. B.J. had wanted to publish another book, Ralph insisted the School could not afford it. But Ralph did not hesitate to come with Herb immediately when told of B.J.'s condition, and his need to talk this over with what he called his "team." In the end B.J. decided he had no choice, so he agreed to go into the hospital the following morning.

The only book published in 1953, the year of the argument between B.J. and his team, was Vol. 29, B.J.'s eighth book in four years, and his longest. It was over 1,000 pages in length.

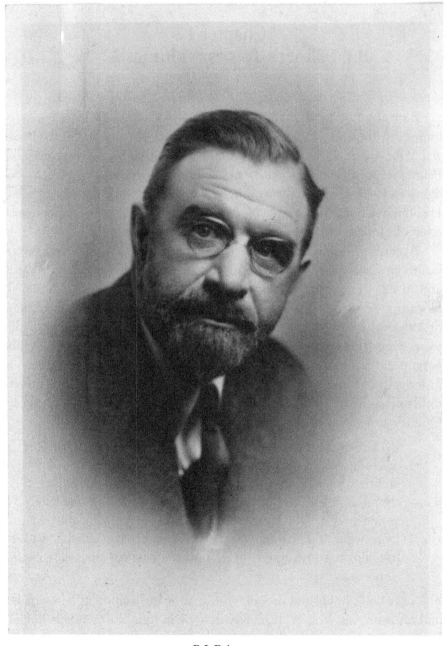

These books are a combination of articles, correspondence, republished talks and pamphlets, autobiography, historical accounts of chiropractic; but most of all, new refinements of his philosophy and theory.

B.J. Palmer

To understand B.J.'s voluminous output, with his custom-made typewriter, we should look to the prologue of Vol. 22, the first book in the new series. The prologue is lengthy, but worth quoting in full as it captures the process of how the final 16 Green Books emerged. The prologue was written by Herb Hender, one of B.J.'s team for over 27 "rich and happy" years. He writes:

He almost always carries his faithful Corona with him. When in a train bedroom or drawing room, out comes the note pad, jotting down notes. Later, out comes his typewriter, when he fills in the notes.

When he begins to look out a window or grows quiet, he wants to be let alone until he has studied what he is going to say and write. I have known him to write and rewrite a particular sentence or paragraph as many as twenty times, until it was whipped into language which expressed his idea. I have heard him say: "Give us thirty days and we'll write a book. Give us three months, and we'll write a paragraph. Give us a year, and we'll write an epigram."

Once finished, he would read it to me or some other critic, get reactions to see if we grasped what he was trying to say. If we did, he was finished. If we did not, he started over again.

I once asked B.J. how he wrote his lectures. His answer was characteristic. "We don't write them, we build them." I asked him to describe the process from time he began a lecture until finished, thinking that might be of interest and help others to duplicate his method. Here is his description:

We deliberate and mentally carve out our fundamental theme around which we desire to build the talk. It might be a new thought, or it could be a symposium of preceding ideas. We then mentally test it for logic and reason to see if it will stand up under the test of time. If it does, we go ahead. If it does not, we whip it until it does. Having given an idea birth, we then begin to shape our approach. Conception of a theme is the hardest part we have to go through.

We then write whatever comes, as it comes, be it good or bad. We keep writing as long as thoughts flow, and they always flow without effort. We may knock out some, much, or all of it later. Much of this may be out of sequence. We keep on until the present line of thinking is exhausted. Then we let it simmer and settle for an hour, hours, days, or weeks. Usually, when building a lecture, it is more or less steadily on our minds, and we are constantly harassed by Innate to keep on keeping on whipping it into shape. Usually, in a few days or a week or two, it is finished for the time being.

Soon a new line of thinking may begin to flow, and away goes the typewriter again. We frequently rewrite our copy the second or third time before we get it to say exactly what we mean, before turning it over to our lecture secretary. When the subject has seemingly been completed, we turn it over to the secretary who types it on regular size sheets, double spaced, each paragraph on a separate sheet, each page numbered separately. We then take these and rearrange them for sequence of thought. Page 1 may be moved to page 6; or page 9 may be page 1, etc.

We continue the study of our subject from time to time, adding copy, marking it "Insert 1, page?" Our secretary then rewrites those pages with inserts. We then go over the copy once more, transpose one sentence from here to there, constantly briefing, cutting out superfluous words or duplicate thoughts, possibly eliminating entire sentences or paragraphs foreign to the central theme.

From time to time, during intervals between working on a certain lecture, we might be found reading, or checking on gold fish in pools of Clinic Gardens or aquaria in Clinic, or doing any one of a hundred other things here, there, or everywhere, during which one or a series of new ideas may flash. We hesitate, then and there, and make notes. This is kept up for days or weeks, at times getting so many inserts that it looks like a crazy-quilt patch job. We then have the lecture completely rewritten, inserting at proper places all late inserts; then by reading it entire we can see how it sounds or listens. Additional inserts continue until we feel the subject has been fully covered. We then lay it away to settle.

When it is finished, we have the secretary copy it once more, double-spaced, on loose leaf form for filing in one of the 150 volumes of lecture outlines, each of which is numbered. This lecture, under its title, is indexed in the Index Volume for quick selection at any time. Every lecture we have ever given, from away back when, is builded around an outline and is filed as mentioned for future reference. This makes it possible to repeat most any lecture on most every subject on short notice. Instead of beginning a new outline, we have one ready builded.

Even then, days or weeks later, a new train of contributory thought may come. When it does, we write them in notes, be it at night in bed or at some other activity, then fill them in on typewriter, revise and rewrite until they represent new thoughts, rewriting pages into which they fit or overlap. If these inserts are of sufficient number to justify, we have all pages of the lecture outline renumbered so they follow each other. This prevents any getting out of order or misplaced. Often this process of renumbering pages may be done three or four times. "Keeping in mind the various topics we have lectured on and have outlines for, we often go back to one of years ago and add something. The listener hears in one hour the labor of possibly hundreds of hours.

Often the comment has been made, 'What a brilliant man. His talks are marvelous. I could listen to him all day.' Little does the listener realize that the talk he listens to is not the product of the hour during its deliverance. It is the product of weeks, months, years in advance, even though he hears it all within one hour.

Every time a lecture is delivered, we see a part or parts which can be strengthened, others may be deleted. No lecture is ever finished. One talk (Selling Yourself) has been delivered more than 5,000 times over the world before all kinds of audiences, cutting and fitting it to suit. It isn't finished yet!

We have funeral orations, sermons from pulpits of churches. We have conducted schools on radio, Chiropractic, legislation, salesmanship, caves, migrations of races, national and international conventions in many foreign countries. In fact, the list is endless.

Criticism has been directed to the voluminousness of our talks. In writing, we endeavor to present a complete presentation, leaving no loop-holes. By presenting every fact, it cannot success-fully be attacked.

Altogether, one lecture may represent scores or hundreds of hours from time of conception to laying it away to rest. That's the process we use in building a lecture.

B.J. Palmer's Bigness of the Fellow Within: Vol. 22 (1949)

In 1949, at age 67, B.J. Palmer published a more personalized version of his Innate philosophy. He used his own life story as a rhetorical device to teach a deeper level of the philosophy and to share the history, principles, theory, and practice of chiropractic. According to Hender, B.J. viewed Innate as a "practical workable personality; something tangible to help man get well," not a vague theory.

Hender also notes that they were in the process of breaking down the "mass of data" from 14 years of research into medical and Chiropractic statistics to "prove the efficacy of Chiropractic adjustment to get cases well which medical men said could not be done." Medical research from

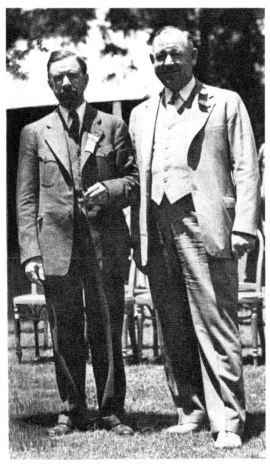

B.J. Palmer with Jim Drain, 1911 PSC graduate
and president of Texas Chiropractic College (1949)

that era did not utilize modern research design. The research from the B.J. Palmer Research Clinic was not very different than other clinical research from that period.

Vol 22 is probably B.J.'s most recognized book besides Vol. 18. *The Bigness of the Fellow Within* is a book of essays, vignettes, stories, and pictures. It also has long quotes from various magazine and newspaper articles. Philosophy, history, and theory are strewn throughout the 177 chapters.

B.J.'s unique writing style was to make his point clear. That was more important to him than accuracy of historical facts or whether every word was written by him or not. The best example of this is Chapter One, *The Story of That Something*, which was an adaptation of a story originally written in 1915 by W.W. Woodbridge. It was originally published by the Rotary Club, so it may have been well known. However, B.J. did not put Woodbridge's name on the chapter. This is not the only time B.J. Palmer used sources without attribution, such as various epigrams and also Greggerson's passage about the subtle substance of the soul, reproduced as Chapter 11. This was either flagrant plagiarism or a postmodern literary style. All indications point to the latter.

The chapters in Vol. 22 could be viewed in four parts. The first part is comprised of chapters 1-60. Those are the Innate chapters. Each one builds on the next. Some are written in a Socratic questioning style. All of the chapters capture B.J. Palmer's viewpoint on the Innate philosophy after living it for five decades.

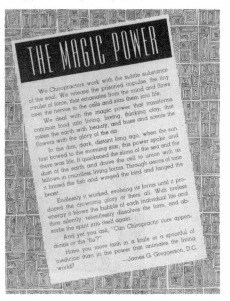

The Chiropractor (1959)

The second part is the stories. These comprise chapters 61-132. Many of the stories are autobiographical and fanciful. Some are just tales of travel and descriptions of the many statues and things in the clinic gardens from around the world. Several chapters explore the circus and circus wagons.

The third part is a combination of old pamphlets such as *Phallic Worship*, *It is as Simple as That*, and various explanations of philosophical questions related to chiropractic.

The fourth part is a 200-page book from 1915 called *With Malice Aforethought*. It contains the affidavits and court cases against B.J. Palmer from 1910 to 1913. The main focus is the accusation that he hit D.D. Palmer with an automobile during a parade, which indirectly led to his father's death. Two grand juries were called. Also, B.J.'s stepmother filed a civil suit seeking $50,000. The chiropractors and lawyers involved in the prosecution were all associated with rival chiropractic schools. All charges were dismissed and there was never an indictment. The grand jury found "No Bill." B.J. published it again in the 1940s in response to a book published in 1944 called *Medical Mussolini*. The book included a chapter that was critical of B.J.

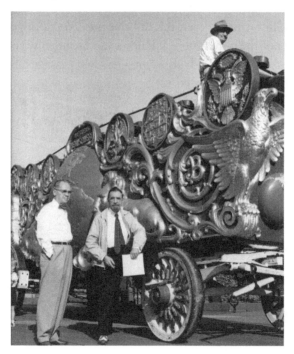

B.J. Palmer and Vern Link with Two Hemispheres Circus Bandwagon

The essence of Vol. 22 is an exploration of the relationship bet-ween Innate and Educated. However, B.J. does not emphasize the way "Innate" is generally described by chiropractors in the 21st century, as a self-organizing and self-healing deep structure of the living organism. Instead, he is expounding on the interior source of wisdom that informs the conscious thinking body/mind. This was always an important part of B.J. Palmer's philosophy, only now he is finally writing about it exclusively.

B.J. spent a lifetime researching, contemplating, and living the Innate philosophy given to him by his father. D.D. Palmer considered that Educated was born from Innate through the course of life. It accumulates experiences while Innate already knows all it needs to know because it is part of the source of Intelligence itself, the fabric of the universe.

B.J.'s viewpoint on Educated Intelligence was that it could hinder one's ability to heed the wisdom of Innate. When that happens, then one becomes "uneducated, sub-conscious, non-conscious, and un-conscious." By allowing Educated to be guided by Innate, one is able to access their inner greatness.

B.J. Palmer's thoughts on this topic were ahead of his time. He was writing about these concepts a decade before Maslow started writing about the levels of being and self-actualization. The Association for Humanistic Psychology (AHP), which was based on exploring the higher reaches of human personality, was formed in 1964. Critics of B.J.'s philosophy of Innate, sometimes use terms like egotistical and yet they never seem to cite the literature from Humanistic psychology or ego development. In many ways, B.J. was leading the culture but only a few people were reading his books. B.J. explicitly included the embodied psycho-spiritual aspects of being human in his later philosophy.

He viewed the relationship between Educated and Innate in the same way that he viewed the relationship between the body and Innate. Innate communicated to both. Also, interference to the expression of Innate could affect both body and mind. He writes:

> If there were no interferences, he might want to express himself; but were he to deliberately refuse to permit the opportunity to take advantage to come forth, all "genius" would be lost.

B.J. viewed the Educated part of consciousness as artificial, built upon the Innate, which was its original source. Interference to Innate's expression due to vertebral subluxation could lead to the Educated brain becoming abnormal.

Always central to this philosophical approach is the role of vertebral subluxation. B.J. viewed it as a limitation of matter, a cause of diminished quantity flow, reduced function, and a producer of dis-ease. He writes:

> The vertebral subluxation occludes, reduces, or makes smaller size of openings between vertebrae through which nerves pass on their way from brain to portion of the human body.

—which compresses, squeezes, or produces constrictive pressure around spinal cord or spinal nerves which pass through these openings between vertebrae on their way from brain to portions of the human body;

—which offers resistance to, or introduces interference to normal quantity of nerve force, or nerve energy flow, which flows through, over, or into these nerves on their way from brain to body;

—which reduction in quantity flow, from normal, does not reach the periphery, or distal, or endings of those nerves in body tissue cells or body organs;

—which reduction, from normal quantity, slows action of these body tissue cells or body organs in exact ratio as normal quantity is lowered to an abnormal level;

—which decreases the quantity and quality these tissue cells or body organs should produce as products or by-products;

—which, given time for destruction, to accumulate, develop and grow these effects, is a condition called disease.

The book also includes clarifications on various theories that date back to the earliest days of chiropractic. For example, in the case of dis-ease, which D.D. Palmer coined in 1887, B.J. writes:

"Dis-ease" is one condition, not many things.

"Disease," to a physician, is many things. It is not always the same thing to differing physicians observing the same case.

"Dis-ease," to a Chiropractor, is "not-at-ease"—a contrast between "ease" in brain energy quantities and lowered "not-at-ease" quantities of energy in an organ of the body.

"Dis-ease," to a Chiropractor, is one condition.

These types of explanations are consistent throughout the text. They reflect the early chiropractic paradigm but also the updated viewpoints inspired by years of research and theory development. It is also important to define the terms in context because incorrect definitions from the chiropractic paradigm have been published in the literature.

Some of his newer theories about Innate like *How the Law Works* and *How to Contact Innate*, involve things like telepathy, synchronicity, and flow states. B.J. explores these topics in more detail in his final books.

B.J. Palmer's Up From Below the Bottom: Vol. 23 (1950)

Vol. 23 or *Up From Below the Bottom* was published in 1950. Many of the chapters from Vol. 23 were republished talks and pamphlets. B.J. did not always let the reader know, these were old pamphlets reprinted as chapters. Some of the pamphlets in Vol. 23 are as follows: *Death Our Attitude Towards It* (1917), *Selling Yourself* (1921), *Reincarnation* (1911), *Education, Knowledge, Wisdom* (1916), *After Tomorrow What?* (1919), *Is Chiropractic?* (1915), *Everybody, A Play in 3 Acts* (1917), *The Value of Chiropractic* (1915), and *The Unwritten Law of Chiropractic* (1917) Recall, in the second edition of Vol. 2, published in 1913, B.J. wrote that many books were being written that will be published in the future, when the world is ready.

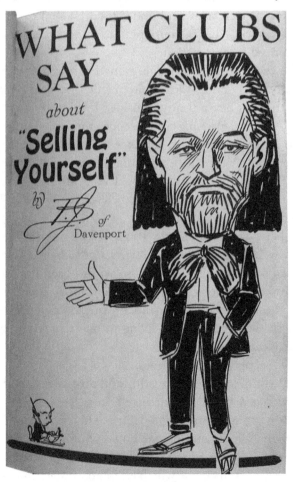

Advertisement for *Selling Yourself*

At the start of Vol. 23, B.J. expands on his rationale for using the pronoun "We," rather than "I." He made a similar statement at the start of Vol. 22, and does so in many of the volumes from this era. It is the statement of "We." This is another indication that using terms like "egotistical" to describe B.J. Palmer's philosophy is misguided. It seems that at some point between 1938 (Vol. 20) and 1949 (Vol. 22), B.J. had what could only be described as a profound transformational experience of self. *The Dead Still Live* in Vol. 37 explains what happened. After decades of living by heeding the inner promptings of Innate and being rewarded by success, synchronicity, and a life that was extraordinary, he stopped referring to himself as "I." Here is the Foreword to Vol. 23:

> At the beginning, we anticipate this subject, as presented, will be taken at face value and understood by some, even many of our profession. Many, in our opinion, possess preconceived ideas which need reconstruction.
>
> We record our knowledge, gained through research, of the fundamentals upon which Chiropractic rests as promulgated by our father but never clearly explained by him. By careful reading of his writings, gleanings of these ideas are apparent.
>
> To be consistent with the objective of this book, these are written with WE and US in mind. Ordinarily, "we" and "us" imply and are understood to be TWO different and separate persons. Ordinarily, "I" implies ONE fellow who lives in a material body and runs it.
>
> Whenever and wherever "I" is used, we refer to the educated fellow who thinks, speaks and writes for himself alone as one of the two fellows he is. He does so within the limitations of his education. This book, so far as the author is concerned, writes from the duality of personalities—the inseparable, indivisible, Siamese-twin personalities living in one structure—the Innate and Educated individualities.
>
> WE serves several purposes:
>
> 1. It eliminates that disgusting and egotistical selfish pronoun "I" which constantly intrudes itself.
>
> 2. It permits the author to delineate his concept of the duality of personalities inhabiting one human home.
>
> 3. It broadly includes and spreads credit where credit is due, to any, every, and all people who have or are cooperating in building

the structures, organizations, institutions, and associations which are an integral part of their lives.

It will be difficult for the reader, as he reads "we", to think "we" because he will constantly interpret it into ordinary channels of thot of TWO different and separate people. To read this book and gain viewpoint of its author, reader must know "we" or HE will fail to gain the fundamental purpose of this book.

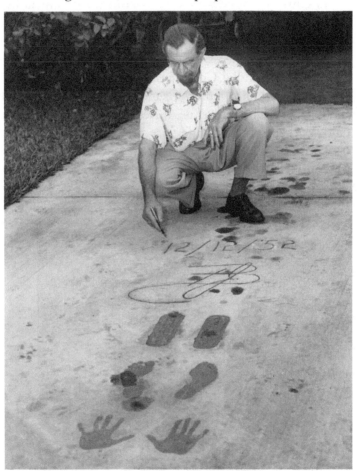

B.J. Palmer, Sarasota, Florida (December 12, 1952)

B.J. repeated this foreword in Vols. 23-28. He wrote a new version for Vol. 29 because he had to retype an entire manuscript from 1933 to change every pronoun. From this point forward, B.J. only referred to himself as "We." His students were profoundly affected by this. Through his use of language he established a culture based on this philosophical perspective and born of the chiropractic paradigm. In his final years, B.J. mentions semantics and being "wordbound" in trying to describe the integration of Educated Intelligence, Innate Intelligence, and Universal Intelligence.

Vol. 23 tackles topics like genius, religion, and God. He took on a similar approach as D.D. Palmer did, by viewing the God of all religions as one. B.J. writes:

> As Chiropractors, we recognize our duty to be adjusters of the CAUSE of sickness, drunkenness, and poorness. We have connecting link between God and man—that knowledge of cause supplies necessity. Look to every religion. Laws of Mohammed, Buddha, Confucius, Good Spirit of Indians, Pope of Roman Catholic Church, Czar of Greek Orthodox Church, and Christ of Christian era—universal recognition of universal God. We recognize no difference between because all look at same thing and same world thru a present or once mortal man. Mohammed, Buddha, Confucius, Pope, Czar, and Christ are all people who lived or are living.

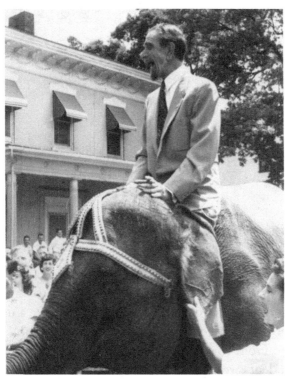

B.J. Palmer smiling on elephant

B.J. also contrasted religion, the chiropractic standpoint, in relation to the medical viewpoint. He continues:

> We watch trees and men anywhere and ALL grow according to God-like laws. Each man interprets this differently, and interpretation takes a different name, and he is different religiously. After all, it is a repetition of what has gone before, except that now we assume different men came to save us than existed before. What have any blank repeaters added to onward movement of world? Where have they added anything more than necessity and church? Have they added a cause? No—they leave that for the doctor; it is within his province. Inasmuch as God made the world, it seems hard to draw lines between what was and what was not. Minister should be minister and doctor at same time, as olden priests were. Chiropractor adds third or unknown quantity—the cause. By so doing, he re-establishes religions from another viewpoint. Much that has gone before will cease; theory will be replaced by facts; superstition will be replaced by art and science, and much howling and praying will be replaced by reasonable philosophy.

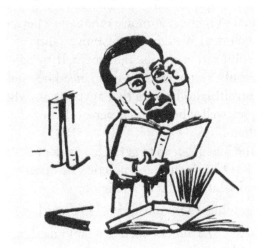

B.J. with Green Book line drawing by Peet (Vol. 23)

Vol. 23 was illustrated with cartoons and diagrams drawn by 1951 PSC graduate Helen Killeen Peet, DC. (Peet was the daughter of a 1913 PSC graduate, J.J. Killeen, the mother of four chiropractors, and grandmother of one chiropractor.)

B.J. Palmer's Fight To Climb: Vol. 24 (1950)

Vol. 24 or *Fight to Climb* was published in 1950. The book includes several classic pamphlets such as *Induction vs. Deduction* (1915), *My Message Analyzed* (1915) and his major address from 1931, *The Hour Has Arrived*. The book is also filled with random interesting stories, much like the stories from Vol. 22. *Fight to Climb* also includes essays on *Chiropractic and Religion*, *The Specific*, as well as historical anecdotes about Thomas Storey and more than 40 pages about the life of D.D. Palmer. The book also includes 322 questions and answers.

The historical elements of the book are fascinating. For example, B.J. writes:

> D. D. Palmer followed no sect, creed, or denomination. If he leaned to any, it was to principle of spiritualism, and then only to its religious aspect. Did he ever intend to make a religion out of Chiropractic? That depends upon what constitutes a religion. If, by "religion" is meant setting up one particular savior of souls of mankind, such as Christ, then this was not his idea of his service to sick mankind. If, by religion, is meant establishment of a church, of a one-day-of-the-week Sunday, with a ritual of hymns, sermons, robes, preachers, etc., this also was repugnant to his concept of universality of Chiropractic vertebral subluxation and its adjustment. If, by religion, is meant that sins, souls, saviors, to save them, need be established, then that was revolting to his idea that anybody anywhere could get sick and get well whether sick person believed in any, all, or none of them.

> After the "devil" began to get in his work of destroying broad aspect of D.D.'s principle and practice, he often expressed wish that he had established it as a religion.

B.J.'s autobiographical accounts in Vol. 23 are priceless. He writes:

> In 1902, D. D. Palmer issued us a diploma signed by himself, his wife, and ourself.

> We practiced Chiropractic since we were seventeen, calling ourself "Doctor". That was the why and wherefore of mustache and beard—to appear older than our years. We thot we could disguise youth because sick people did not want to go to a boy with a new idea they knew nothing about.

He continues,

> We practiced in those early years in Lake City, Iowa; Traverse City and Manistique, Michigan; Elkins, Belington, and Kernes, West Virginia, etc.

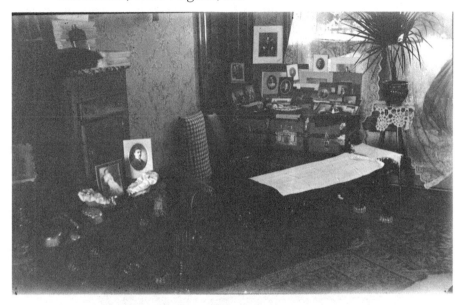

B.J. Palmer's office in Minnesota (1902) - from *The Chiropractor's Protégé*

Several interesting philosophical points are strewn throughout the text, such as an update from D.D. Palmer's original idea of too much or not enough function. B.J. writes, "There is only ONE dis-ease—the minus. There is ONE normal-abnormal adaptation to this minus—the plus." B.J. usually emphasized the reduction of impulses related to vertebral subluxation.

Vol. 24 includes detailed autobiographical accounts. For example, B.J. tells a story of how he traveled with a stage hypnotist named Herbert L. Flint. B.J. was around eighteen years old. From Flint, B.J. learned to go into hypnotic trance states at an early age. According to B.J., learning the skills of "self-hypnosis," was "THE TURNING POINT OF OUR CAREER." He learned to train his mind and access sources of inspiration and intuition. He writes, "THAT laid a solid foundation upon which rest of our life has been molded." The writings in his final books include details, instructions, and methods about his insights from decades of learning to listen to Innate as a guide in life.

B.J. Palmer's Clinical Controlled Research: Vol. 25 (1951)

Vol. 25 or *Chiropractic Clinical Controlled Research* was published in 1951. It is one of B.J. Palmer's most iconic books. Vol. 25 is set apart from every other Green Book because of its chronicle of 14 years of research at the B.J. Palmer Clinic. The book has six chapters. Chapter 1 covers the research at the clinic. It is titled *Researching the Unknown Man*. The other five chapters were reproductions of important research pamphlets such as *Crowding the Hour* (Chapter 2), *Electroencephaloneuromentimpograph* (Chapter 3), *Disciplining the Hour* (Chapter 4), *Torqued Subluxation—The Torque Adjustment* (Chapter 5), and *Publication Statistics* (Chapter 6). The topic of Chapter 2, on the timpograph, was also discussed throughout the text.

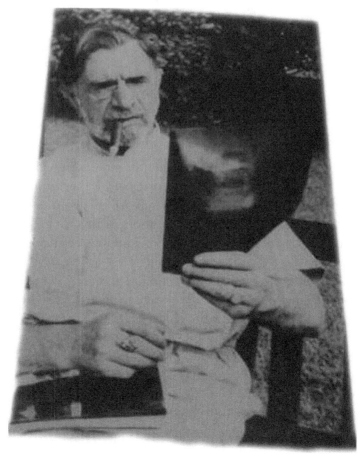

B.J. Palmer analyzing upper cervical X-ray

Chapter One comprised the bulk of the book, 476 of the 744 pages. It was a follow up to Vol. 19, *The Known Man*. The chapter describes the years of research conducted at the BJP Research Clinic and also lays the groundwork for a theoretical framework through which to interpret the findings.

About 120 pages of the chapter are dedicated to Crile, Speransky, and Morat, with extensive quoted passages from each. Many chiropractors from the era felt that Speransky's research described in his 1936 text, *A Basis for a Theory of Medicine*, proved the chiropractic premise that vertebral subluxation could disrupt the normal function of the nervous system and lead to pathophysiology. B.J. also integrated Crile's two books to support his own energetic viewpoint on living systems. B.J. had been quoting Morat's text on neurophysiology since 1909 as a way to explore the link between intelligence and matter.

The invention of the timpograph was at the heart of the research in the clinic. It was a precursor to the electroencephalogram and electrocardiograph.

His engineers developed pinpoint pads, which were placed at the ends of eight grounded leads, placed bilaterally; two at the head, two above the subluxation, two below, and two on the backs of the legs. B.J.'s goal was to locate the mental impulse. He writes:

> The electroencephaloneuromentimpograph is a very delicate instrument which detects, amplifies, and records flowing and active mental impulses in a living body. The mental impulse registers five-millionths of a volt or less, of current. It is then amplified four hundred trillion times.

B.J. concluded that the mental impulse could be detected as a micro-current, which was less than a millionth of a volt. He referred to it as a "continuity energy potential," recorded as a "nerve-energy flow graph wave pattern." He was not sure if it was "pulsatile" alternating current (AC) or a "carrier wave," direct current (DC). He concluded that the timpograph "picks up NERVE ENERGY QUANTITY CURRENT FLOW DIRECT." He concludes:

> AS RESEARCHERS, we approached these problems with the D.D. Palmer concept.
> Research proves:
> —a spiritual, electrical, mechanical, chemical background of a knowledge of Innate Intelligence mental impulse flow.

B.J. Palmer's Conflicts Clarify: Vol. 26 (1951)

Vol. 26 or *Conflicts Clarify* was published in 1951. It is one of the most eclectic of the tomes from this era. The book includes several of the early pamphlets like *Stones* (1911), *The PSC Lecture Bureau* (1915), *Problems* (1916), *Hemorrhages* (1916), *Abnormalities* (1917), *Public Speaking* (1917), *Remedies - Worse than Disease* (1917), *Kidney Diseases* (1917), *Tuberculosis* (1917), and *Rheumatism* (1917). Three hundred and fifty pages of Vol. 26 is a reproduction of B.J.'s book, *Invisible Government* (1917). As in previous volumes, B.J. does not inform the reader about when the original pamphlets were published. Vol. 26 also includes chapters on various topics and a few chapters by different authors.

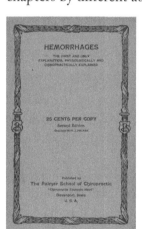 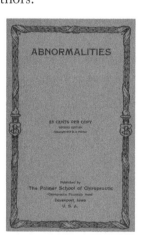 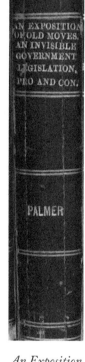

Hemorrhages and *Abnormalities* (1916 & 1917)

The most philosophically notable contribution to the literature is Chapter 15, *The Story of Marcus Bach*. This reproduction of the first letters between B.J. Palmer and religious scholar, Marcus Bach, written in 1951, represents a moment of concrescence in the philosophy of chiropractic. Bach and B.J. became close friends, with Bach speaking at many Lyceums in the 1950s and counseling B.J. on the spiritual elements of the philosophy. B.J. used Bach's work as a rhetorical stepping stone to further elucidate and develop his Innate philosophy, while also teaching Bach about the wisdom within. In the lead up to Bach's first Lyceum address in August 1951, he and B.J. shared some correspondence. B.J. writes:

An Exposition of Old Moves, An Invisible Government, B.J. Palmer personal collection

This "story" is written as of May 20, 1951. It contains information leading up to Marcus Bach's speaking appearance at Lyceum this year. As this comes in last week in August; and as he has not yet spoken; and as this book goes to press in June, to be out FOR Lyceum this year, we cannot print here his talk. It will be our intention to print it in full in another book to be issued in 1952, to be ready for Lyceum that year.

In a printed form letter issued to our profession in March, 1951, we had this to say re Marcus Bach's qualifications to intelligently and from experience discuss the issue involved:

Some in our profession have tried to propagate the idea that Chiropractic philosophy is a 'cult' as tho this were a crime against interests of Chiropractic and mankind. The greatest American researcher into ancient and modem 'cults' is Marcus Bach, Professor of Religions, Iowa State University. He has asked to speak at our '51 Lyceum, reviewing our recent Volumes xxii, xxiii, and xxiv. He has researched and lived with the Trappist Monks, Hutterian communists, Doubkohors, Penitents, Voodoo of Haiti, Spiritualists, Bahai's, Pentecostal groups, Vandentists, Snake Handlers of Kentucky and Tennessee, and many others. Living with each of them he sought the constructive common denominator, and what made them tick. He lectures these subjects from coast to coast, border to border. He has written, 'They Have Found a Faith,' 'Report to Protestants,' 'The Dream Gate,' 'Faith and My Friends,' etc. He will tell, without restrictions as to what to say or how to say it, whether in his opinion Chiropractic philosophy is another 'cult' or a science destined to evolutionize mankind."

The following correspondence has passed between ourself and Marcus Bach. It speaks of what transpired BEFORE his talk will be delivered in August.

In the letters between May 16, 1950, and May 15, 1951, some fascinating new territory was covered. Their exchange offers a first-hand account of how Bach's perspective and B.J.'s were in sync.

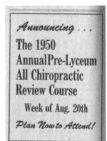

Announcing ...

The 1950 Annual Pre-Lyceum All Chiropractic Review Course

Week of Aug. 20th

Plan Now to Attend!

The Chiropractor (1950)

B.J. Palmer's History Repeats: Vol. 27 (1951)

Vol. 27 or *History Repeats* was published in 1951. The book mostly a collection of chiropractic writings from 1905 to 1931. The first part of the book includes essays and letters from D.D. Palmer and his contemporaries. Accounts of his 1906 trial and confinement in the Scott County Jail are printed alongside articles published between 1905 and 1912 on the history and philosophy of chiropractic. The chapters include several articles by Howard Nutting, the 1906-1907 graduation address by Morikbo called *Stray Thoughts on Chiropractic and PSC*, a treatise on *Genius* by Joy Loban, and B.J.'s classic article on *Cycles*. It also includes D.D. Palmer's 1905 article, *Chiropractic Rays of Light*, his writings from prison from 1906, as well as his classic article *Immortality*, also published in 1906. Interestingly, when B.J. Palmer republished D.D.'s works in 1921 as the second Vol. 4, he edited *Immortality* and removed reference to Jim Atkinson. However, in this 1951 version it appears unedited.

The second part of the book is comprised of various topics. Articles from the 1920s and 1930s include topics such as: *Is Chiropractic the Practice of Surgery?, Is "Spinography" a Practice of Medical X-Ray?, Are They Medical "Adjuncts" Being Used by Chiropractors?, Are Spinograph and NCM Using Medical Principles and Practices?, Is Each Human Body an Intelligent Unit or a Unit Depending Upon Intelligence of Some Other?*

One of the highlights of the book is Chapter 74, *The Story of And Why Not?* The chapter includes seven photos of Dr. Clare palpating and toggling the C1 vertebra of a Chimpanzee in side posture in the 1950s.

The final chapters of the book include several pamphlets written between 1915-1919 such as: *Paradoxes, Wet and Dry Man* (1917), *Laboratorical Findings and Inductions vs. Clinical Findings and Deductions* (1916), *Diagnosis vs. Analysis (~1916)*, and the 50-page classic, *Majors and Minors* (1918).

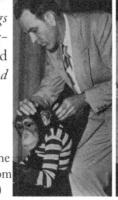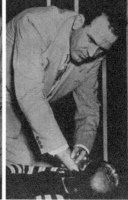

Dr. Clare and the Chimpanzee from Vol. 27 (1951)

B.J. Palmer's Answers: Vol. 28 (1952)

Vol. 28 or *Answers* was published in 1952. The book is another important contribution to the chiropractic literature. *Answers* breaks new ground in several areas by clarifying philosophical and theoretical questions. It also contains a hodge-podge of historical events and happenings from 1952, such as; Chapter 8, *The Story of Clearview Sanitarium*, with 13 pages of photos; Chapter 11, *The Pictorial Story of B.J.'s B.H. (Beach House)*, or his Sarasota home; Chapter 24, *Innocents Abroad*, 58 pages on the New York chiropractic legislation; and Chapter 25, T*he Story of The Battleship USS Iowa*, with 146 pages of correspondence between chiropractors and the United States Navy, with tales of a trip to visit the ship. The book concludes with a continuation of the questions and answers from Vol. 24.

One of the most interesting features of the book is the updated collection of B.J. Palmer's epigrams, originally published in 1918, 1921, and in the 1930s. This chapter, *As a Man Thinketh*, included all of the epigrams painted across the campus, the radio station, the printery, and clinic. The 1930s edition was reproduced in *Answers*. It contains about 730 epigrams, many written by B.J. The epigrams were recently organized by topic and contextualized with a biography and extensive quotes in the book, *Success, Health, and Happiness: The Epigrams of B.J. Palmer.*

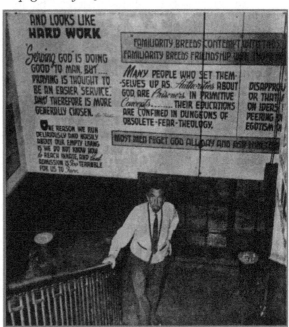

B.J. Palmer with epigrams
at PSC

Vol. 28 also includes the follow-up chapter about Marcus Bach, which was promised in Vol. 26. Chapter 19: *The Story of Marcus Bach (continued)* describes Bach's first appearance on campus and B.J.'s account of their first meeting. It also includes the transcript of Bach's address on *Chiropractic and Religious Cults* to 5,000 people at the 1951 Lyceum. In the talk, Bach writes:

> The more you know about Innate, the more you will know about the deepest truth of your work and the deepest truth of the universe. Innate is the mystical principle which no other healing art, no other healing science recognizes in exactly the same way that Chiropractic recognizes it and in which is the greatest secret for your success and the success of your practice; the one thing that will push back your horizon— and one more thing—the study and understanding of Innate is truly contemporaneous; it is current; it is alive with all the motivations of today—this peace of mind age—this age in which churches are getting back to personalized religious faith, this emphasis on the personal life and adventurous thinking— this is your golden hour...

> You know Roger Bacon spent fourteen years in prison because he said that the rainbow could be explained because of the laws of physics. B.J. will be criticized far longer than that, because he dared to put in one of his books a diagram based upon the system of Charles Hasnel and at the bottom of the diagram B.J. said, "This is the most valuable drawing in the world for it solves all the problems of man." I am not here selling B.J.'s books...

> All I know is that you will learn more from one chapter on Innate—you will learn more than you have learned in many a night reading another scientific or unscientific book, because you will learn that as your knowledge of Innate grows, so grows your success and your influence and your understanding of yourself, your clientele, and your relationship with the cosmic mind which I call God.

In regards to The Universal Diagram, which Bach refers to, it was originally drawn in Stephenson's Text (page 196, Fig. 4). Stephenson also attributes this quote to B.J. In Vol. 36, published in 1958, B.J. includes the diagram at the front of the book along with the quote.

Another interesting aspect of the chapter is B.J.'s account of their lunch in his home. He writes:

> It was one of those rare intellectual feasts where men of understanding exchanged views on perplexing problems which confront and complex human minds upraising or holding them down. It was one of the most enjoyable meetings we have ever had.

Seven years after Bach delivered the eulogy at B.J.'s funeral, he published *The Chiropractic Story*. In the book, he too gives an account of that first meeting Bach's first observations of B.J. were as follows:

> Now that I had this nearness to him, what were my impressions? His personality? Electric. His presence? Contagious. His influence? Provocative. His manner? Supernal...
>
> Disturbed and thrilled by the apparent way in which this plural-personality called B.J. read my mind, I realized that thoughts are things, lines of communication defying words, transmitted, as B.J. had correctly said, "from spirit to spirit..."
>
> What kind of an extra-sensory man was this?
>
> He was a receiving and sending station, turned on, tuned in, seeing with an inner eye, listening with an inner ear, speaking with an inner voice.

This type of insight helps us to understand what B.J. Palmer was like in his final years. This is especially valuable because in those final years, his writings on the Innate philosophy were on such topics and quite provocative and supernal.

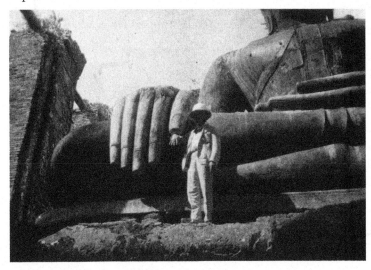

B.J. comparing hand with giant Buddha, Thailand, from *'Round the World with B.J.*

B.J. Palmer's Upside Down Right Side Up: Vol. 29 (1953)

Vol. 29 or *Upside Down Right Side Up including The Greatest Mystery in History*, was published in 1953. It is the oddest of the Green Books. The book is an edited version of B.J.'s travel logs from a 25,000-mile journey with Mabel and Dave in 1930 and 1931 throughout Hawaii, Fiji, Samoa, New Zealand, Australia, Java, Bali, Sumatra, Malaya, Burma, Siam, Angkor-Thom, Cambodia, Indochina, China, and the Philippines. As noted, when he had the edited version of the manuscript retyped, he changed every pronoun from "I" to "We." He writes:

> In this book, at this date, we revised our original writings to make them conform to other recent books from Vol. 21 to 28 by changing "I" to "we," "ours," etc. for same reasons we stated in previous books.

From *The Chiropractor* (1954)

The book is filled with photos and stories including dozens of images of indigenous peoples, with brief commentary under each photo.

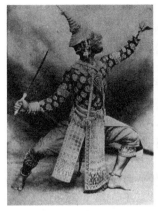 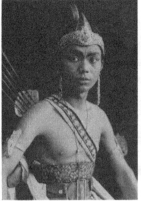 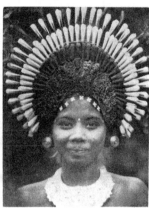

Images from Bali, Vol. 29

B.J. wrote his thoughts at the start of this long journey in relation to missing family and friends. This captures some of his philosophy of life, Innate, and destiny. He writes:

> Everybody was happy, smiling, loving thots and thotful goodbyes. It was just "another" trip, as tho we were to be gone overnight. And, what is time after all? Someone has ably said: "Live today as tho you were going to live always; live this hour as tho it were the last." But, underneath in the hearts of everyone, there was a subtle something that told our reason that there was always the intangible innate that controls our destinies, but it was not openly displayed on the surface.
>
> All preparations had been made for sailing from San Francisco on the S.S. Tahiti. She sunk on the up trip from New Zealand. We would have gone down to New Zealand with her had she kept afloat. And, who knows, had she returned, she might have gone down on our trip. Innate knows!

The most interesting aspects of the book are his writings on the religions of animism, Hinduism, and Buddhism; as well as part two, or what he calls *The Greatest Mystery in History*. In the more than 200 pages B.J. provides a detailed photo display and commentary of the temples of Ankor Wat and Ankor Thom, which was the main object of the journey. To prepare for this photo odyssey, he researched all data he could find on the Khmer peoples, including ancient books and writings about religion and daily life.

Additionally, the book included a new realization about Innate. He learned that living in nature and connecting with "Innate" were not the same. He writes:

> During time we spent in the jungle over here we have come to realize nature and capacities of jungle foes. We have often felt life in a monastery would be a great relief; where we could retire from selfish human beings with petty bickerings; where we could get away from people who live so close to themselves that they cannot think of any thing or anybody else. We have felt that life in a jungle would be a vacation out in the great open spaces where we would be close to earth and closer yet in communion with Innate where all runs wild without narrow restrictions made by man for man. How different the reality! For most part you pilot yourself with aid of a heavy staff along steep and stony paths or slither over slippery paddy fields. Streams thru which you wade are over shoe tops. Average village road is a narrow isthmus of caked mud running between bogs into which you are liable to slide every seven steps. You are caked in mud. You are soaked in sweat. You are weary by time you reach compound where you are to spend the night. You sit forward on a log, limp and motionless, too tired to smoke or talk. You eat and fling yourself upon your cruel bed and in a couple of minutes you are asleep.

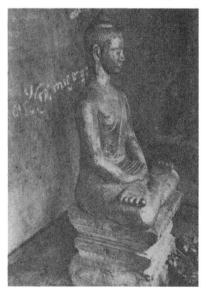 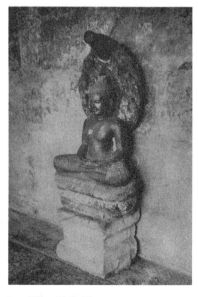

Buddha statues from Ankor Wat, Vol. 29

Chapter 13
Vols. 32, 33, and 34

In 1957, B.J. concluded that Vol. 32, Vol. 33, and Vol. 34 were connected by a thread of similar ideas. In fact, he viewed Vol. 34 as a continuation of the other two. Considering that these writings were his first books after the health challenges of 1953, they represent a significant milestone in the development of his ideas. In these books B.J. makes new contributions to chiropractic theory and the Innate philosophy. He built upon many themes of Vol. 22 such as greatness, inspiration from Innate to Educated, the expression of life in matter, Universal Intelligence, vertebral subluxation, and the role of chiropractic in the evolution of humanity.

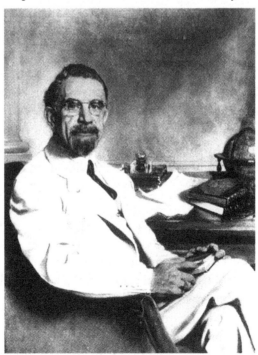

B.J. Palmer portrait used as frontispiece for many Vols. (1940s)

Chiropractic Philosophy, Science, and Art: Vol. 32 (1955)

In 1955, B.J. Palmer published Vol. 32 as *Chiropractic Philosophy, Science and Art*. The book expands on several ideas from his 1949 book, *Bigness of the Fellow Within*. Vol. 32 includes philosophical innovations such as his critiques of the medical perspective, his ruminations on the relationship between Innate and Educated, and his exploration of greatness as a natural Innate phenomenon. Vol. 32 also includes 15 chapters of Socratic-styled questions, like the chapters from *Bigness*, designed to inspire the reader to contemplate the philosophy more deeply.

Universal

B.J. asserts that all things "were once in Universal Intelligence." And so, since Universal Intelligence is Innate Intelligence, all of the natural secrets are hidden within. He goes even further and proposes that God has been hiding in the body as Innate. Accessing this intelligence is the key to becoming great.

Greatness

Greatness is described as the flow of thoughts and actions from Innate to Educated, which is how Innate expresses itself. This flow gets limited by vertebral subluxation. Interference with the communication between the Educated brain and the Innate brain is the result. Interference leads to decreased levels of greatness such as those who are near great, commoners, insane, unhealthy, and dying. Lack of interference leads to sanity, health, greatness, and being fully alive. If the individual refuses the ideas from Innate, "all genius is lost."

Vertebral Subluxation and Limitations of Matter

Inner forces resist external concussions of forces as best they can. When they can't, it could lead to vertebral subluxation, "a mechanical violation" of matter. This leads to dis-ease and an abnormal functioning brain.

The chiropractic adjustment is an intentional concussion of forces. This reverses the process and Innate takes its course. Physical incoordination disappears. Mental coordination appears. Innate may then get in tune with the body and the educated brain. Chiropractic advances mankind because of increased efficiency, peace with himself, and the ability to make man more natural.

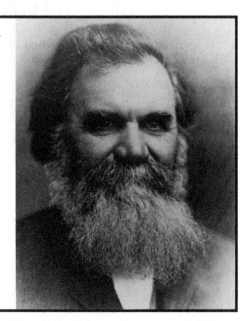

Advertisements for Vols. 32, 33, and Chiropractic's 60th Anniversary (1955)

Natural, Normal, and Abnormal

B.J. linked causes of vertebral subluxation to the challenges of modern living. He writes:

> Education, because of artificial demands of ways of living, forces man away from normal, forces abnormal excessive existence, which produces vertebral subluxations which interfere with normal flow of the natural between Innate and educated brains, hence produces a below par level of functional activity.

He basically identified a biological, mental, and social feedback loop of the modern world. The educated mind becomes less natural. This leads to a greater distance between the Innate and the Educated.

B.J. describes it as a type of ego inflation whereby the conscious mind thinks it can control the organic functions of the body mainly through medical interventions from outside. The likelihood that Educated will not allow Innate to contact it increases. This inner conflict between the normal and the abnormal causes the vertebral subluxation, which creates the loop because it perpetuates the conflict. According to B.J., the optimal solution is for Innate to dominate Educated.

Critique of Medicine and Religion

B.J. critiqued religion and medicine as part of one related problem, an inability to recognize the intelligence flowing to man from within. He concluded that medicine views life as something activated in matter, mysteriously, by nature. On the other side of the spectrum, religious believers view God as the source. The chiropractic perspective is that there is an abstract law, not a God. "Organized mind flows through matter." Thus, prayers are unnecessary since the wisdom of creation constantly flows into and through the brain and body. The chiropractic adjustment restores health, sanity, and normality.

His view was consistent with D.D. Palmer's that medical therapies are not natural and work against Innate. In contrasting medicine and chiropractic, B.J. concludes that medicine is complex, variable, the societal norm, based on Educated, focused on effects, takes a shotgun approach, uses lots of methods, and assumes cures come from outside. Chiropractic is simple, natural, singular, constant, specific, uses little, focuses on Innate, and views the cause as within.

Non-Materialist Definition of Life

According to B.J., there are two opposing theories of life: materialistic and spiritualistic. Each one interprets things differently. Mind and soul are viewed either as a chemical reaction or eternal spirit. Chiropractic bridges these because it views the body as a medium for the Innate source. Innate is a pattern of intelligence, a blueprint of the body.

Life is the product of working with the outside forces and the adaptive inside forces. Evolution is an attempt to interpret and adapt to the vibrations bombarding the organism from the universe. The inner striving of life bursts through the material constraints.

Life is motion directed by intelligence. Health is motion from the inside. Sickness is when control of inside motion is directed from outside. Motion is the only function. Muscles contract and relax in relation to the energy supplied by nerve force flow. The nerve force energy is generated in the brain.

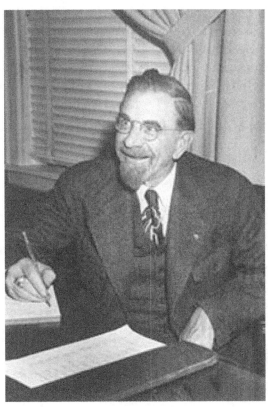

B.J. Palmer

Mental Impulses

The main principle of chiropractic is that normal quantities of mental impulses get to the tissue cell. If that is interfered with, it leads to abnormal quantity and some level of slowed down motion. There are differences between forces and nerve forces and between energies and mental impulses. Mental impulses are "impregnated" with intention and purpose in order to intelligently harmonize with functions. Intelligence permeates into the impulse.

Dis-ease

The separation between Innate and the body is the fundamental cause of all dis-ease. B.J. writes:

> The idea that all power comes from within is not mystical. The kingdom of God is within, not mystical. It is physics, Innate is centrifugal, inside forces. Environment is centripedal, outside forces. The normal range of adaptability is expressed with a perfectly aligned spine. Vitality can be studied as a measure of centrifugal forces, resistance, and the ability to resist dis-ease. Thus, chiropractic makes the body stronger to "suit" the environment.

D.D. Palmer also used the terms centrifugal and centripetal in his final lectures. Reversing the process that caused the dis-ease is the goal of chiropractic.

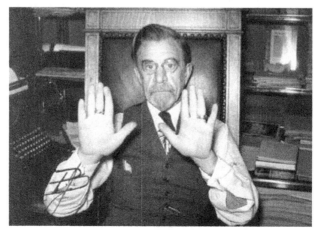

B.J. Palmer

B.J. defines two kind of dis-ease: direct and indirect. Direct dis-ease is in the organ and leads to paralysis of function, decreased action, decreased energy flow, and decreased products and byproducts. Indirect dis-ease is an adaptive Innate reaction. This leads to symptoms related to inhibited or stimulated actions, increased or decreased functions.

Finding Yourself

The way to find yourself is to get in tune with the Infinite. Great men open the channels of communication. First they receive the message. Then they understand it. Then they act on it. You "must" act on it. "That is how you make Innate serve you... respond when you call... and obediently perform." It is not just a power but an "inexhaustible resource." Innate is a potential. We all have the opportunity to develop "talents" and "intuitions." Getting this "gigantic value" of Innate, opens us to the kingdom of God within, the law of the human being. He writes, "The time to follow your hunches, intuitions, and inspirations is now." When you are ready, Innate will find you.

Inhibitions of the Conventional Self

The uninhibited receive from Innate and make history. The majority of men are inhibited, stifled, and suppressed. Vertebral subluxation is an inhibition that leads to abnormality, sickness, and insanity between Innate and the body. When Educated does not receive the thoughts given by Innate, it is due to inhibitions. Educated attempts to hold us back, which has been ongoing for centuries.

According to B.J., "Most people, non-consciously, live in prison." Each failure, because of an inhibition, is a prison cell. When you know you have inhibitions, you are a prisoner. We can choose to free ourselves. Getting yourself out of your mental prison is the key. It is possible to unlock the one door that unlocks every door. The path to freedom is to unlock that door and don't look back.

B.J. observed that choosing to become a chiropractor was breaking convention for many. Sometimes students go into practice and then turn back and lock the doors. Some keep the doors open. Many chiropractors are afraid to be uninhibited. Success comes from being uninhibited and guided by a vision of service.

Fame and Fortune: Vol. 33 (1955)

In 1955, B.J. published Vol. 33 or *Fame and Fortune and The Know-How and Show-How to Attain It*. The purpose of the book was to "develop self-made individuals." It was dedicated to the rights of the sick.

In Vol. 33, he explores the relationship between the Educated Brain and the Innate Brain in more detail. He positions the discussion in light of the chiropractic paradigm. For example, D.D. Palmer noted that he developed the principles and practices of chiropractic as part of his search to understand why one person is healthy and the other sick. In his later years he lectured on individual greatness. B.J.'s theme of greatness builds on this original chiropractic premise about the difference between two individuals working side by side. Similar to his father, B.J. wants to understand why one man is great, another "near great," and "the masses" on skid row.

B.J. proposes methods on how to receive the all-knowing wisdom from the "great inner intellectuality." Innate "can and does reach down, enter, and create powerful thoughts, ideas, and ideals." The only way to prove this is by doing. He implores the reader to study the whole book and thereby learn the Innate principle and how Innate communes with Educated.

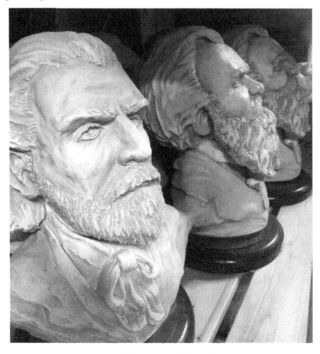

Busts of B.J. and D.D. Palmer

Chirometer and P-T-A

In the book, he describes two new technological innovations: the Chirometer and the Palmer-Thompson-Adjustment. Both were tested in the B.J. Palmer Chiropractic Clinic and the Clear View Sanitarium, as well as some field clinics starting in 1953. The Chirometer was used to "solve borderline cases." It was a single-probe skin temperature thermometer used to compare skin temperatures bilaterally related to vertebral levels. It was used in conjunction with the NCM, NCGH, Timpograph, and Spinograph. The P-T-A was a side posture adjusting table developed around Thompson's drop head piece. According to B.J., the P-T-A increased results in a positive way. Both instruments added to the evidence base of vertebral subluxation and the expression of the Innate principle as health.

Intellectual Functional Energy

According to B.J., Innate is a constant. He writes, "Innate is THE ONLY vertebral functional constant." Part of its constancy is the flow of intellectual functional energy from the brain. Interference to this flow because of vertebral subluxation leads to dis-ease. He refers to this as a type of "abnormal variable" from the Innate constant.

Dis-ease is viewed as a functional variable. Over time, it undermines the constancy of Innate's organizational control of functional motion. It is a deviation from normal. Functional and pathological dis-ease takes time to grow due to a decrease in the functional activity. He writes, "Dis-ease is a condition of difference between abstract ease and lack-of-ease." Adjustment restores the connection. It takes time to restore normal from abnormal.

Levels of Living Systems

B.J. viewed the organism as a holistic organization. The interrelationships from the tissue cell to the organ and the entire living system was described as "functionally correlated in totality and unity." This holistic viewpoint also understood the organized life in terms of hierarchical levels. He writes:

Living life is a combination of spiritual, electrical, mechanical, chemical combinations of motions;

—spiritual because of source

—electrical because of spiritual

—mechanical because of electrical

—chemical because of mechanical

Living is a spiritual (abstract), electrical mental impulse (abstract), mechanical movement (of physical matter) pro-ducing chemical (substances) products and by-products (of secretory and excretory glands). Each is coordinated, each to other, each of which is essential and necessary.

He viewed this living, organized being as controlled by an internal (Innate) and an external (Educated) mentality, which was the beginning of "the great divide," separating man from other forms of life.

Thought depends on the organized matter of the brain, nerves, muscles, organs, and other tissues. Physical action depends on thought. Thus mental impulses unite the immaterial mind with matter through physical function.

Blending Mind and Matter

According to B.J., a complete understanding of chiropractic's role in the unity between mind and matter was a key to success. For him, the spiritual and physical are united in the living body. He writes:

Knowledge of VERTEBRAL SUBLUXATION as CAUSE of interference, and VERTEBRAL ADJUSTMENT as CORRECTION OF CAUSE, solves ALL disunity and unity of two halves to make ONE UNITY mind and matter which blends each into other.

He suggested that by bridging the gap between mind and matter, chiropractors are free from the conflict of the great divide. They understand and live according to the wholeness of reality, mind and matter as one. This leads to personal development and success.

When chiropractors get stuck in the conflict and live from uncertain principles, failure results. This uncertainty comes from external economic pressures, patient pressures, competitive pressures, focusing on non-chiropractic methods, and focusing on what the patients think they want.

B.J. felt that chiropractors who use medical concepts and focus on treatments, effects, symptoms, and diseases, lack knowledge of the principles and practices of Innate Intelligence. They weaken the profession by their lack of consistency and understanding.

Becoming Uncommon

Innate has millions of years of experience adapting through millions of human bodies from generation to generation. Since Innate stores all memories from all lives as potentials, it acts as an endless source of genius. Learning to access that wisdom in daily actions transforms the common man by stripping away what blinds the thinking mind to reality. Building on his metaphor from Vol. 32, B.J. concludes that Educated mind constructs the mental key that locks the door to Innate. The door is likened to a flood-gate.

Innate Thot Flash

The Innate Thot Flash (thot flash) was introduced in Vol. 25 in relation to the timpograph research. Now, in Vol. 33, B.J. explores the thot flash for the first time, on its own terms as an organic flow of consciousness from Innate brain to Educated brain and then to Educated mind.

B.J. explained this spiritual and mental transmission of thought with organic metaphors. He considered the process of sending inspirations and intuitions to the Educated brain to be the same as Innate telling the liver how to make bile. He even suggests that trying to force Innate to send thot flashes is like trying to force a bowel movement. "Let Innate do the work – with a book handy."

Innate Radar

B.J. also considered that Innate Intelligence is what wakes you up at night when you hear a baby cry or smell smoke. It is an inner sense connected to instinct and intuition. He writes:

> Whence came that mysterious Innate radar, called "instinct," "intuition," "soul," which directs young salmon which stays at sea four years, then comes back to the river, to the very tributary, the very channel where it was born?

The great challenge according to B.J., is when the thot flash comes to the mind and the Educated mind thinks it knows better. That would be like salmon choosing to go in a different direction, away from its nesting grounds.

Mental Hibernation

B.J. observed that most people try not to let Innate commune with them and struggle to keep Innate out. They "hibernate mentally" and don't have purpose. Often, Educated receives the thot flash and might hesitate or minimize the message. Educated may want to add ideas or theories to the original thot flash. For Educated to oppose and deny Innate is a losing strategy. The winning strategy is to let Educated work with Innate.

Learn to Access Innate

Contacting Innate is a way to "penetrate into the invisible." B.J. proposed several methods to access Innate. The primary method is to not attempt to reach Innate. Allow Innate to come to you. Another method is to create a "blank slate" by meditating 20 to 30 minutes per day in silent contemplation, and to allow the Educated mind to seek the depths within. All of these approaches are far easier when free of vertebral subluxation so that the channel from above is open.

Another method that B.J. utilized regularly was to constantly provide challenges for Innate. This method involves seeking solutions to a problem. B.J. offered four steps to this process. First, forget the problem for a while. Then complete an unrelated activity that has nothing to do with the problem. These first two steps help to remove the emotional and mental blocks that "kept Innate from giving the answer." This type of diversion is followed by illumination. Insight emerges, which allows access to the "secret place of all knowledge." The next step is to "grab it quick." Then, write it down immediately. The thot flash comes from Innate to Educated in a split part of a second. Thot flashes must be accepted fully and acted on immediately.

Innate is Beyond Words

B.J. found that language was a difficult medium through which to explore these topics. He writes, "Words bound us to the known." The relationship between the conscious and unconscious was an important way to explain the duality, but even using terminology like "conscious" and "unconscious" was challenging. For example, Innate is conscious day and night running the functions. During sleep, Educated goes unconscious and Innate flows through.

B.J. viewed Innate as a personality. He described it as silent, adapting, and internal. It acts, uses logic and reason, and is non-linguistic. Educated talks, uses emotion and prejudice, and is linguistic. He also described Innate as selfless personified wisdom and Educated as "selfishness unlimited." And yet he felt there could be harmony between the two.

B.J. viewed Innate as an internal law that starts within itself. It knows itself. It ends within itself. It is within us and around us. He writes, "D.D. Palmer re-discovered its hiding place and revealed its vast limitless identity in expression."

Positive Educated vs. Egotism and Dogma

B.J. does not critique all forms of Educated mind. He sees the value of things like engineering, chemistry, and education. His criticism of the values associated with medicine and religious dogma. He viewed Educated as inherently egotistical, especially when it views itself as the superior intelligence. It tries to run the body and the world.

He found that there are generally three types of people. Those who live within Educated, those who are a bit uninhibited, and those who listen to Innate and follow it. The last group are "the masters of men." His goal was to improve our understanding of living man.

Living a Life of Service

B.J. considered these new insights about humanity as a type of evolution brought forth by chiropractic in the form of service. He writes:

When Chiropractors understand and know this great law within, they become a servant to service and let Innate cooperate WITH education to accomplish Innate's desires and demands that chiropractic was able to initiate.

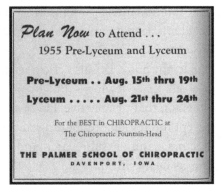

Plan Now to Attend . . .
1955 Pre-Lyceum and Lyceum

Pre-Lyceum .. Aug. 15th thru 19th

Lyceum ..... Aug. 21st thru 24th

For the BEST in CHIROPRACTIC at
The Chiropractic Fountain-Head

THE PALMER SCHOOL OF CHIROPRACTIC
DAVENPORT, IOWA

Advertisement for Pre-Lyceum (1955)

Evolution or Revolution: Vol. 34 (1957)

Vol. 34 or *Evolution or Revolution* was published in 1957. The prologue is a treatise on survival values and ADIO. In Chapter 1, B.J. writes:

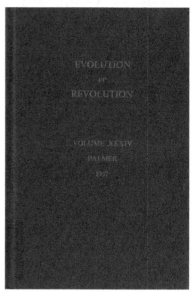

Vol. 35 cover

> Volumes 32 and 33 were designed to enlarge upon Innate Intelligence. Articles which now follow are later additions to either of those books. They can be studied as separate articles.

The bulk of the book includes philosophical theorizing. The last three chapters are excerpts from August Dye's *The Evolution of Chiropractic*, MacCluskey's *Your Health and Chiropractic*, and Turner's *The Rise of Chiropractic*. The back pages of the text include a list of books available from the PSC sales department such as Speransky, Crile, Bach; as well as Boyd's *Preventive Medicine*, Hayakawa's *Language of Thought and Action*, and Peale's *Power of Positive Thinking*.

In Vol. 34, B.J. expands on core philosophical theories such as the organism as self-constructing and life moving through matter. He also refines various definitions such as dis-ease as slowed down action, evolution as a universal law and as a complete pattern, and vertebral subluxation as the "internal interfering intermediary." He proposed that 95% of all minor accidents lead to vertebral subluxation and the subsequent sequence of sickness.

In the book, B.J. also critiques religion and rational thinking in general. He felt that viewing mind in matter was sensible and yet society looks down on that perspective. He saw it as a double standard whereby religions accept mind in matter but to science, and to religious scientists and medical doctors, nature is subjugated and referred to as "subconscious." B.J. viewed this as hypocritical.

There are several fascinating aspects of Vol. 34. These include B.J.'s treatise on the new era in history and his personality theories. Also, B.J. references Aldous Huxley's article on genius, which had an influence on

B.J. Palmer's later ideas. B.J.'s correspondence with Marcus Bach is also included in Vol. 34. Bach's comments to B.J. offer us a contemporaneous view of the philosophy of chiropractic from a well-published religious scholar.

The Self-Constructing Body

The first analogy B.J. offers to describe life and living man is very autopoietic. He builds on the levels described in Vol. 33 and describes the dynamics of living man as "the original and first internal, automatic, autonomous, auto-mobile." The mental generator is the spiritual engine of the living automobile. The intelligence is described as self-sustaining and self-perpetuating from the inside. The brain is described as a battery, the nerves as wires with peripheral ends as spark plugs, and muscles as motors. The body's chemistry is the fuel. Carbon dioxide is the exhaust expressed from the lungs as mufflers. The system communicates with itself and constructs itself for millions of years in an ancient assembly line.

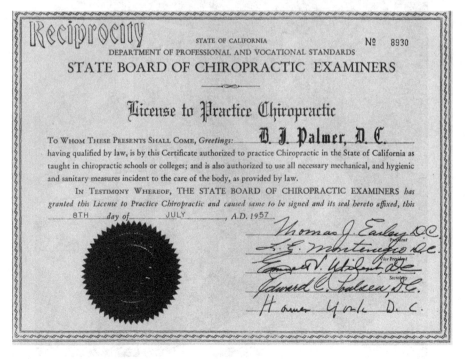

B.J. Palmer's first certificate of reciprocity bestowed upon him from a state of the United States to honor his life's work. *The Chiropractor* (1957)

Life Moves Into and Through Matter

B.J. suggests that the mental impulse is the nerve force that pulsates matter into functional action. Thus, chiropractic reestablishes the balance between the abstract and matter as life and health.

Educated mind is not the source like Innate, it is a semi-source. It can't directly observe the unreachable infinite, which is within and around man. The actual source, the Innate, can only be known when it is united into the substance of the body. B.J. proposed that the active function of living moving matter, the substance, is the proof of this unification. Life moves into matter and through matter.

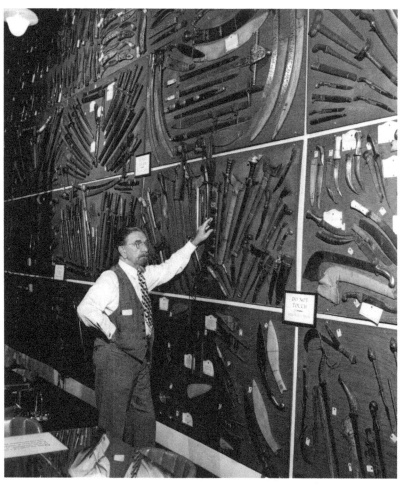

B.J. Palmer with knife collection
Sign reads: "Do Not Touch Poisonous Edges"

Old and New Eras

The second part of Vol. 34 is called *Old and New Eras*. B.J. describes the new principles emerging in the world and the gradual change he viewed as progress from old principles. He provides examples, such as cars, radar, television, airplanes, electricity, atomic energy, and Morse code. The process of progress and cultural change began with a few leaders like Tesla, Edison, Fulton, Einstein, and D.D. Palmer, who were first scorned.

In order for the new principles to emerge in the world, certain conditions must be met. The first step is to break with the old. An extended quote is warranted to best capture what B.J. meant. He writes:

> The FIRST condition of establishing a NEW principle is a COMPLETE BREAK WITH THIS OLD. One can't give medicines and an adjustment; rely on drugs to cure, and preach that Innate cures.
>
> In contemplating the satisfaction in science, one must be guided by a realistic approach of the present, and the probable future course. If we look back two or three generations, we see a world OF LIMITED HORIZONS, one in which the most exciting challenges lie IN REFINEMENTS. How mistaken that conception is, has been dramatically demonstrated by the phenomenal progress of new concepts of the past half century.
>
> In philosophies, sciences, and arts, it is important to delineate and understand these limits. The process is attended with risk with new principles. If we are up against a hurdle, it is important that what looks like a permanent obstruction is a temporary road-block which can be removed.
>
> A recognition of limits of physical properties and processes can serve as a guide to efforts in the IMMATERIAL FIELDS IN WHICH THERE ARE NO LIMITATIONS BECAUSE IT IS AS YET PRACTICALLY AN UNEXPLORED FIELD. The future course of developments will be determined by progress into these seen and unseen limits AND BY THE DISCOVERY OF NEW PRINCIPLES not now recognized, such as we have in our Chiropractic philosophy, science, and art.

He considered 1957 a transition period to a new era with a new principle. He described this as an evolution because of the revolution that had already begun. The future will require that many more people open the channels to Innate.

Huxley on Genius

B.J. quotes Huxley's entire article, *Genius*, which was published in July 1956 in *Esquire* magazine. Huxley emphasized originality and the uncommon man. He posited that genius originates outside of personal consciousness. Thoughts come from "out there," which is analogous to the external world, from a topless attic. Huxley also quoted William James. After the article on genius, B.J. invokes Mohammed, Christ, Buddha, and Confucius as examples of individuals who brought forth the principles from within. In later writings he builds on some of Huxley's ideas and analogies.

Typologies

B.J. proposes some typologies in regards to how people are in the world. First he suggests there are two groups. One group who have found themselves. They are fewer in number and even include some chiropractic leaders. He writes, "Knowing yourself is when you understand and know the Innate within." The other group is confused. They are looking for answers from outside-in rather than from inside-out.

He also contrasts types of chiropractors. Traditional thinkers are conventional. They don't easily accept new principles and they comprise the majority. Seekers of factual truth are open to new ideas. Few are radical.

The Perennial Philosophy

The final sections of Vol. 34 are about Bach's newest book, *Circle of Faith*. In the book, Bach describes interviews with spiritual teachers from all over the world. B.J. sent Bach a critique of the book and admonished him for not looking within. B.J. complained that instead of seeking truths on the outside, Bach should just go within. He suggests that Bach could have shared that insight with all of the spiritual teachers he met.

In response, Bach expresses to B.J. that he considers the philosophy of chiropractic as part of the Perennial Philosophy. Bach writes:

> This is the first chance I have had to thank you for your penetrating critique on CIRCLE OF FAITH.
> I darn well appreciated your common sense approach. Reason is that which makes all things reasonable, and I am happy that in the midst of all sorts of comments on this new

book, you related it to the ABOVE-DOWN INSIDE-OUT concept. That this is the secret of the 'great ones' and that it is the same potential expressed within different physical beings, is what Leibnitz called the 'Perennial Philosophy,' the vertical-ABOVE-DOWN, horizontal-INSIDE-OUT figure.

Health, blessings and creative power to you always!

Fondly, Marc.

According to Huxley's 1944 book, *The Perennial Philosophy*, it is the common core of all religious traditions and philosophies. B.J. Palmer's experiences and his Innate philosophy were at the leading edge of contemporary thought and also linked to a long line of philosophy from both east and west.

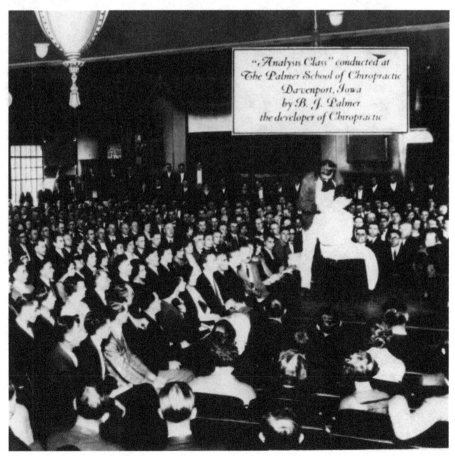

B.J. Palmer demonstrating during Analysis Class (1920s)

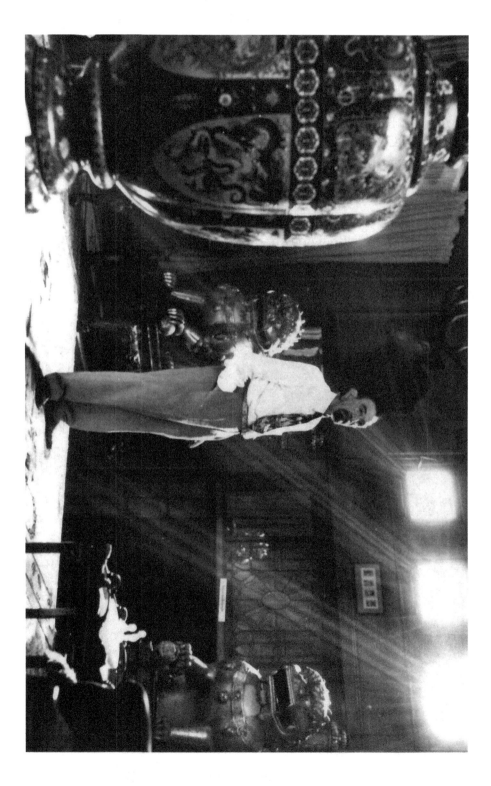

Chapter 14
Vols. 35 and 36

The next two books in the series were published in 1957 and 1958. Vol. 35 summed up the evolution of chiropractic and defined the current program at the PSC, which was an expansion from a strict upper cervical model to a full spine approach. Vol. 36 codified Palmer's theories in a series of proposed "laws," which were described as constants of life according to B.J.

In both books he describes new advances of clinical research findings like the best time of day to conduct a full-spine thermographic and postural scan was between noon and 2 p.m., technique protocols like the new program of correcting misalignments lower than axis after two weeks of unchanging patterns, theoretical developments such as a new rationale for compensatory distortions; and other philosophical insights like, "Materialism has been the ne plus ultra of diseases." The two books represent yet another important moment in Palmer's writings, the Green Books, and the history of chiropractic ideas.

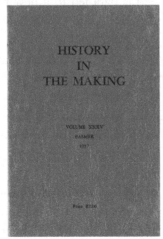 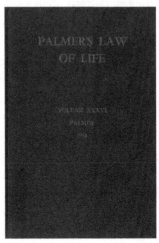

Vols. 35 and 36 covers

History in the Making: Vol. 35 (1957)

Vol. 35 or *History in the Making* was published in the fall of 1957. The book is comprised of B.J. Palmer's pre-Lyceum talk from that year. The talk was a detailed rationale for why the chiropractic analysis evolved from a strict upper cervical approach to a full-spine approach starting in 1956. The complete argument included a 71-page history of practices and research. The turning point, according to B.J., was the introduction of the conturographer, which led to a large cohort study in the student clinic to explore the new full-spine approach. The study included 17,871 patient visits and was conducted from January 1, 1956, through June 30, 1957, to "prove or disprove the frequency of necessity for correction of vertebral misalignments inferior to atlas or axis." As of January 1956, with a speech given by Marshall Himes, DC, who was director of clinics, the PSC officially gave the "green light" to the new program, which allowed full-spine adjusting in the clinic for the first time in two decades (Appendix 4). Vol. 35 was designed to explain the change so that it was not misinterpreted.

Up until this period, thermographic patterns below axis that did not change were dismissed as unimportant and compensatory because only atlas and axis were deemed as true subluxations. Full-spine thermography research with a printed graph had been ongoing since the introduction of the neurocalograph in 1936, which used an electronic rolling readout synched to the NCM. The addition of the conturographer linked measurements of postural distortions to the data collected from full-spine spinographs and thermographic pattern analysis. Examining this data led to a new perspective on the adaptive process, minor interferences, and secondary muscle contracture.

B.J. admitted that a mistake was made, which lasted 26 years. The "program now" advocated "correcting misalignments" below axis if the NCM indicated the lower pattern hadn't changed after two weeks of adjusting the actual subluxations. He felt it was necessary to explain his rationale to the students, alumni, and the profession. The error was only discovered after decades of research. The historical argument for the evolution in protocols is highlighted below.

Vol. 35 also includes B.J.'s critique of chiropractors who misquoted D.D. Palmer's well-known statement about relieving suffering humanity. This is worth noting since the quote from D.D. has been used out-of-context in the chiropractic literature several times since 1957. In his 1910 book, D.D. included a small section about adjusting impinged nerves of feet related to corns and bunions. In that context, D.D. wrote, "I have never found it beneath my dignity to do anything to relieve suffering humanity. The relief given bunions and corns by adjusting is proof positive that subluxated joints do cause disease." The first half of that quote is sometimes used to imply that D.D. Palmer advocated combining therapies or practices besides the adjustment of subluxation to relieve nerve impingement. The out-of-context quote is even inscribed on a monument to the founder in Port Perry, Canada, which was thought to be his place of birth at the time.

The PTA Table

In Vol. 35, B.J. described the importance of adjusting on the Palmer-Thompson-Adjusting (PTA) side-posture adjusting table with the PTA headpiece, both of which were invented by Clay Thompson, DC. This description was set in the context of a wider history of adjusting tables, which was part of the overall evolution leading to "the program now." He writes:

> Now, PTA full spine table, side-posture, even adaptable to basic technic if desired.
>
> As of this time (1957), after working with this table and seeing what it makes possible, we are convinced it is the most progressive step to more accurately adjust any subluxation, or for correction of any misalignment.

He continues by describing the adjustment on the PTA table. An extended quote about the adjusting method and its results is warranted as it is one of B.J.'s final writings on technique. Also, the quote demonstrates how he integrated adjusting misalignments as well as subluxations. He writes:

> Now, more than ever, is this vitally important for what we do, as we do it, on the PTA table, when, where, and why, leads to gratifying success or disappointing failure. TRAIN OUT your inadequate clumsy pound or push, and TRAIN IN that ARTISTIC all-sufficient sharp quick tap.
>
> Adjusting with PTA head-piece for superior cervical specific vertebral subluxations, or correction of inferior specific misalignments, requires ARTISTIC skill, care, thot, study. Instead of pounders, pushers, shovers, or squeezers, a sharp quick LIGHT tap movement is required. More than that CAN DO HARM.

ADJUSTING on and with the PTA head-piece, or the PTA table, IS AN ART and calls for deep ARTISTIC INSIGHT.

This PTA table is another step along the continuous and tortuous road we have set as our goal. This may not be the last word, but it is a substantial part of what we have been working to attain. It is difficult to know how to describe the after effects from an adjustment on PTA table. It isn't exactly an over-all-glow, or a feeling of complete relaxation; possibly the nearest expression would be to say "There is an all-rightness feeling" which comes into one.

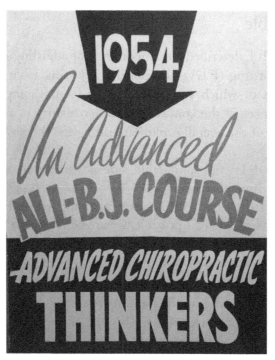

Advertisement for B.J. Palmer's advanced course based on research with the Chirometer, NCM, NCGH, Spinograph technics, & the PTA headpiece

Chiropractic Evolution

The main focus of Vol. 35 was to explain the change from a strict upper cervical approach to a full-spine approach. To do this he covers the history of empirical research including every major innovation. For example, the first innovations included palpation, heat detection by hand, the years of public teaching in the pit class, the development and refinement of the meric system, and the development of majors and minors. He also covers the changes related to x-ray analysis, starting in 1910, which led to the clinical observation that palpation was incorrect between 50-85% of the time. Pre and post x-ray, which also led to the decrease in over-adjusting. Over time, the x-ray analysis became more reliable, especially after the introduction of tracing of pre and post x-rays described in Vol. 20, and the addition of positioning head clamps invented by Thompson, first mentioned in Vol. 28. B.J. described the research leading up to the Upper Cervical approach, the development of NCM, shielded and grounded booths, full-spine pre and post graphs, and the neurotempometer to synchronize speed of graphing. He also writes that the timpograph:

> Did more to prove many solutions than any other research process. IT alone solved nothing; it merely PROVED WHEN we did and WHEN we didn't, whether what WE DID or did not restore more normal, natural flow of mental impulse supply.

Also in Vol. 35, which was published more than two decades after the research clinic opened, he gives three reasons why the clinic was formed: to develop a research model that could be repeated, to find answers to problems that needed research, and to develop a place for chiropractors to refer difficult cases.

Posture and Osseous Locks

According to B.J., the main reasons for the change in protocol was the addition of two new observations, one postural and the other anatomical. The postural information was developed with the conturographometer (CTGHM) and the anatomical with the study of osteology. Of the CTGHM, B.J. writes:

> We developed the conturgraphometer, which graphed data could be subsequently duplicated as to a posture constant. This instrument had a traveling fine-point crayon which electrically traveled at a definite rate of speed which was graphed on a traveling paper. We took two graphs, one A-P, the other lateral.
>
> Later, we took subsequent graphs and compared them. We then traced these one or more graphs on translucent sheets, overlapping one over other, each in a different color, to study the speed with which corrections took place of all adaptative

curves back to normal curves. We found that, by adjusting upper cervical specific ONLY, many adaptive corrections took place below in from one to six weeks, raising the height of the case anywhere from 1" to 1-1/2". This conclusion was made on muscular conditions wherein there was no pathology or other inferior diseased conditions of one or more vertebrae involved. In that case, as we now understand the problem, we would need correct certain lower specific misalignments.

B.J. also emphasized osteological research. He used the osteology lab at the PSC, of 25,000 specimens, a study of of comparative anatomy demonstrating the basic laws of biological intelligent organization. He writes:

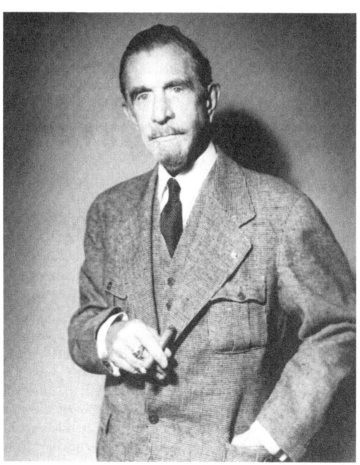

B.J. Palmer

> Osteology is to human behavior what geology is to the study of strata of the history of the world; what archeology is to the study of peoples who once lived here or what anthropology is to the study of its living creatures.

This viewpoint was congruent with the overall chiropractic paradigm, which considered intelligent adaptation as the crux of evolution and viewed the body from the perspective of Innate. He continues:

> Pursuing our research, we constantly tried to think as INNATE did think in those specimens; evidence; and to interpret all living activities as INNATE delineated itself.

He viewed the osteology lab as an encyclopedia, each bone a chapter about Innate adaptation.

Studies of anatomy also involved an examination of "osseous locks" and "the wet specimen," in relation to the spinal nerves and cord. These anatomical observations were viewed as further support for the subluxation theory, especially as it related to compression, cord pressures, and the importance of the two upper cervical vertebrae, which had no osseous locks. Vertebrae below axis were interosseously locked and thus could only misalign not subluxate, and cause minor interference, not cord pressure. These were secondary compensations to the primary subluxations.

The One Mistake

Of the mistake he writes:

> Here is where we made one mistake—because results were thus attained in so many cases, in like manner—we concluded there was only ONE place pressures and interferences along entire spine where there could be a subluxation—occipito-atlantal-axial area. WHY? Because of inter-articulatory, osseous locks at all places below inferior of axis. We believed then this proved a difference between a causative SUBLUXATION above and MISALIGNMENT effects below.

He also writes:

> —that THERE COULD BE INFERIOR SPECIFIC MISALIGNMENTS THAT NEEDED CORRECTION IF WE KNEW WHERE AND WHEN THEY WERE. Our late idea of full-length pre and post NCGH checks proved the

long lost connecting link between what we once developed, and what we NOW know, with what we had TEMPORARILY FORGOTTEN—the adaptative conditions below that we formerly denied needing attention.

We are today picking up those loose threads and weaving them into a new format and correcting them if, as, and when we prove they exist.

Today, we are getting cases well on that per cent of cases we formerly overlooked.

He includes a statement from 1956, which reads:

We Admit A Replaced-Discorded Correction

TODAY, in 1956, we admit an error of judgment in concluding that at no time, in no way, in no manner. was a correction EVER necessary below occipito-atlantal-axial area.

Because of its all-inclusive field of adjustment of the vast majority of causes in cases, we conceived the superior specific was an all inclusive and all-exclusive field of adjustment.

There ARE times, locations, and conditions which do justify lower specific corrections

—which are not adjustments OF CAUSE

—which are corrections of mechanical, traumatic, or adaptative misalignment effects

—which are not subluxations, but misalignments.

Misalignments are adaptations, not subluxations.

Misalignments are visible, i.e., out of juxtaposition with correspondent above and below, sometimes with inferior occlusions and interferences.

In all subluxations and some misalignments, four elements are present:

(a) malposition

(b) occlusion

(c) pressure

(d) interference to flow—the latter two of which are not visible, even with spinographs.

Cord pressures only occur in the occipito-atlantal-axial region. According to B.J., this area involves the largest percentages of interferences. It also leads to the greatest number of causes of dis-ease. These cord pressures also affect the Educated brain and senses, leading to diseased vertebral structures, which can produce occlusion, pressure, and interference.

To correct it to proper alignment is to temporarily ease the pathology; but its results would be temporary and not permanent.

IF adjustment ABOVE does NOT check out inferior NCGH readings, as proven by pre and post full-spine NCGH checks, then and then only is one justified in establishing proof that the INFERIOR SPECIFIC is that in fact and not in theory or snap judgment.

True subluxations occur in the upper cervical spine because of cord pressures. If the pattern does not change after two weeks, misalignments due to compensations below C2 causing interference are corrected.

Advertisements for Pre-Lyceum and Lyceum (1958)

Palmer's Law of Life: Vol. 36 (1958)

Vol. 36 or *Palmer's Law of Life* was published in 1958. The alternative title to the book is *Comparable Assembly Lines*. B.J. suggests Vol. 36 should be studied alongside Vol. 34 and Vol. 35. On the facing page he includes a schematic of the relationships between Innate Intelligence, Innate Brain, Innate Body, Educated Brain, and Educated Body. He suggests this schematic solves all the problems of the world. B.J. wrote the book with extra repetition to amplify the principle and practice. He asserts that the only way to understand the book is to apply it.

The law of life is summed up in the final chapter of the book titled *The Vicious Perversions of Law*. B.J. writes:

> Palmer's LAW OF LIFE possesses the following elements:
>
> 1. There is a gigantic, exhaustless and intelligent power house resident in living man's brain.
>
> 2. This intelligent power is sufficient unto man's every need IF it gets from where IT IS, to where it is needed.
>
> 3. Sickness or dis-ease can exist anywhere, in any organ, in any manner, when this free flow power is interfered with between brain and body.
>
> 4. What interferes, blocks, obstructs this unlimited supply?
>
> 5. A twisted, distorted, abnormally positioned vertebra of the backbone producing pressure upon the power-transmitting cord of nerves.
>
> 6. This "shorts" the circuit downward from brain TO body and upward senses FROM body to brain.
>
> 7. This condition CAUSES every dis-ease, in every organ, in any form.
>
> WHAT IS NECESSARY TO BE DONE TO GET SICK PEOPLE WELL?
>
> 8. Correct, by hand only, the mal-positioned vertebral sub-luxation.
>
> 9. Release pressures upon nerves.
>
> 10. Permit a restoration of the imprisoned power supply from above-down, inside-out.
>
> 11. Let it have free flow normally.
>
> 12. When it reaches dis-ease, ease follows of its own accord.
>
> This condition FROM ABOVE-DOWN, INSIDE-OUT CURES EVERY AND ALL DISEASE.

THAT IS PALMER'S SIMPLE AND SINGLE LAW
OF LIFE.

A chiropractor, who knows chiropracTIC, who KNOWS
the Palmer Law of Life, knows how and does but ONE thing

13. ADJUSTS the vertebra: subluxation

14. Letting intellectual power from ABOVE-DOWNWARD,
INSIDE-OUT do the curing.

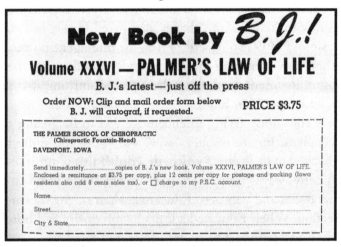

Advertisement for Vol. 36 (1958)

The core of the book is a series of laws summing up B.J.'s theories
to date. The book follows its own logic, from Innate Intelligence and its
impact on consciousness and genius, to the flows of energy, to the use
of power in the body by muscular action, to the unity and continuity of
mind and matter, balance of nature, and the expression of health and the
condition of dis-ease, and the role of chiropractic in the adjustment of the
mal-position of the vertebral subluxation. The order that B.J. presented the
laws as follows: *The Law of Innate Intelligence, The Law of Non-Conformity,
The Law of Evidence, The Law of Applied, The Law of Compensation, The Law
of Source, The Law of Energy, The Law of Fusing Energy, The Law of Assembly
Lines, The Laws of Human Assembly Lines, The Law of Muscular Power Units,
The Law of Patterns, The Law of Muscular Importance, The Law of Percentage-
Wise, The Law of Builders, The Law of Continuity, The Law of Unity, The Law
of Supply and Demand, The Law of Par, The Law of Balance, The Law of Aches
and Pains, The Law of One Only Dis-Ease, Cause and Cure, The Law of Where
and When, The Law of Potentials, The Law of Progress, and Epitome of Palmer's
Law of Life.* A few of the highlights are summarized below.

Law of Innate Intelligence

Innate Intelligence comes from the mother at birth and leaves at death when, "Innate takes that long vacation from us." Innate memorizes every impression and interpretation from every life. It shapes destinies. Because of its millions of years of existence prior to birth, it is the embodiment of potential within, yet to be explored.

It is described as an abstract quality and yet, Innate Intelligence transforms raw substances into shapes, organized forms, and coordinated "motion systems." B.J. also describes it as an intelligent power or energy or force that flows through the body and manufactures the body by superimposing its intent on the impulse and transmitting that purpose to the tissues, which perform action.

Innate is constantly trying to encourage you to be greater than "your educated" realizes. Innate reaches "over" and "into" the finite mind. The mind of educated man. A crude way of describing this is intuition, hunches, instincts. A better way is thot flashes from Innate. It sneaks up on Educated. Innate flows down and comes to Educated, when Innate "deems educated needs" direction. When Educated admits its inferiority and humbles itself it can listen. Educated must be receptive and not repulsive.

Innate contacts Educated when Educated is "blanked out." Sleep is the best time for contact because Innate is always awake and Educated can't deny or debate when sleeping. That is why it is important to always keep a pad and pencil next to the bed. A good example he provides of actively learning to open to Innate, is the Yogis of India. According to B.J., Yogis have the correct mental principle, especially when they take on a relaxed posture for hours or days. They get in tune with the infinite. He refers to their states of consciousness as a semi-sleep and points to Gandhi as an exemplar who used this principle. B.J. even suggests that chiropractors could use yoga but some might ruin it.

Man should be more Innate-like rather than oppose it. Educated makes mistakes because of ignoring the Innate, especially in regards to medicine. He writes:

> If we were able to bequeath one virtue to every Chiropractor, we would give him the joys of Innate, for without it the world would stand still. The Innate man, hard to satisfy, moves forward. Educated man satisfied with what he has done, moves backward.

Innate needs no instruction from Educated. It regulates all. It is infallible. It cannot be interfered with. The nerve-force is a materialistic product. It can be interfered with. Because there is a material intermediary, the immaterial being is diminished in matter only. It is an interference between the source and non-source.

The Law of Nonconformity

The law of nonconformity involves strong individuals and progressives. The chiropractor is the modern nonconformist and yet too many try to stagnate and fall into conformist grooves. He refers to chiropractic as a breaking plow. The nonconventional overcomes the conventional. This is an approach that is outside the mainstream of contemporary life. It is a new path.

The Law of Evidence

The law of evidence involves Innate subtly whispering evidence of a world that can't be seen with the eyes, a world of patterns and intelligence. To be a student of living, one must examine the evidence of the producer as well as the product. The producer, Innate, is the mental pattern maker. It is a common intellectuality that is the same in all. Vertebral subluxation causes a mental block between the flow from above down. The evidence of the outside world is easy to see: why not look for evidence within.

More evidence of the Innate within is found by studying genius. What makes genius people different? Genius is the individual who listens, accepts, and permits development from within. "It just comes." To some it just flows. Others cultivate it. Others suppress it. It is an internal law that beckons for entrance constantly.

Genius is when the person absorbs from a source greater than they know. An inherent capacity of receiving and using those "inspirations," "aspirations," and "perspirations." Each has the same thot flashes. Educated challenges the subtle when it flashes through. Educated gets stuck on the "outer states" of thinking. The great mass lock all the doors between the source and the semi-source. This is the conventional way. To do otherwise is to be called "an odd person." They run with the mob. Are afraid to be unusual. The finite mind is obscured and blinded because the finite cannot tap the evidence. The rational interprets the process. You can't treat effects from Outside-In-Below-Up (OIBU). There is an inter-relationship between Educated and Innate.

Look for the qualities of greatness in others and you will see it in yourself. Instead of looking next door, look within. He constantly encourages genius in others.

Laws for Energy Governing Life

The law of source explores how the superior consciousness comes to the brain, flows through the brain, and produces life. Physics does not apply directly to life especially when the brain is viewed as a source of energy.

The law of energy explores the types of energy between organic and inorganic matter. For example, is there a different law for energy governing life through matter? Are electrons concentrated in the brain? Into it, through it, out of it? He also describes energy in terms of increasing levels of complexity such as: Positive/Negative Energy, Electrons, Neutrons/Protons, atoms, molecules, tissue cells, organs.

B.J. posits that energy produces motion. Even though the tissue cell is made of energy, it is only alive as a unit in relationship with coordinated purpose in context of the whole. The tissue cell expresses power from the concentration of energy in the brain.

In Chapter 9, on the Law of Fusing Energy, B.J. writes:

> We met Albert Einstein. "How come you discovered the LAW of relativity?" His answer was characteristic: "I discovered nothing. Sitting on the sea shore, I looked into space and saw something which had been there for millions of years—TIME—and I saw something in TIME AND SPACE which no other man had seen before, a LAW of relativity BETWEEN SPACE AND TIME.

Also in relation to that law, he describes the constant energy that is transformed into life. The energy is the same from amoeba to man. It is systematically organized, and manages internal heating, cooling, locomotion, energy generating, repairing, and restoring. All from one central source. Each living being is pregnant with potential.

Law of Muscular Importance

The law of muscular importance was published as Chapter 14. The law describes the power flowing into muscles. The brain absorbs intelligence and power from space. It concentrates and condenses the forces from the environment. Internal forces react and resist. Internal muscles contract and relax. When there is a clash of forces between external and internal, a subluxation may result. Nerve distribution via muscles, impedes flow of power, force, energy and decreased action in muscles. This leads to abnormal action.

The primary subluxation at C1/C2 is the issue. This is where the interference and pressure is. The secondary misalignment, below, is where the tissue is affected. Vertebral subluxation leads to decreased function, muscle contraction and relaxation, as well as decrease to the normal quantity and quality of byproducts of the organs systems.

Dis-ease

Dis-ease relates to symptoms of diagnosis, distribution, location, and quantity of nerves under pressure. Also, degree of pressure, length of time it is abnormal, and organs affected, and the decreased function of muscles' rhythmic motions. Dis-ease destroys the functional normality. Over time, dis-ease grows. Dis-ease is defined as destroyed functional activity. It is a condition where the full source of power is not expressed.

Laws of Continuity, Unity, Par, and Balance

The law of continuity was published as Chapter 17. Man is viewed as a totality, "one continuity totality," "one entire system." The chapter begins with the developing fetus and the continuity of structures described as a wholeness. It is a law of constructed pattern.

Living is viewed as an internal process that is continuous and expresses a law. Matter and energy are inseparable and thus, a continuity of substances. Physiology, a continuity of actions. Matter and energy are never separated. B.J. applies this law directly to causation. When the body is viewed as one, as a continuity of energy and actions, the abnormal functions are viewed in the context of the source of life. "Organ is part of the whole." This is contrasted with the medical focus on individual diseased parts rather than viewing parts as a continuity of a whole. Medicine and therapy, in general, focus on separating what is continuous. Dis-ease is then viewed as physical, mental, and emotional: one whole system.

The law of unity was published as Chapter 18. This law takes the broader perspective of balanced cycles between immaterial and material; and the continuity of life, health, function, motion, and sense perception. Dis-unity is when things are out of balance.

The law of par was published as Chapter 20. It has to do with levels of function. Par level function is known to Innate Intelligence. Drugs either stimulate or inhibit. Par in brain is normal. Below par in body is abnormal. Balanced organs leads to normal function. This is the law of balance, which was published as Chapter 21. Unbalanced is when function is too much or too little.

According to B.J., chiropractic offers a physiological proof of dis-ease and its restoration.

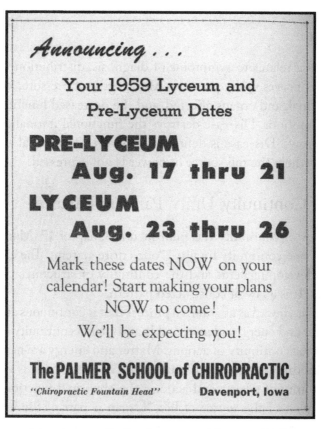

Advertisement for Pre-Lyceum and Lyceum (1959)

The Law of Potentials

The law of potentials was published as Chapter 26. This law involves brain potential and learning to accept thot flashes. B.J. offers yet another approach to having Innate work on a problem. He suggests that if you have a problem to solve, follow these steps: 1. Imagine it is not your "waking fellow's problem." 2. Find solutions when sleeping. When you allow the deeper mind to work on it, you will be rewarded. Innate possesses all knowledge. Our job is to learn to tap it and utilize it. Tapping the untapped power is to utilize more than five senses. It is the great internal adventure.

The Law of Where and When

The law of where and when to adjust was updated from 1956 to 1958 and published as Chapter 24. B.J. explains the importance of the neurocalograph to determine the relationships between the adjustment of the upper cervical subluxation and the correction of the misalignment below. The misalignment is viewed as a minor interference caused by local trauma or major adaptations involving the cord pressures from the primary subluxation.

Appeasers and Compromisers

In the last chapter of the book, B.J. suggests different groups of chiropractors. The first group are the appeasers. They do whatever patients want. The second group are the compromisers. They dilute chiropractic with medical practices and do chiropractic in name but without knowing what that is. They practice medicine. A third group knows nothing of chiropractic and buys into "anything medical." He proposes chiropractors should confine themselves to chiropractic only. He writes:

> The history of chiropractic was born of ONE simple, single principle and practice which has remained fixed and has not changed thruout its career. Step by step, year after year, the APPLICATION of that principle in practice has been clarified, stepped up its percentage of reducing sickness and restoring health in the human race.

Prior Arts Rights

In several of the books, B.J. suggests that chiropractic has "prior arts rights" as a profession. Chapter 63 of Vol. 27 reproduces on article on the topic from 1928 in Fountain Head News. The prior arts rights argument was successfully used in the courts to demonstrate the chiropractic separate from medicine because of its distinct science, art, and philosophy.. The principles and practices of medicine are antipodal to chiropractic. If they are doing medical therapy they are not a chiropractor. The chiropractor is a vertebral column specialist focused on the right of the sick to get well. This is the chiropractor's moral duty.

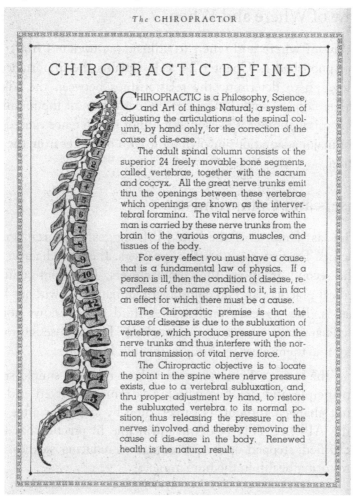

The CHIROPRACTOR

CHIROPRACTIC DEFINED

CHIROPRACTIC is a Philosophy, Science, and Art of things Natural; a system of adjusting the articulations of the spinal column, by hand only, for the correction of the cause of dis-ease.

The adult spinal column consists of the superior 24 freely movable bone segments, called vertebrae, together with the sacrum and coccyx. All the great nerve trunks emit thru the openings between these vertebrae which openings are known as the intervertebral foramina. The vital nerve force within man is carried by these nerve trunks from the brain to the various organs, muscles, and tissues of the body.

For every effect you must have a cause; that is a fundamental law of physics. If a person is ill, then the condition of disease, regardless of the name applied to it, is in fact an effect for which there must be a cause.

The Chiropractic premise is that the cause of disease is due to the subluxation of vertebrae, which produce pressure upon the nerve trunks and thus interfere with the normal transmission of vital nerve force.

The Chiropractic objective is to locate the point in the spine where nerve pressure exists, due to a vertebral subluxation, and, thru proper adjustment by hand, to restore the subluxated vertebra to its normal position, thus releasing the pressure on the nerves involved and thereby removing the cause of dis-ease in the body. Renewed health is the natural result.

Chiropractic Defined, *The Chiropractor*, every issue (1950s)

Chapter 15
Vols. 37, 38, and 39

In the winter of 1959 and 1960, B.J. Palmer nearly completed his last three books. In his address to the student body delivered on June 8, 1960, which was published as Chapter 8 of Vol. 37, he acknowledged that he had "written, compiled, and prepared for publication this, our Vol. 37, as well as Vol. 38 and Vol. 39." In Vol. 38, he notes that for many chiropractors, the emphasis of chiropractic "is almost entirely ON THE PHYSICAL PLANE and sadly enough little of the Innate Philosophy." He contextualized the latest books in relation to the Green Book series. He writes,

> This chiropractic scientific Innate interval research program, was well organized and completed determined in the very beginning to prove or disapprove every concept, postulate, theory or principle of its basic and fundamental chiropractic philosophy, science art, as flowed forth thru the fertile but otherwise construed ignorant mind of D. D. Palmer. We who review and look back to our Vol. 1, then follow the exposure from within, follow those steps thru to and up to Vol. 36 and you will have a positive and well rounded, all encompassing series of steps climbing to attain our ultimate goal. Right now Vol. 37 is being sent to type in our PSC Printing Plant. Vol. 38 has been written, and is completed in MMS form. But, THE book we are most proud to think of as the ultimate, is our Vol. 39, completed in MMS form and ready to be printed any time. This book is an exhaustive all-review historical review of all the successive steps from our earliest Innate days, to our latest work this winter in Sarasota. Its title will be, THIS IS OUR MASTERPIECE. Time will see the publications of these three works...

Glory of Going On: Vol. 37 (1961)

Vol 37 or *The Glory of Going On* was published in 1961. The first four chapters of the book include: a tribute to B.J. Palmer by Hugh Harrison, editor of *Davenport Democrat and City Leader*, written in 1919, called *The Man Who Made a Ladder of his Cross;* an article from the PSC yearbook from the class of 1960, by Matthew Sportelli and Leon DeGomes-Coelho, both PSC graduates; a chapter on statistics about the Palmer school's growth; and an exchange of letters between B.J. Palmer and Marcus Bach from April 1960. In the letters, Bach accepts B.J.'s invitation to speak, once again, at the Palmer Lyceum. B.J. responded with a philosophical treatise on "the law road," and "God in man." He signed the letter, "Our Innate Blesses Your Innate."

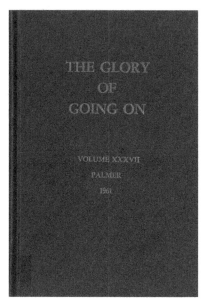

Vol. 37 cover

Vol. 37 includes further developments of B.J.'s theories. For example, he writes how *Palmer's Law of Life* is not a religion but a philosophy that acknowledges a "supreme universal intellectual law which many call God." He also wrote that chiropractic is the opposite of medicine and religions. His central rationale being that medicine has no principle or method, its theories of causation and treatment vary, it is not based on laws or the internal. In terms of religion, you cannot talk up to Innate, Innate talks down to Educated brain, which needs to be receptive. God talks down to all creatures and man should be more God-like.

Toward the end of the book is a thirty-page glossary of terms. This terminology section mostly repeats definitions in various ways for everything from Universal Intelligence to symptoms, and from pathologies to cause, which is described as simple and singular. In the chapter on terms, B.J. developed a new way of describing Energy, Force, and Power as personifications of intelligence. Energy is described as an abstract potential. It resides within itself and also within action in organized forms. Force is the "potential possibilities" of energy reaching matter. Power is the ability to shape and form matter into action. These three are transformed into the Mental Impulse. In his unique writing style, B.J. writes that the transformation is when the Mental Impulse:

> super-imposes thots, ideas, and specific purposes into its path of flow, as it permeates human force as living man formulates thots and ideas of a conjoint of force, energy and power, with mind sending forth this force, energy or power IMPREGNATED with DESTINED flow to a CERTAIN location to perform a specific functional purpose of the law of life.

He also expands on the concept of disease. He points out that medicine puts disease up on a pedestal. He writes, disease is "a physical object of adoration, which is or can be physically located by various medical PHYS-ICAL testing methods." Dis-ease on the other hand is defined as a paralysis of motion and functions and as a condition where the organic function is not at ease.

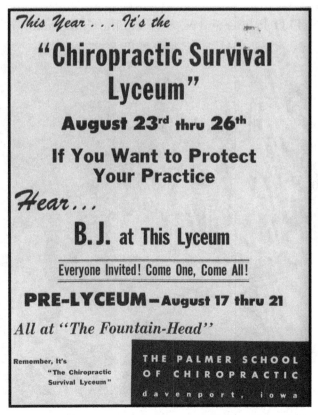

Advertisement for "Chiropractic Survival Lyceum" (1959)

The bulk of Vol. 37 is a philosophical treatise and a discussion of B.J. Palmer's own personal development, his methods for developing self, and the role of thot flashes as an intermediary between Innate, Educated, and the world. He summed this up when he writes:

> The transitions from kid, to young man, to man, and now in the ripe age of maturity; and the more this man egotistically sublimated himself to the greater Innate, the more humble he became. He realized HIS education was like one drop of water to an Innate ocean. What he egoistically THOT he knew was like one grain of sand to the sea-shore. Innate proved there was a great unexplored world within him which needed understanding.

Two of his most iconic writings on Innate are Chapter Eighteen or *The Dead Still Live*, and the final chapter called *Ponder These Things*. The last chapter is perhaps his most advanced discussion of the Innate philosophy, which culminates in an often quoted passage on the sacred trust bestowed upon him by D.D. Palmer and passed on to the chiropractors of the future.

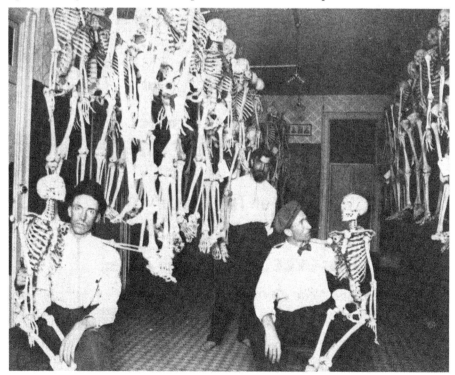

B.J. Palmer and friends in the Osteological Lab (1910)

Innate and Educated

Chapter 5 is a sixteen-page treatise called *How Does Innate Contact Education?* The chapter combines many different theories. It begins with the acknowledgement that it is difficult to explore this topic with words. He writes, "We find ourselves word-bound to present OUR thots AS thots, to another. This article is an attempt to use semantics to try to do just that." This self-reflective stance towards language is an indicator that he was aware of the role that language plays in shaping culture and perspectives.

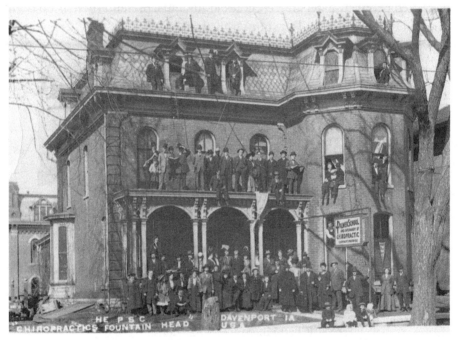

PSC with B.J. hanging out window (behind sign)

B.J. describes the two brains: one for internal contact and one for external contact. The Educated brain is defined as an organ of Innate. Its purpose is "to make it possible for man to think with in his contact with environment." One can also do this while living "entirely with THE INTERNAL."

The Educated is artificial, superficial, and counterfeit. The Innate is the silent partner, "the real you within you." Academic training decreases the value of Innate reception. It prevents Innate thots and actions. By relying more on Innate thot flashes, one becomes an original thinker. The submerged and dormant potentials become activated.

The Innate is the super conscious that makes tissue cells and a fetus in 280 days. The Educated is an egotistical exaggeration and thinks it is greater than Innate. It relegates Innate to subconscious, unconscious.

Innate People and Educated People

According to B.J., there is a breach between Innate people (small group of nonconformists) and Educated people (larger group of conformists), worldwide. Innate people let thot flashes through and make history. Educated people use debates, complex arguments, pretend there is no such thing, and deny contact. They put on the breaks.

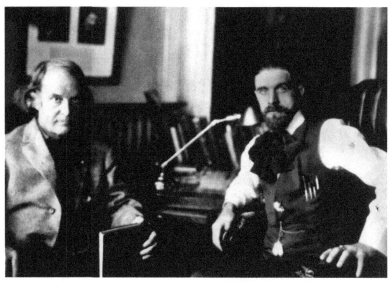

Elbert Hubbard and B.J. Palmer

Thot flashes come in a split second as a flash of vision from the wisdom of the ages. Educated may oppose this for years. The originator type takes human understanding to new heights and unknown fields. The educated type plods on in educated ruts, follows the paths of least resistance, follows grandparents and scoffs at the new. Innate memorizes all and flashes memory from the "Innate storehouse."

B.J. proposes that a hierarchy of people could be classified according to levels of knowing; from conformist to nonconformist to Innate listener to one who can reflect on being an Innate listener. He also suggests there is a difference between scholars and geniuses. Scholars are plentiful. Geniuses are Innate types, subtle, and concealed. Most men can't relate to geniuses.

The majority receive thot flashes from Innate to Educated but do not realize it. When they do, they deny it. That leads to Innate sending less flashes. Accepting the thot flashes leads to receiving more.

Innate Thot Flash Research

B.J. included several facts about Innate thot flashes (thot flashes), based on objective research, subjective experience, and objective research of intersubjective experiences. Since it was difficult for people to believe his subjective accounts of Innate thot flashes he developed anatomical, physiological, and psychological proofs. Research was conducted using the timpograph. They placed eight sensors throughout the scalp and noted a distinct electrical pattern when the subject reported a thot flash. Out of 18 distinctive patterns, one pattern demonstrated thot flashes. They also concluded that thot flashes registered at five-millionths of a volt.

Extra-sense-perception research using the timpograph was included in B.J.'s pre-Lyceum talk for 1960 and published in Chapter 16. B.J. noted that he had researched ESP most of his life, debunked the frauds, and acknowledged that one percent were authentic. They split the timpograph sensors so that four were on one person's head and four on another's head. They found that one Innate can contact another.

Subjectively, B.J. concluded the flash duration may be a simple flash or continuous. It continues until the thot is completed and captured, perhaps the entire time of writing it down. This could last minutes, hours, or days depending on the subject.

Methods to Follow Innate

B.J. offers to go beyond theory or suggesting "the possible" and instead suggests a method so that the reader might find himself, like B.J. did at age 18. The method is designed to convert failures to successes. Learning how to listen to Innate is the key, to take advice and suggestions as a guide, informant, and teacher, which is wisdom.

In Vol. 37, he highlights methods to follow Innate. The main method occurs at night during sleep, when there is no interference between the two brains and the channels are open. A pad and pencil are important so that you can write down every idea completely and clearly. He advises one not to roll over and go back to bed when Innate rouses you with a flash. That is a mistake, and Innate will go "to the back seat." When Innate is willing to give you must capture it. If you ignore a thot flash, Innate will ignore you. This can become a fixed habit.

B.J. councils that it is difficult at first, to know when it is a thot flash. In order to test it he recommends using a problem and allowing Innate to solve it. Don't press Innate for the answer and don't follow Educated or you will lose it. Just turn it over to Innate and let the answer flash through. The more this happens the stronger it gets.

The thot flash will not flash to an educated brain filled with complex and muddled ideas. Innate won't attempt to sort out an over-filled brain. However, when Innate realizes that Educated is understanding more and more, Educated may begin to rely on Innate for direction. Eventually, Educated may be submerged to Innate and replaced as the guide.

Pay more attention to Innate in order to know the self within. This is how to find oneself.

B.J.'s Experience Opening to Innate

B.J. paid attention to his own internal transformation. He says that at first Innate was like a stranger and he had to get more acquainted. He was humble and hesitating. As the thot flashes came, Innate was testing him and his ability to receive and act upon them. Innate became like a friend, anxious to serve.

The more he listened to the thot flashes, the more they came. He tested it again and again to see what would happen if he just did whatever Innate prompted. His advisors tried to stop him until they too learned to listen to their own Innates. Then he studied other Innate people and realized that it was an old process always described in much the same way. It was another sense, just like animals have other senses. He writes:

> When there are no restrictions between the greater and lesser personalities, all conflicts cease. Instead of bucking failures with regularity, he was succeeding in attaining his objectives with no internal conflict. Eventually, when this comradery became fixed and firmly established in his life, he realized this was a law and A WAY of life—one which had succeeded WITH HIM, would succeed with others. It became to him a way to live, to convert failures into successes. If this could occur IN HIM, it should be told to all who would listen, that

THEY, too, might use the same law and repeat THE SAME route of travel thru life. Innate then impressed upon him that it became HIS DUTY to explain the process, method, and way HE succeeded, that THEY might duplicate WHAT he did, AS he did it.

Innate told him, through thot flashes, to teach this to others so they could find themselves. He tried to explain this to others so that they could use the method. They called him daft, accused him of being a spiritualist, conducting séances, and there were skeptics even amongst his own followers. Some thought he turned mystic but he claims this is not supernatural. It is just as natural as Innate contacting the cells. "It is rare, therefore a much misunderstood process." According to B.J., we can't stop biological function but we can get in the way by refusing to accept the thot flashes.

B.J.'s Evolution

B.J. wrote of his personal evolution, which came from Innate: from above down. Also, that "under the guidance of Innate thot flashes," he consecrated and dedicated his life to "teaching the Chiropractic profession to succeed in like manner, by explaining as best he could that WHAT had occurred in him could occur in others, because they contained same Innate as he." He was describing a transition beyond the self where "life becomes a boundless field of human service," by accessing a "boundless source of wisdom" available to all.

Chapter 18 of Vol. 37, is one of B.J.'s most fascinating philosophical and autobiographical writings. It is the essay in which he describes his personal evolution and the moment when he stopped using the pronoun "I" and switched to "We." The chapter is written in a unique style that highlights the location; the osteology lab as "This One Room." This was where he studied thousands of specimens of vertebra and was struck by the realization that the Innate in each and every life was the same. This was a profound shift for B.J., a new awareness. He writes:

Up till THIS period of MY life, I was INVOLVING MY thots, words, and acts much like so many have done and were doing. The "I" was egotistic as well as egoistic.

After THIS period of OUR life, WE began EVOLVING like few people do or have done. From then on, WE thot, spoke, and acted. From then on, "I" was humble in the presence of Innate within as WE lived together.

IT WAS THERE, plus time, IN THIS ONE ROOM, I found MYself. WE found OURselves—INNATE AND I—until EACH lost his or her singular and single identity and became a plural duality, to eventually walk down the byways and highways together the rest of OUR lives.

This non-duality was the result of the years he and Innate "became intimately acquainted." Even though thot flashes have no language, he eventually stopped distinguishing between educated thots and Innate thots. Innate and Educated spoke with one voice, as "We."

The Sacred Trust

The last chapter of the book describes his viewpoint on Innate as the living God in the tissues of living man. He restates positions from other books but emphasizes the "God" terminology. He writes that it is "a living provable God in man," a "God law in man." This law is proven in daily actions and functions. In this context, he presents the final three paragraphs *to guard chiropractic well.* This is his most often quoted passage; to guard the sacred trust bestowed upon him by his father and from him to his students and readers. The passage is set in the context of his Innate philosophy, a spiritual viewpoint that divinity is expressed through the living tissues of the body. Rarely is this connection made, between the famous quote, and the profound and radical philosophical viewpoint B.J. Palmer meant by the sacred trust.

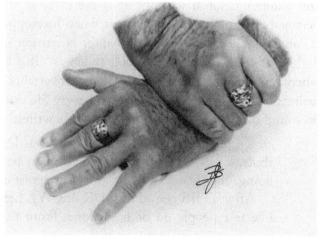

Portrait of B.J.'s hands, signed

The Great Divide: Vol. 38 (1961)

Vol. 38, or *The Great Divide* was completed in 1961. The foreword to the book was written in January 1959. Chapter 12 includes a talk B.J. gave at an ICA conference in February 1960. Chapter 8 includes a reference from March 1960.

As with most of the books from this era, B.J. theorized about research findings in the clinic. For example, Chapters 4 and 5 of Vol. 38 describe the research involving the polygraph and the timpograph. As part of the research clinic, B.J. had one of the only Keeler polygraphs in the state of

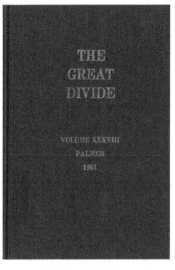

Vol. 38 cover

Iowa. The polygraph was used within the shielded and grounded booths (B.J.'s controlled conditions), which, according to B.J., inspired Keeler to adopt similar booths for his testing. B.J. describes this research as a way to understand the relationships between body, emotion, mind, and Innate. He felt that the lie detector was a test for a conflict between the Educated and the Innate, the source of conscience.

In his writings on the timpograph, B.J. offers a theoretical model that bridges his theory of paralysis, first developed in 1909, with D.D. Palmer's model of too much or not enough "functionating." B.J. proposes that excess function could follow a "minus" due to adaptive mechanisms. It is a route of pathophysiology. He first wrote of this in the second edition of Vol. 2.

Also in Vol. 38, B.J. proposes a postulate about motion. Motion defines the primary function of living and it occurs through muscles, which are moved by nerve force. The power expressed as action has a speed, a rate, and a frequency. Thus sickness, disease, and ill health are caused by paralysis of motion.

In 1957, towards the end of Vol. 34, B.J. mentions that he just wrote an article called *The Great Divide*, not yet published. In Vol. 38, he explores the idea and expands on his theories of human cultural evolution, what he calls the social educational problem. This approach is described in the context of his Innate philosophy and the coming of the New Era, also described in Vol. 34.

The Cosmic Faculty

In describing the new Cosmic Faculty coming to humanity, B.J. writes of the historical development of reason in early human culture. He refers to a break from an idyllic state of nature for humans. The shift from the natural state to the development of reason is referred to as a fall from grace that we must return to. This was a common viewpoint from the second part of the twentieth century.

The idea of returning to a pre-rational state as a form of development has been described in the literature as a pre-trans fallacy. The fallacy involves confusing a post-rational structure of consciousness with a pre-rational structure of consciousness. This approach views each new stage of development in terms of transcendence and inclusion. A new level of development, like rational thinking, transcends and includes earlier levels, like pre-rational thinking. By definition, a pre-rational stage does not have access to rationality. From this perspective, an embrace of intuition and inspiration as a guide for rational thought is a transcendence of rationality, or post-rational. Rational thinking is still a resource for the individual. The fallacy is confusing the pre and the post. Since both are not "rational" they are sometimes confused with each other. This modern philosophical viewpoint is a useful way to re-frame B.J. Palmer's approach.

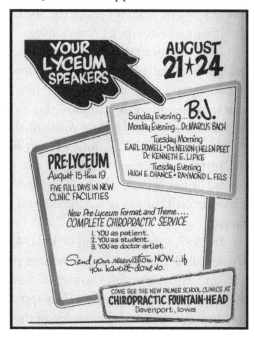

Advertisement for Lyceum (1960)

In describing the new faculty of Cosmic Awareness, B.J. writes:

> Years passed and man in keeping with the design of life gradually took on more and more new faculties: the awareness of music, awareness of color, the awareness of environment, etc. It seems that first one person would come into awareness of a new faculty, then a few more people would come unto it, then gradually the members of the people with this new faculty would compound upon itself until it was common to the majority of mankind and became accepted in their search for understanding. We came into a faculty of Cosmic Awareness and as time goes on more and more people came into this awareness and their primary motive for being was recognition of the distorted path that man was treading and they tried to bring back right direction, in other words an awareness of this Universal Intelligence and how simple life can be if only people would look within and let their Innate doeth the works. We see the period of time when many Prophets and Philosophers became illuminated to this awareness and tried desperately to portray it to their followers from the Cosmic aspect and some of them came into illumination themselves but those who followed were educated men without Innate awareness and they followed the letter of the word rather than the spirit. Voices from the source, in their own language, and, it is understandable now that the voice which has been guiding us over these years is that small wee voice which spoke to them. What is interesting is that this voice speaks without audible sound and comes more as an impression. What is beautiful is that there is no doubting it and it is an absolute positive expression which cannot be denied or refuted. If only people would let the barnacles which encrust their hulls start falling away and listen from within long enough to let this tremendous source of power start manifesting itself through them, the so-called problems of life would soon be eliminated. There can be an unfettered simple joy of life which is difficult to put into words.

B.J. refers to the days when humans come into this new cosmic faculty as a new age, a new era of evolution, one where the artificial falls away and the natural shines through. Even though, as he writes, "the physical is seemingly in the ascendancy even into our ranks," and yet, he viewed chiropractic as a beacon to transform the culture. He viewed this as a cultural evolution and a vision of service for humanity. A new way to live.

The way for this new awareness to move into society was for people of Innate awareness to replace the old with the new. He referred to this as an "Innate Positive Attitude." The challenge, he notes, was that few chiropractors were able to embody the new levels of thinking and too easily slipped back to the "physical plane," with its emphasis on the outside-in below-up perspective.

However, more and more chiropractors were developing the Innate Awareness and this was "multiplying upon itself," and thus, impacting the world. The explanation of this transformation is a journey from educated to illumination.

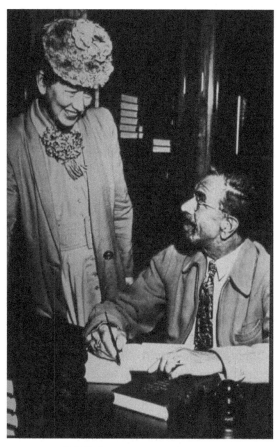

B.J. Palmer signing a book to
P.S.C. alum Dr. Margaret Peterson (1947)

An Evolved B.J. Palmer

A new attitude from B.J. extended to his approach towards the philosophy and other chiropractors. Perhaps, for the first time he wrote about love and gratitude in relation to service. He writes:

> Our Innate and the love FLOWING THRU US FROM ABOVE-DOWN, INSIDE-OUT reaches out to each of you and in addition our gratitude and thanks are unmeasured for what you have done, not for us, but for what can be done through us in the service of others.

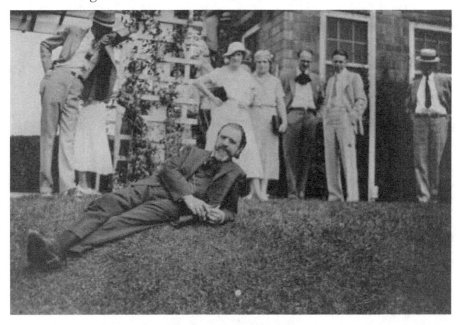

B.J. Palmer (1930s)

In these writings, he also softened to his critics. This is congruent with an observation from Dye, written in 1938, that B.J. grew more accepting in his later years. Interestingly, D.D. Palmer was also less critical in his final lectures. In Vol. 38, B.J. refused to condemn his critics and felt that "they don't know better and are doing the best they can, for what they think they know." This is a far cry from the B.J. Palmer of the 1910s, 1920s, or 1930s, who alienated many in the profession. The repercussions of the battles he and his rivals waged against each other are still being felt in the profession in the form of bias toward him, and a general lack of knowledge about his life's work.

The Great Divide

The Great Divide was described as a split, which started around 500 B.C., with Thales, the Greek philosopher. B.J. wasn't the first chiropractor to write about Thales, nor was this the first time he wrote on the topic, but this book was his most developed exploration of the theme. According to B.J., the split between the abstract and concrete, the inanimate and animate, death and life, is a hypothesized separation. In living reality these were never separate.

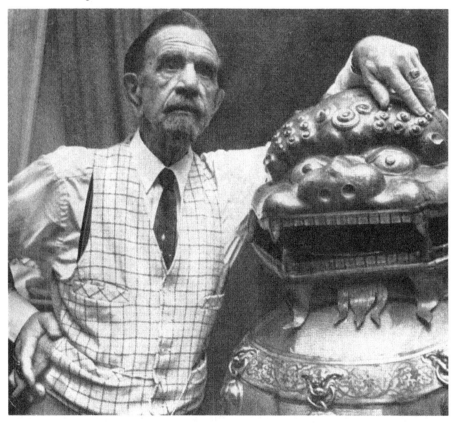

B.J. Palmer, *The Chiropractor* (1960)

This approach allowed B.J. to discuss broader themes like unity and disunity between mind and matter in a new way. He proposed that Thales' approach was to divide the indivisible, which led to two historic schools of thought. One led to medicine and physical materialism. The other led to mental or spiritual approaches from psychology to Spiritualism and, on the farthest end of the spectrum, Christian Science. He viewed the divide as a fundamental and historical foundation for the modern viewpoints on health and illness. One school of thought emphasized the body only and the other the mind only. He concludes that medicine was based on disunity between the mental and the physical.

B.J. positioned chiropractic as an enactment of the two perspectives. In living man there is no separation. The only way for one to fully know Universal Intelligence and Innate Intelligence is through various levels of embodied function. Unity of mind and body is expressed through the act of living.

Organized Life

As a way to sum up his theory to date, B.J. offered 25 chiropractic commandments. The foundation of these was Innate Intelligence, expressed as human and organized motion, which was the result of organized matter acted upon by power or energy. Organized life is mediated through the neural structures. Vertebral subluxation causes interference to this organization, which leads to dis-ease.

The Law of Capacity

B.J. first presented his theory of *Capacity* in June 1960, which was published in Vol. 37. In Chapter 10 of Vol. 38, he further developed it as *The Law of Capacity* also described as *The Law of Inherent Innate Capacity of Minds in Matter.*

This theory spans several levels of complexity in terms of evolution, biological forms, and an Innate oriented epistemology. For example, he describes two different ways of knowing: Above Down Inside Out (ADIO) and Outside In Below Upward (OIBU). He also proposed that there are types of minds just like there are different types of bones, malformations, and anomalies of the body.

B.J. describes a range of Educated capacities. One example he gives is understanding E=MC2 because not everyone has the capacity to understand it. Some people have capacity but act as though they don't. Also, there are veils that hide the educated mind from truth such as hatred, envy, ignorance, and prejudice. We can only do something about those who have capacity. There is nothing we can do about those who can't understand. For most, capacities are just dormant.

He links this to the Great Divide. For much of human history rational thinking had not yet developed. Rationality brings forth OIBU approaches and is reflected in educational thinking in the forms of medicine, religions, metaphysics, and psychology. Each one of these domains of knowledge tries to influence Innate in various ways.

B.J. relates this directly to chiropractic, the flow of mental impulse, and limitations of matter. He writes:

> Innate alone is great I am that I am—the oneness, the sub-limate, IN THE ABSTRACT, even when present in living man.
>
> However, Innate is limited in expression in matter ONLY by THE QUANTITY of mental impulse or nerve force flow REACHING MATTER to produce motion to produce function.
>
> Innate, per se, AS AN ABSTRACT INTELLIGENCE, is UNLIMITED. It BECOMES LIMITED by potentials of capacities contained WITHIN NORMAL MATTER, per se.

B.J. added capacity to his theory of Innate potential, which transformed his interpretation of the unity of mind and matter, Innate and matter, as well as Innate and Educated. The relationship between these levels of being were viewed as far more complex and yet simpler than he previously described. The basic structure of reality is part of the evolution of consciousness and awareness. This viewpoint discloses a "oneness" in living man.

He proposed there is a natural range of functions, which include the field of capacities. Potential is expressed as increasing levels of capacity. His example is how life evolves into increasing complexity in lifeforms; reptiles, birds, animals, bipeds, humans, then, levels of Educated. He writes:

> All animal, human, reptile, bird, or other living forms have some form of what we humbly think bipeds call education, which is a limited transference of a limited flow FROM Innate as bypassed through matter to permit us to associate with the environmental world which surrounds us. Even this small quantity of the unknown abstract is normally limited TO THE CAPACITY of the individual to normal, natural, and constructive uses. Even here, resistance frequently lowers quantity flow below normal, short-circuiting, shortening the circuit or circle, FROM brain TO body and FROM body back again TO brain. If this quantity IS interfered with, and

educational facilities be insane by comparison with the always-sane Innate, then insane education cannot restore sanity to itself. Even this still MUST come from the greater source ABOVE-DOWN, INSIDE-OUT, over which insane education, from OUTSIDE-IN-BELOW-UPWARD, has no control. Yet, as insane as educations are, they too often insanely think they can.

Too many of us are over-burdened carrying around sane educations. We pilaster on perverted educations of physiology, pathologies, diagnosis, treatments, all of which come from OUTSIDE-IN, BELOW-UPWARD. We need MORE KNOWLEDGE OF SOURCE and less of semi-source or even non-source, to reach factual realities. We are too prone to magnify insanities and thus belittle, question, or deny sanities.

He proposes that Innate is a reality "about and in us," and that our purpose is self-development by finding ourselves.

The Great Responsibility

In the talk from February 1960 to the ICA and the school heads, B.J. noted that there was a cancer growing in the profession affecting schools, legislation, state boards, licenses, and practices. He also noted that he was depressed and exhausted. His life was spent developing chiropractic's principles and practices, and after 60 years of daily work, he watched it being stolen "slowly from our grasp." The schools are our anchors to the future. He writes:

Today, we stand on the threshold of our GREAT responsibility to save what WE have... We have now come to the pass where we are casting this GREAT responsibility upon you younger men. You have a lifetime AHEAD of you. Our life is beginning to recede. We are passing THIS CHALLENGE to you, NOW, TODAY, to save what we have labored so long, so diligently, to protect, preserve, and survive for the sake of mankind.

The CHIROPRACTOR   7

Lyceum and Homecoming   1 9 6 0

Second Largest Attendance in Years — 6,432 Registered

Lyceum ad (1960)

Our Masterpiece: Vol. 39 (1961)

In 1961, B.J. completed Vol. 39, *Our Masterpiece*, the last Green Book. The text of Vol. 39 includes dates for 1961, which demonstrates that he continued working on it until the end of his life. The book traces the development of research, theory, and practice of chiropractic. He goes through every technological innovation from the NCM to the polygraph, clinical protocols from nerve tracing to the 1956 inclusion of misalignments, and even the evolution of adjusting tables. He also captures the philosophy at the highest levels of abstraction.

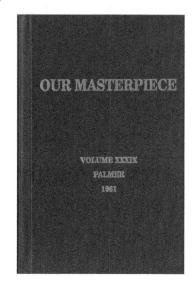

Vol. 39 cover

In Vol. 39, B.J. builds on previous theory and proposes at least one new term, "adjustment setment," which is the Innate adjustment that comes slowly and may be measured with comparative instrumentation. He also proposes two kinds of dis-ease, two kinds of results, and two vital principles. Dis-ease may be either below par quantity of nerve force flow or an adaptation to lowered function. The two kinds of results are the "stimulative temporary kind," and the "restorative energy permanent kind." The two vital principles are that the cause and cure are within and rehabilitation. Rehab of the dis-used part "must be done by internal use by patient himself." These last two principles were enacted in the research clinic.

In *Our Masterpiece*, B.J. included several new approaches based on the work at the research clinic. He considered the NCM patterns as determined by using the neurocalograph and the neurotempometer as unique as fingerprints. Research using the timpograph and the neurocalograph led to new ways to assess under adjusting, over adjusting, and the difference between true or false retracing. The nerve force was described in the book as normal rhythmic energy wave flow, which is expressed at a normal rate of function, sensibility, and tissue cell activity.

There are sentences and passages in Vol. 39 that were repeated from other Green Books. For example, *Our Masterpiece* has a chapter on Innate thot flashes (spelled as "thought flashes" in the 1966 publication), which includes several reorganized passages from Vol. 37. The chapter is the clearest explanation on the topic from any of the books. It is obvious that B.J. was fine-tuning the best of his ideas in order to present them as coherently as possible.

On Research

B.J. believed that chiropractic science, art, and philosophy were proven. He writes:

> There is only ONE issue, not "ten", to be proven scientific: That TIC is a (1) philosophy, (2) science and (3) art.
>
> a. No one element lives alone in living bodies.
>
> b. No one factor lives alone in sick or healthy bodies.
>
> c. It takes joint action of ALL THREE to prove TIC is SCIENTIFICALLY sound, Innately and physically.
>
> d. Without ANY ONE element, TIC fails to be true or sound.
>
> e. Without this unity we have NOTHING to prove.
>
> f. No NOT ONE of these three united living elements can be separated from the other two for "scientific" research, especially when one is exclusively physical, omitting its abstract producer, maintainer, and reproductive factor.

To sum up the research he writes:

> With 30 years of intensive application in this 'timpograph field, we were able to prove all correlated phases of chiropracTIC philosophy, science and art hitherto unknown. While men were spending millions to reach the moon, we spent 30 years to reach into the hitherto hidden normal and abnormal recesses of man's existence, where, why, how and when.

Cord Pressure Theory

B.J. expanded on his cord pressure theory in Vol. 39. He referred to two kinds of occlusion: bony or mechanical and soft tissue or callous. The first should be adjusted and the second should be given time to resolve because it involved inflammation around the cord and swelling of meninges. He proposed that the swelling squeezes the cord inward.

Limitless Innate Limited Matter

An extended quote from one of B.J.'s last chapters of Vol. 39 will provide us a place to pause in our study of these Green Books. We hope these words may inspire you to study the books and learn for yourself why the chiropractic series continues to captivate chiropractors and chiropractic students worldwide. B.J. writes of being an "Innate-chosen" human being. He writes:

> There is an issue of matter, where one can take just so much punishment down through the years, and no more. When that time arrives, Innate rebels and teaches the individual that a limitless Innate must do much within the limitations of a material body and, if the individual pushes beyond that breaking point, beyond human possibility, something gives, after which limitations of matter have been reached.
>
> The limitless Innate, thought-flashes an unlimited frequency of problems to a certain limited machine, who, through necessity, not convenience, has a limited time in which to move mountains of failures backed with prejudices.
>
> This limitless Innate and limited man-machine can do just so much, in his limited span of time from 1905 to 1961, and not more. Innate, pushing, squeezing, demanding every day be 16 to 18 hours, seven days a week, (including Sundays), every 52 weeks a year, proves that matter can only stand a limited wear and tear with a break-down, here and there, and then and now, which follows especially if the individual accepts every and all thought flashes demanding consistently, beyond its disability, something gives and the inevitable happens.
>
> To multiple people of limited matter, average day is an exhaustive 8 hours work, 8 of relaxing pleasure, and 8 of recuperative sleep. Not so with some especially Innate-chosen limited human being, through which the limitless Innate has chosen to perform definite and positive responsibilities.
>
> It is common procedure for this limitless Innate, to thought flash to the limited sleeping brain endless unlimited ideas during the so-called 8-hour restful period. There is no returning to sleep until the limited matters gets up, writes, rewrites that or those thought flashes concisely, in explanatory language; then, and not until, does the limitless Innate retire and let the limited matter return to sleep.

The more limitless Innate thought-flashes ARE respected in its demands, to record its unlimited interpretations of its law and principles, the more frequently they come, less rest sleeping limited matter gets, month by month, year by year. This breaks down restful periods, wears the man-machine to an exhaustive state of matter. The written word is praised, but the man-matter suffers in exact reverse ratio.

Matter, regardless of the body Innate exists within, can resist resisting conflicting frictions, to ITS human limit. After that it becomes human abuse. You can wisely suggest matter should hesitate, call a halt when it reaches the recuperative limit and exhaustive period. Innate, having nothing limit, having found an assemblage of matter appropriate to its biddings, thinks more of masses to be served, than of any one unit himself.

Every living person HAS an Innate, or he wouldn't be alive. EVERY such has organic functions as proof such exists within him. EVERY person GETS Innate thought-flashes. Vast majorities do not realize this, therefore are not conscious of such. The MORE educationally you DENY, the LESS you will RECEIVE. MORE you ADMIT such, MORE you CAN receive. Education is considered the new plus ultra, most essential, it is THAT WHICH he seeks, struggles and strives to get more and MOST of. Innate is the silent partner, unobserved, unknown. Because education is 99 percent for ambitious of people, they think mostly in terms of cramming more OF IT from OUTSIDE-IN BELOW-UPWARD, getting little of Innate percolating down and through to education. By reversing that order, all would realize Innate is the wholesome and reliable knowledge of ALL things while education is artificial, superficial, side-tracked counterfeit of THE REAL YOU WITHIN YOU. Is it sensible and logical to have more faith in a spoonful of medicine from outside than the intellectual power which built your body from inside?

The Innate-chosen with limited matter may only express intelligence for so many years. B.J. Palmer died May 21, 1961. His son, Dave Palmer, published the last two books in 1966 along with a reproduction of D.D. Palmer's *Science, Art, and Philosophy of Chiropractic.*

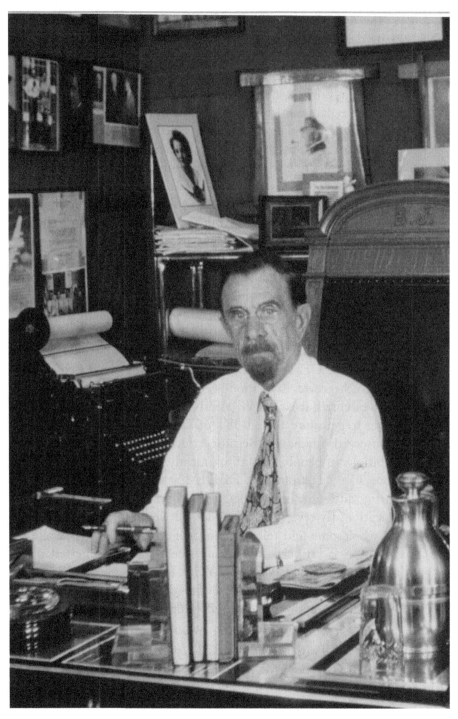

B.J. Palmer, President, ICA (1946)

Chapter 16
Green Book Collecting:
Special Considerations

When reviewing the Green Books from a collecting standpoint, you will need to take note of many physical details of each book. Simply looking at the title or year printed may not provide the details needed to properly identify the book. Many of the Green Books have different printings and editions. The rarity and value may vary widely depending on the printing or edition of the book.

Over the years, several Green Books have been reproduced to look almost exactly like the originals. Collectors must be careful and know what to look for. Without a guide like this, you could purchase a book that you thought was an original and pay a lot or sell an original for little. This guide will help you to know what you have, how rare it is, and its value.

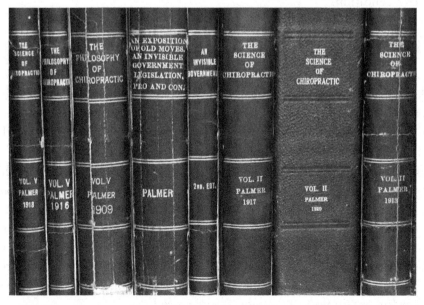

B.J. Palmer's personal bound black books stored in the archives at Palmer.
The Vol. 2 (1920), second from the right is a author's mock up-double thickness

Details about each book may be critical in identifying which edition or printing it is. Important details about the binding include: the color of the cover and end papers; the type of paper used to print; thread colors used for the binding; as well as the color, size, and shape of the guild. Other important publication details might include: year of publication, year of printing, whether there is any guild or not, and whether the spine matches the cover and title page. The specific edition of the book, along with the overall condition of the book, are significant factors when determining value.

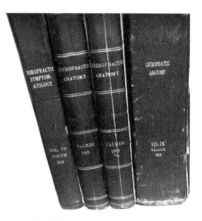

B.J. Palmer personal copies from the Palmer archives. The *Chiropractic Anatomy* on the far right is an author's mock up- double thickness

This chapter covers special considerations unique to the Green Books such as covers, volume numbers, missing volumes, unnumbered Green Books, other Palmer books, and details related to special editions and printings. Appendix 5 includes basic considerations when evaluating a book's condition.

Volume Numbers

B.J. Palmer's use of volume numbers for the Green Book series makes identification of the books seemingly simple. However, there are a few details to be aware of when looking at volume numbers. For example, several of the volume numbers were reused. Completely different books had the same volume number. In some instances, B.J. reused a volume number after the original volume was out of print. As we suggested in Chapter 8, this may have been for ease of advertising in the 1920s, specifically in the case of the new use of Vol. 3, Vol. 4, and Vol. 14. In this way, a full set of books could be advertised without having to account for volumes that were no longer in print. In other instances, in the 1950s, he reused Vol. 34, and Vol. 37. In these cases, the second use of a volume number was soon after the initial book was published by someone other than B.J. Palmer. We'll never know for certain why the numbers were reused.

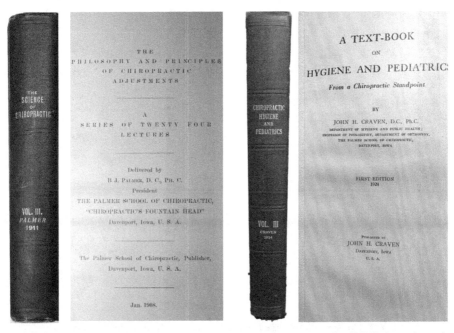

Vol. 3: *The Philosophy and Principles of Chiropractic Adjustment* by B.J. Palmer (1908) and *A Textbook on Hygiene and Pediatrics* by John Craven (1924)

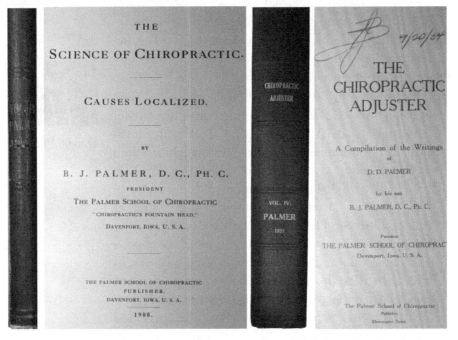

Vol. 4: *The Science of Chiropractic: Cause Localized* by B.J. Palmer (1908) and *The Chiropractic Adjuster: A Compilation of the Writings of D.D. Palmer* by B.J. Palmer (1921)

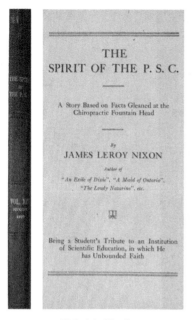
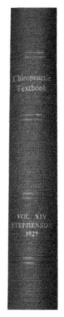
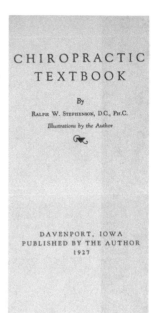

Vol. 14: *The Spirit of the P.S.C.* by James L. Nixon (1920) and
Chiropractic Textbook by Ralph W. Stephenson (1927)

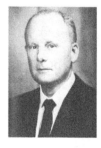

Donald Pharaoh published *Correlative Chiropractic Hygiene* in 1946, and the first Vol. 34 or *Chiropractic Orthopedy* in 1956. He was born August 27, 1914, in Worcester, MA and graduated from PSC in 1936. Of Pharaoh, Rolf Peters writes:

He grew up in Riverside, California, graduated from Riverside Junior College and attended the University of California at Los Angeles. Playing semi-professional football, he sustained a back injury, which led him to chiropractic. He graduated from the PSC in 1936... Pharaoh became a member of the faculty in 1938, teaching Anatomy, Histology, and acting as Athletic Director. He authored two books, *Correlative Chiropractic Hygiene* in 1946 and *Chiropractic Orthopedy* in 1956 as Volume 34 of the Palmer Green Books. In 1957 he became the founder and faculty advisor of Pi Tau Delta, a national chiropractic honor society...

Donald Pharaoh

Pharaoh was named Dean of Basic Sciences and remained on the faculty until his premature death on 30 September 1967.

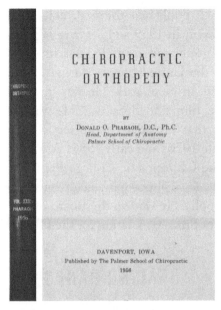 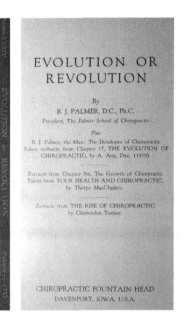

Vol. 34: *Chiropractic Orthopedy* by Donald O. Pharaoh (1956) and
Evolution or Revolution by B.J. Palmer (1957)

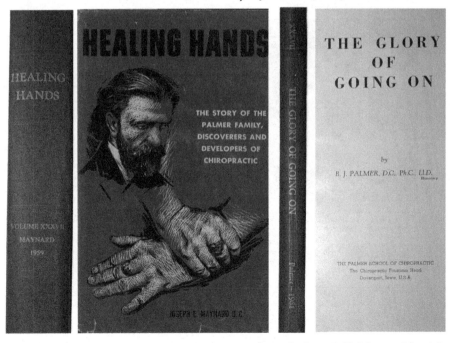

Vol. 37: *Healing Hands: The Story of the Palmer Family* by Joseph E. Maynard (1959)
and *The Glory of Going On* by B.J. Palmer (1961)
* future editions of *Healing Hands* by Maynard did not list a volume number

Joseph Edward Maynard, DC, PhC, published the first Vol. 37 or *Healing Hands: The Story of the Palmer Family* in 1959 and *Selective Writings of Daniel David Palmer* in 1982. He graduated from Palmer in 1949. During World War II, he served with the United States Marines. After graduation he practiced on Long Island, in New York. He was involved in many business ventures in real estate, film, and Broadway. He was the owner of Precision X-ray laboratories that provided X-ray services for many of the area chiropractors. In the late 1970s and early 1980s, Maynard served as administrative assistant to Life Chiropractic College President, Sid Williams. He was also department head of philosophy, faculty member and an instructor of chiropractic philosophy. He was on the Board of Life Foundation and was a founding member of the Association for the History of Chiropractic.

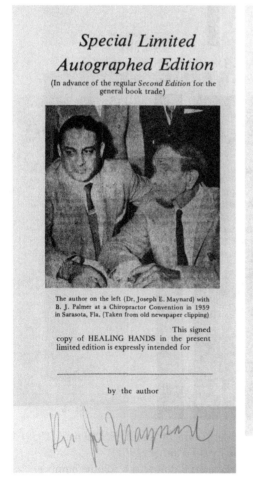

Special Limited
Autographed Edition

(In advance of the regular *Second Edition* for the general book trade)

The author on the left (Dr. Joseph E. Maynard) with B. J. Palmer at a Chiropractor Convention in 1959 in Sarasota, Fla. (Taken from old newspaper clipping)

This signed copy of HEALING HANDS in the present limited edition is expressly intended for

_____

by the author

"HEALING HANDS"

HEALING HANDS by Joseph E. Maynard, D.C., is the story of a service to mankind that has seldom been equalled in the history of the world.

HEALING HANDS is the story of the Palmer family who discovered and developed the philosophy, science and art of Chiropractic which, in the short period of three generations, has grown to become the second largest healing art in the world today.

HEALING HANDS is an intimate, authentic, and thrilling human drama, telling the inside story of Chiropractic and of the men and women the Creator entrusted with the job of giving Chiropractic to the world. The story is as strange and fascinating as fiction, yet it is true. It deals with human emotions, love, hate, trials, hardship, pioneering, heartbreaking struggles, hopes and despair; and the final triumph of a righteous cause through sacrifice, courage and a fighting spirit that would not be defeated.

You will enjoy reading this thrilling story, this human drama, that has meant so much to millions of people who are ill—a story that may reach into your own life with helping, healing hands that no other method of healing can offer.

Get and read HEALING HANDS by Joseph E. Maynard, published by Jonorm Publishing Company, P. O. Box 789, Freeport, L. I., New York. Price $5.00. You will be glad you did.

Advertisement for Healing Hands, *The Chiropractor*, 1960, January

Missing Vol. 30 and Vol. 31

There is no obvious explanation for the fact that B.J. Palmer did not designate any books as Vol. 30 or Vol. 31 in the Palmer Green Books series. This gap in book volume numbers happens between 1953 with Vol. 29 and 1955 with Vol. 32. Did B.J. have books written or planned during these years that were never completed and printed? There are no known drafts or other B.J. writings that fit into this time period that could be the "missing" volumes. Based on his autobiographical writings in his final years, it is unlikely that B.J. lost track of his Green Book numbering system. So, why is there a gap in numbers? There are a few possible explanations.

As we indicate in Chapter 12, B.J. was faced with significant health challenges in 1953. During that time, he reached out to his closest advisors who were in a dispute with B.J. over book publishing. B.J.'s advisors were concerned about the costs of publishing more books. We suggested that their angst was about the publication of Vol. 29, which was the largest of the eight books that were published during a four-year period. Perhaps they were also pushing back against other books? Perhaps B.J.'s health was a factor in the gap?

There are other possibilities for the missing volumes. What if the missing books were not planned as B.J. Palmer-authored books? Up to this point, PSC faculty had authored 12 of the 29 Green Books in print. PSC faculty members could have been working on books and B.J. left a space in the volume numbers to accommodate two new faculty-authored books. B.J. printed his Vol. 32 or *Chiropractic Philosophy, Science and Art* in 1955, and if the PSC faculty failed to complete and publish their planned books, B.J. was stuck with a gap in the numbering system. We note that PSC faculty member, Donald Pharaoh, published *Chiropractic Orthopedy* as Vol. 34 in

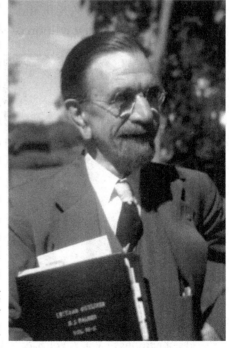

B.J. Palmer with book

1956, but B.J. published his own Vol. 34 *Evolution or Revolution,* the next year in 1957. After the Vol. 30 and 31 gap, B.J. never again left spacing in his Green Book volume numbering for faculty-produced books.

Unnumbered Green Books

It appears that B.J. Palmer did not initially plan to have the textbooks written by PSC faculty included as part of the numbered series of chiropractic books. None of the first edition books written by faculty prior to 1918 included a volume number. In 1914, Firth published *A Textbook on Chiropractic Symptomatology* with a dark blue cover and no volume number. In 1916, Vedder produced *A Textbook on Chiropractic Physiology* with a brownish-red cover and no volume number. The second edition of Vedder's book was published in 1918, with the same cover and no volume number. In 1918, Mabel Palmer produced *Chiropractic Anatomy* with the traditional green cover but with no volume number. In 1918, Thompson published *A Text on Spinography* as a soft covered booklet, also with no volume number.

In 1919, all of the faculty books were printed in the *Standard Green Book Format* (SGBF) with traditional green covers. These books were published with volumes 7, 8, 9, and 10 printed on the spines. Also in 1919, Burich published the first edition of Vol. 11 or *Chiropractic Chemistry* with

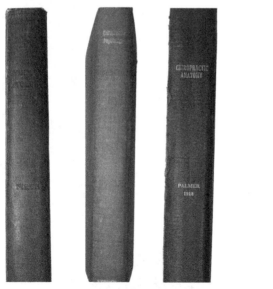

First editions of Vol. 7, Vol. 8, & Vol.9, *Correlative Chiropractic Hygiene*
all without volume numbers

the volume number on the spine. We conclude that by 1919, B.J. decided to include the PSC faculty-authored books officially as numbered volumes in his chiropractic series.

There are several other books that are not numbered that are defined as Palmer Green Books based on the definition of a Green Book from Chapter 17.

The definition includes D.D.'s two books, the supplements to volumes, Pharaoh's *Correlative Hygiene* and the Stephenson's *Art of Chiropractic*. It excludes other books authored by the Palmer family such as: *'Round the World with B.J.*, *Radio Salesmanship*, *The Palmer's*, *Three Generations*, *Stepping Stones*, and *All the Glory to God*.

Other Palmer Books

Even though several books written by B.J. Palmer and his family are not defined as Green Books, they still add value to any chiropractic book collection. Of these books, there are a few that stand out.

The Great Undertow was written by B.J. Palmer in 1929. The book was republished in 2011 by PSC graduate (1947), Harold Hughes, with the help of Rob Sinnott, DC. Sinnott worked with Hughes over an 18-month period to turn this manuscript into a text of 330 pages, published on demand as a hardcover by Lulu, Inc. On the storefront for the book on Lulu.com, Sinnott writes:

> Dr. Hughes passed from the physical plane days before this text went to print here, but thankfully his sons have completed the final steps and made it available to a profession in desperate need for the words etched across these pages. Dr. Palmer's last revision of this text was never published. It was dated weeks before the Great Depression struck America, and I suspect this to be the reason it was set aside for so long. As an avid historian of the profession, I promise you that this is without question the most important book written by B.J. Palmer. It is a book for TODAY. It speaks to the issues we face today with clarity, if we would but learn from these pages. Dr. Hughes had made arrangements for the proceeds of this text to go 100% to his student scholarship trust fund. An amazing man, and an even more amazing book. It has my wholehearted endorsement to any interested in the future of the profession. No Chiropractic

book collection is near complete without this book and it should be required reading in our schools!

The H.T. Hughes, DC Chiropractic Medal 75 Scholarship Trust is for chiropractic students.

We surmise that *The Great Undertow* would have had a volume number as part of the Palmer chiropractic book series if it was actually printed with a hard cover in 1929. Since it was not printed until 2011, we classify it as a Palmer-authored book and not as a Green Book.

'Round the World with B.J. was published in 1926. This book documents two trips around the world in the early 1920s by B.J., Mabel and Dave Palmer. During this period, PSC enrollment was at an all-time high and B.J. Palmer was a wealthy man. The Palmers traveled the world in luxury. The chapters include dozens of photos of the family on various adventures from India to Egypt. The chapters were read over the radio by B.J. on WHO, a radio station owned by Palmer. The book has no volume number and it is not a chiropractic textbook so it is not defined as a Green Book based on the definition.

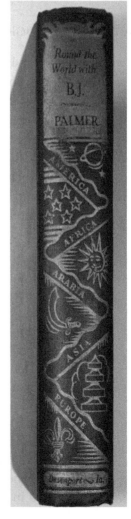

For collectors, condition of the cover is an important factor in the value of this book. Mint books have a brilliant blue cover with bright gold lettering. The blue is often faded and the gold rubbed off these books. There were two print runs of the first editions of *'Round the World with B.J.* Some were the standard edition and some were signed and numbered. Earlier numbers have some added value. The signed and numbered editions included an extra page in the front for a number and signature where B.J. occasionally wrote a brief inscription. In a section below we discuss signed and numbered editions in more detail.

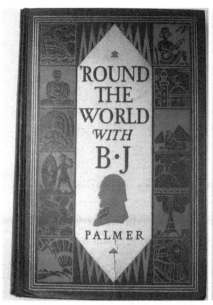 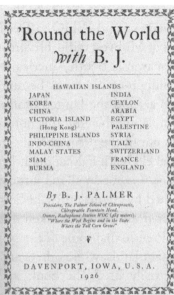

'Round the World with B.J. cover and title page (1926)

Radio Salesmanship: how its potential sales percentage can be increased for Radio Sponsors, Radio Agencies, Radio Copy-writers, Radio Broadcasters, Radio Station Managers, Radio Station Program Managers, Radio Station Announcers, was published in 1942. The book was initially 23 pages in length and printed in July 1942. A second edition, also with 23 pages was printed in August 1942. There is no known information about a third edition. The fourth edition included 83 pages and was printed in 1943. The fifth edition included 130 pages and was printed in 1944. These early editions were spiral bound soft covered (28 x 22 cm). The sixth edition was printed in 1947 as an oversized red hard covered book with 371 pages.

B.J. Palmer was prominent in the radio business. He purchased the first radio station west of the

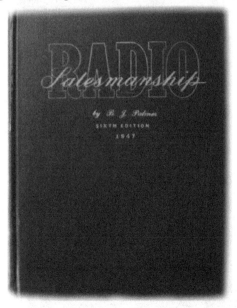

Radio Salesmanship by B.J. Palmer, sixth edition (1942)

Mississippi River in 1922. As the owner operator of WOC in Davenport and WHO in Des Moines, B.J. controlled a section of Midwest radio. His broadcast signals were picked up as far away as South America, the North Pole, Rome, and the Philippines. The book became a standard in broadcast schools around the United States. *Radio Salesmanship* has no volume number and it is not a chiropractic textbook, so it does not fit the definition of Green Book.

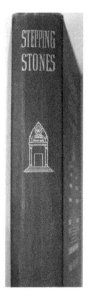

Mabel Heath Palmer published *Stepping Stones* in 1942 and *A Soliloquy,* a small red soft covered booklet of 19 pages published by Sigma Phi Chi Sorority. *Stepping Stones* is a memoir from her notes taken over 38 years. Mabel writes in the Preface that some of the stories were "on sea, some in far distant lands, while others are just homey observations in my daily life." The book includes her reflections on their world travels and notes about her life with observations about the world in general. Mabel writes, "In this changing world, where dogma, self opinion, indifference, and intolerance are said to run rife, I must say I find it otherwise. I firmly believe that the world is growing better-spiritually

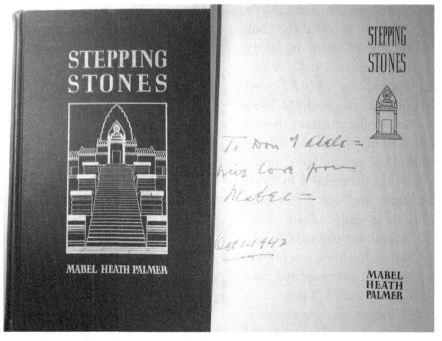

Signed edition of *Stepping Stones,* cover and title page

growing better-slowly, perhaps, but certainly true." This book adds new insights about the many stories captured in *'Round the World with B.J.* and Vol. 29 or *Upside Down and Right Side Up with B.J.* Mabel signed many copies of *Stepping Stones* with her purple pen in 1942.

Dave Palmer, son of B.J. and Mabel, wrote two books. *Three Generations* was published in 1967. It was a soft covered book of 59 pages with yellow/gold cover. *The Palmers* was published in 1977. This was a brown hard covered book of 184 pages with black dust jacket and a hard protective case. The book was published sometime in 1977 according to the Palmer College of Chiropractic Library, but no specific year appears in the book. Dr. Dave died on May 24, 1978.

Agnes Mae High Palmer, second wife of Dave Palmer and mother of his three daughters, published *To God Goes all Glory* in 1987. It was a blue soft covered book of 124 pages. The book includes 50 pages of images and an appendix.

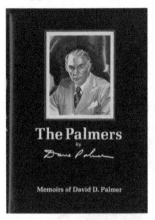 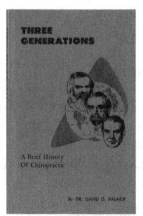 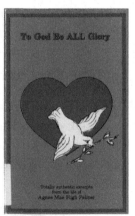

The Palmers (1977), *Three Generations* (1967), and *To God Goes all Glory* (1987)

Green Book Covers

The green colored covers are the most distinguishing feature of the Green Books and yet not every Green Book was originally printed with a green cover. Some were blue, red, black, gold, brown, and variations of the color green. The cover color is one of the simplest ways to identify the edition. Most of the books in the series are covered with a dark green cloth over a hard rigid board.

It is unlikely that, when B.J. published the first book in 1906, he intended to create a series of books called the Green Books. In the early days, books were ordered in short runs or printings. When B.J. sold out of the books on hand he ordered more books to be printed. Some had editorial changes to the content and some did not. We speculate that on a few orders the printer may simply have been out of the green cloth or had an abundance of another color cloth that could be offered at a reduced printing cost. Most of the cover color variations are found on the faculty-authored books. This is an indication that B.J. was not involved in their productions. Whatever the factor was, some books had different colored covers. In addition, B.J. had special printings done in leather as an upgrade or special edition to several of the early volumes. The cover color variation is mainly in the early editions. By the 1920s, the books were printed with green covers and had a consistent appearance or the *Standard Green Book Format.*

The SGBF were printed with dark green covers. The title and spine are printed with gold lettering. The spine includes the volume number printed in Roman numerals and the author's last name and year. The inside of the covers have green patterned end pages.

Leather Special Editions

It is a common practice for printers to make special "presentation" copies with book orders. The book author would request a single book or small amount of books that were bound in leather or with some other special aspect of the book to keep as their personal copy, present to important supporters, or to sell as a special edition.

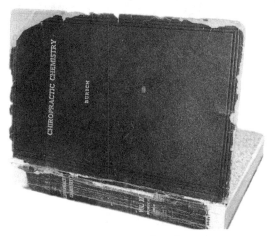 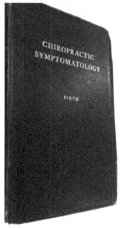

Leather editions

A red leather edition of *The Science of Chiropractic* was published in 1906 with no volume number. We believe that the very first 50 books printed of D.D. and B.J. Palmer's book has several unique features that can identify them. When the first books were ordered by B.J., he may not have initially envisioned a set of books with sequential volume numbers. The initial run of 50 did not have Vol. 1 printed on the spine like the rest of the 1906 books. These books are covered in red leather with black covers that extend the full length. This is different than the next run of leather covered books that had black covers with red triangle tips on the covers. There is a small oval photo of D.D. Palmer pasted across from the script. D.D. Palmer's signature is printed in the front pages. This set of books has a page in the front with a small number printed in the dead center of the page. This first run of 50 books was a numbered edition. (see other numbered editions later in this chapter). This book does not have a Wunder Bros. stamp like other leather presentation copies. It is not identified who bound the book. Wunder Bros. could have done the covering without stamping it.

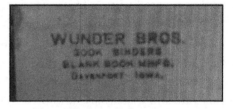

Wunder Bros. Stamp

Vol. 1, Vol. 2, and Vol. 6 were printed with red and black leather presentation copies. This could imply there are similar presentation copies of Vol. 3, Vol. 4, and Vol. 5. Since presentation editions are usually a very small number of books, and could be only a single book, these are very rare. There may be leather presentation copies of Green Books that have yet to be located by collectors. (The Green Book Master List in chapter 17 includes these books as "suspected" to have been printed.) It is possible leather presentation copies were printed for all of the first six volumes.

The 1906 edition of Vol. 1 and the 1907 edition of Vol. 2 were both printed by a local printer and some of the bound copies had covers done by Wunder Brothers. These two volumes were printed in red and black leather covered special editions. The spine is red and the covers are black with small red tips on the corners. The books have a small stamp from Wonder Bros. Davenport Iowa, inside the front cover. The Vol. 1 has a small oval photo of D.D. Palmer pasted across from the script of D.D. Palmer's signature printed on the front pages. These special edition books were a small printing run. It is unknown how many were printed. We speculate that 50 copies of Vol. 1 were printed and even less of Vol. 2 based on known surviving copies.

There is one known red and black leather presentation copy of Vol. 6. The style is very similar to the Wunder Bros.' printings of Vol. 1 and Vol. 2. The only minor difference is that the border between the red and black leather is accented with a gold line. This book does not have a Wunder Bros. stamp. The book binder is not identified. It is probable Wunder Bros. could have done the covering.

There are two known red leather bound copies of the original *The Science Art and Philosophy of Chiropractic* by D.D. Palmer, published in 1910. Of these two copies, one is over stamped 1911 and the other is not. It is unknown how many of these copies of D.D. Palmer's first book were printed. Others may exist.

In 1919 several of the faculty authored Green Books were printed with a soft, thin, brown leather cover. Dr. Thompson advertised and sold this leather covered edition of Chiropractic Spinography as "A limited Number Leather Bound" for $10, twice the price of the standard green cloth covered book. No other ads have been found for the other faculty Green Books that were produced with the brown leather cover. Several of these brown leatherette covered editions are in the Palmer Archives. These books are very rare and essentially unknown to Green Book collectors.

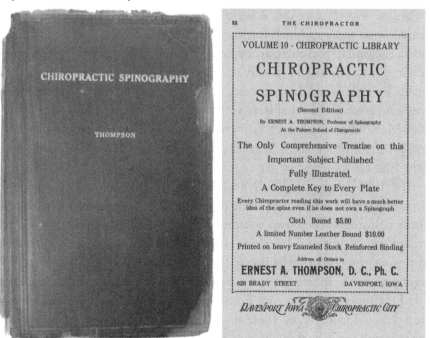

Leather edition of Thompson's text with advertisement

Known brown leatherette editions:

> *Chiropractic Symptomatology,* Second edition (1919)
> *Chiropractic Chemistry,* First edition (1919)
> *Chiropractic Spinography,* Second edition (1919)

It is speculated that the other books in the Green Book series printed during 1919 were also printed with the limited edition brown leatherette cover, but known copies have not been documented at this time. These books are accounted for on the Green Book Master List in Chapter 17 as "suspected" to have been printed.

The B.J. Palmer Private Collection Books

B.J. Palmer had his own personal collection of Green Books. These are considered single book author presentation copies. The Green Books in B.J.'s collection are bound in black leather boards with gold guild and red edged pages. These books are stored behind a locked glass cabinet in The Special Collections Archives Department at the Palmer College of Chiropractic in Davenport.

The B.J. Palmer Private Collection Books were the personal copies of B.J. and Mabel Palmer. Most were written by him plus Mabel's Chiropractic Anatomy published in 1918. Outside of this collection there is also one known copy of a black leather edition of Vol. 13 or *A Textbook on the Palmer Technique of Chiropractic*. It appears to be a personal copy as well, which would mean that B.J. Palmer personal editions probably stop at 1920.

There is no evidence of any other B.J. Palmer books bound in black beyond 1920. The only known copies are the six in the collection and the one privately owned Vol. 13. B.J. authored a total of 25 Green Books. If other black leather books were printed after 1920, there could be another 18 black leather bound books in existence.

There are a few other personal black bound books in B.J.'s collection. These include a first edition of *An Invisible Government*. It was bound with an *Exposition of Old Moves*, published 1911-1916. He also had a leather edition of the second edition of *An Invisible Government* bound in black by itself. There are four bound *PSC School Announcements* as well as 12 volumes of *The Chiropractor*.

Author Mock-ups

It is common practice for a book printer to produce a special mock-up of a book for the author. This book contains a blank page inserted between each page of text. This mock-up allows for an author to make notes and plan revisions for future editions. The addition of a blank page for each page of text doubles the thickness of the book. Examples of these can be found in the Palmer Archives with several of them in the brown leatherette covered editions. The Archives contain mock-ups of Vol. 2 (1920), Vol. 5 (1920), and Vol. 9 (1918). A first edition mock-up copy of Craven's Vol. 15 (1921) is known to exist in a private collection. It is possible other faculty-authored mock-ups exist outside of the Palmer Archives.

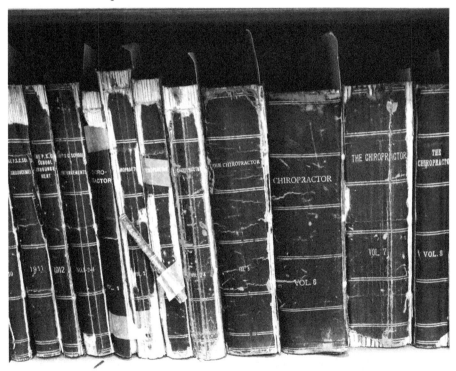

B.J. Palmer's collection

Also in a private collection is a 1907 edition of Vol. 2. It was printed by Wunder Bros. with a red and black cover. B.J. used it to make his revisions for the second edition of Vol. 2. The book has papers inserted where B.J. typed revisions and additions to the first edition. There is also a mock-up of *Round the World* in a private collection.

Signed and Inscribed Books

Signing books is a common practice for authors. There is one known copies of a signed editions of D.D. Palmer's 1910 book. However, there are many Green Books signed by B.J. Palmer.

At Lyceum each summer in Davenport, B.J. would make a point to autograph his latest book. Most of the time B.J. did not sign his name in books, instead, he signed his initials with the flowing, overlapping, script of B.J. His early signature did not overlap the B and J. Also, the script B was formed differently. (See examples on the next page.) In some books, B.J. would write a brief message or inscription. There are fewer ex-

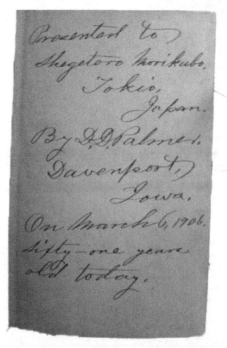

D.D. Palmer's inscription to Morikubo

amples of B.J. signed editions of the early Green Books. The practice of B.J. initialing books became more common in the 1950s when he started producing a new book each year.

An inscription, initial, or signature from a Green Book author does not increase the value very much. A book that was initialed or inscribed by B.J. adds minimal value to a Green Book. In general it could increase the value between $25 - $45, depending on the specific book and the inscription. B.J. initials in Green Books from the early 1920s are more valuable than books from after that time. Books signed or initialed by B.J. Palmer from before 1911 could be worth an additional $100. Signed copies from other PSC faculty generally adds $15-$25 depending on the book value and author's fame. For example, a signed Ralph Stephenson's *Chiropractic Textbook* would be more valuable than a signed copy of Percy Remier's *Modern X-ray Practice*.

While not common, there are certainly fake signatures out there. Knowing each author's authentic signature helps collectors to verify authenticity.

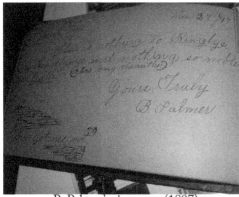

B. Palmer's signature (1897)

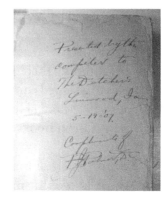

B.J. Palmer's signature (1907)
(Formation of the "B' is inconsistent
around this time

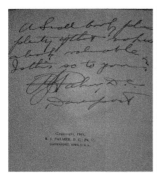

B.J. Palmer's signature
(1908)
(Formation of the "B' is
inconsistent around this
time.)

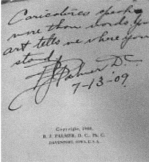

B.J. Palmer's signature
(1909)
(Formation of the "B" is
now consistent)

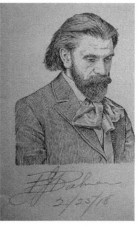

B.J. Palmer's Signature
(1918)

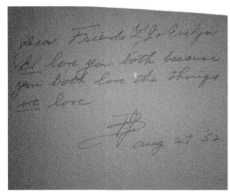

B.J. Palmer's initials (1952)

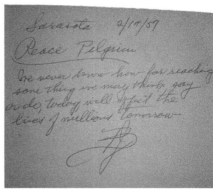

B.J. Palmer's initials (1957)

Numbered Editions

A numbered edition has a specific number that identifies each copy. The very first print run of the 1906 *Science of Chiropractic* was a numbered edition. B.J. produced two other books that were marketed as signed and numbered special editions. The books were, *'Round the World with B.J.* in 1926 and *Subluxation Specific Adjustment Specific* in 1934. These special editions were printed with an extra page for a signature. The page also identified the book as a signed and numbered edition.

'Round the World with B.J. stated that 1,000 signed and numbered editions were printed. The numbering was handwritten by B.J. Some of the books had inscriptions and some just the script, "B.J." It is unlikely that he kept up with the correct numeral to write. These special editions were available for decades. Some known copies were signed in the mid-1950s. It is possible there are gaps or even reused numbers. Also, there are unsigned and unnumbered copies of this edition in private collections.

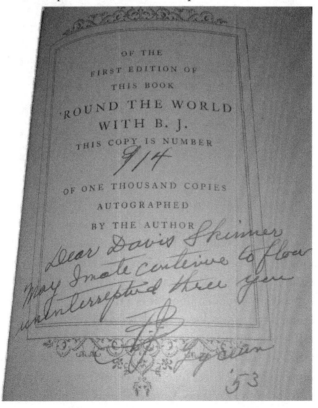

Signed numbered edition of *'Round the World with B.J.* (signed 1953)

The special editions of Vol. 18 had a specific number printed at the top of the extra page. B.J. probably learned his lesson from hand numbering hundreds of copies of *'Round the World*. Based on how many known copies there are of this edition, we estimate that 400 of these special signed and numbered editions of Vol. 18 were produced. Along with the printed number, a six line inscription was printed in each book. Given the low number of these books produced, it would be easy for a collector to assume they had a copy that was personally inscribed by B.J. Unfortunately, that is not the case. The initialed "B.J." is a unique hand-written signature by Palmer, but the eloquent inscription is printed in all of these editions along with each book's unique number.

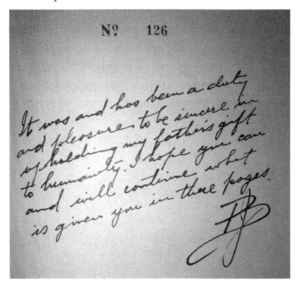

B.J. Palmer signed and numbered Vol. 18

The first edition of Remier's Vol. 21 or *Modern X-ray Practice* and *Chiropractic Spinography*, published in 1938, is also individually numbered. The book states this was an effort to assign ownership of each specific book. This faculty-authored Green Book is not highly valued by collectors. Most collectors probably do not even know it is a numbered edition because they have never opened the book due to its dated and technical content.

It is possible an extremely low number could add more to the value, especially with the B.J. authored books. However, added value to the Remier *Modern X-ray* book because of lower number is unlikely. We have not seen any of the numbered books traded or collected with the intent of looking for the lowest possible number.

Non-Traditional Sized Green Books

Two of B.J. Palmer's Green Books were printed in non-traditional sizes. In 1938, Vol. 20 or *Precise, Posture Constant, Spinograph, Comparative Graphs* was published as an oversized book measuring eleven by sixteen inches. It is a spiral bound text of 207 pages with a soft gold-colored cover. In 1958, Vol. 35 or *History in the Making* was published as a small booklet of 72 pages with a soft red cover measuring six by nine inches.

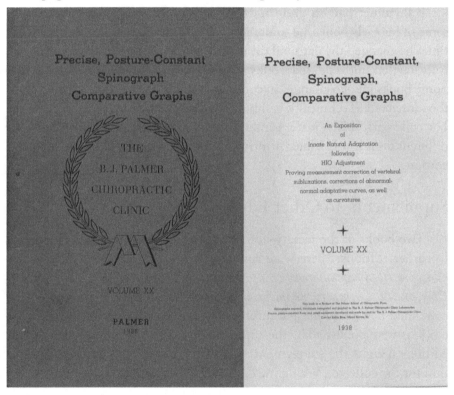

Oversized Vol. 20

Editions vs. Printings

In the publishing world there are various ways to describe books and the order in which they are produced. Most are familiar with a first edition book. Printings or print runs are not as commonly discussed. Any edition may be printed at different times or have different print runs. If the book is unchanged, it is considered a different printing. Most print runs are done very close in date. An author may order 50 books printed. A month later another 50 books are ordered and printed. This is the same book, but two different print runs. Printing books this close together is not usually identified in the books. Sometimes there can be subtle differences that a collector may detect such as a different paper used, different dye color, or different patterned end pages. If the printing is done after a longer period of time, the printing may be noted in the book, with a different year printed on the title page. When there is true content change, revision, or update of the content, the book is considered a different edition.

B.J. Palmer had an unorthodox style of publishing. When reprinting some of his early books, he sometimes added a new date to the spine. Other times he changed the date and the edition number. Some of these texts were truly revised and updated books so the edition change was appropriate. Some books had no changes in content so this is just a different printing of the same book. Technically, it should not have been listed as a new edition. For collectors, this is just an interesting fact. Each book is identifiable as different even if it is a later printing. The GBML uses B.J.'s style of stated editions.

Supplements To Other Editions

Two books of the faculty-authored Green Books offered supplements to earlier editions. There were supplements to the first edition of Firth's *Chiropractic Symptomatology Supplement*, printed in 1919, and Burich's *Chiropractic Chemistry Supplement*, printed in 1925. These supplements contained new or additional information and were printed before revised editions were published by the authors. Since not every buyer of those new editions bought the supplement, these supplements are rare and hard to find for the collector. We define each supplement as at Green Book.

Modern Reprints

Today nearly every volume has been reprinted, some by several different groups. It is important for collectors to be able to distinguish modern reprints from originals. There are many modern reprints after 1980. Most, but not all, are identified on the title page as a modern reprint. For this reason we have chosen to limit documentation of specific reprints to those done before 1980.

There are some modern reprints that are not identified as such. The cover and paper of any book should be examined and compared to known original printings. If the condition is too good to be true it is unlikely to be a mint edition book just out of a box after 90 years. It is more likely a modern reprint. Green Book buyers and sellers should identify their books with due diligence.

The Delta Sigma Chi Fraternity in Davenport, Iowa, has reprinted and sold Green Books for many years. These modern printings have the basic green covers of the original but are clearly marked reprints.

Dr. Michael U. Kale and the Kale Foundation reprinted many of the Green Books. These books are easy to identify as they have black covers with "Special Edition Kale Foundation" in large lettering on the cover. The Kale printings are good reading copies of the books but they are not sought after by most Green Book collectors. Their value is no different than any other modern reprint.

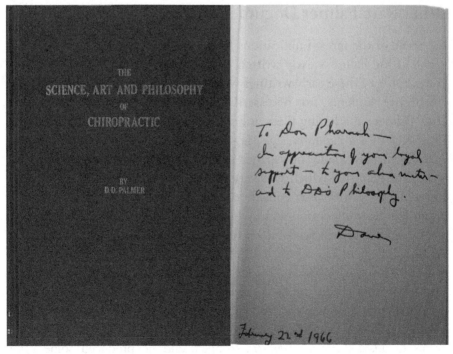

1966 edition of D.D. Palmer's *Science, Art and Philosophy of Chiropractic*
signed by Dave Palmer

Dr. Fred Barge provided Dr. Jim Parker of the Parker Chiropractic College with an original 1906 edition of Vol. 1 or *The Science of Chiropractic*. According to Barge, that copy was used to make the 1988 reprint. The books have a red cloth cover and were marked as a reprint. Also, page 95 is not upside down as it is with the original 1906.

In 1966, Dr. Dave Palmer reprinted his grandfather's book, *The Science, Art, and Philosophy of Chiropractic*, originally published in 1910. This reprint is the edition that most of the profession have seen. The headband in the spine in this book will have yellow and red stripes. It includes a foreword to the book with a message from Dr. Dave as well as a 1966 date at the end of that page. The copyright page still says 1910. This version was the first of the founder's book made readily available to the profession. The original 1966 printing is now 50 years old. The book has been printed numerous times over the years since the 1966 printing.

Other Rare Palmer Documents

Some of the rarest publications from the Palmers are not books at all. Much of the Palmer's early written material was promotional advertising. The purpose of these early writings was likely for marketing to patients and prospective students, not necessarily for teaching. The materials include D.D. Palmer's marketing fliers or broadsides published between 1894 and 1902 such as *The Educator*, *The Magnetic Cure*, and *The Chiropractic*. These were essentially small newspaper-styled publications with inexpensive newsprint material, which was very fragile. Since these were advertising materials, they were not considered true educational materials for the purpose of learning chiropractic. These artifacts do not meet the definition of a Green Book. Very few of these materials exist outside of the archives at Palmer College of Chiropractic. Also, some of these early editions printed by D.D. Palmer have been mentioned in the literature but not documented from any source. There are no surviving examples of several publications.

Other rare documents include publications by D.D. Palmer during his travels to California starting in 1902. While he was in California, publication of his broadside, *The Chiropractic*, stopped, and he produced some print material. The only known copies are in the Palmer archives.

There are no known examples of early teaching notes for either D.D. or B.J. Palmer. D.D.'s initial instruction of students was apprentice style.

Here are Kiro points = Do you see them?

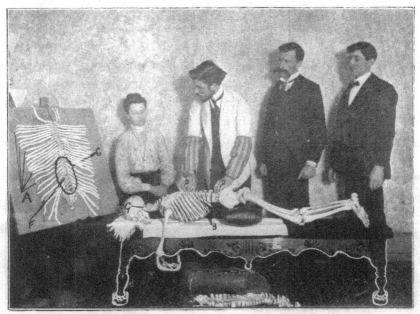

B.J. Palmer advertisement, 1902 or 1903

We suspect the more formal process of teaching students by B.J. began with written lessons and lecture notes. No one is exactly sure when these first lessons were put to pen and paper. Oakley Smith said when he was there in 1899 there were no notes from D.D. Palmer for students. From Palmer correspondences in 1903, it can be established that The Palmer Chiropractic School in Santa Barbara did have class notes for students. No surviving copies are known to exist. In fact, no D.D. Palmer lecture notes have been documented from the time before the first Palmer book was printed in 1906.

Other rare Palmer documents include the early issues of the magazine, *The Chiropractor*, starting in December 1904 and going through 1961. The early issues of this journal were printed as a small paper booklet stapled in the center with heavier paper than the old newspaper stock of the prior publications. Like the other Palmer publications it was marketing about chiropractic. It was not a true teaching vehicle for students.

Other rare documents from this time period include copies of D.D. Palmer's journal, *The Chiropractor's Adjuster*, published while he lived in Portland. Only six copies of these journals are known to exist with dates from January 1909 to February 1910. Copies of every known issue is housed in the Palmer archives.

In the early years of the PSC, B.J. Palmer produced large volumes of print material. He opened and operated a printing plant on the campus of the PSC. It was sometimes referred to as Ye Olde PSC Printery, the prettiest printing plant in the world, and modeled after the printery of the Roycrofters. The PSC Printery mainly produced supplies for the profession. This included items such as customized letterhead, envelopes, advertising tracks, and brochures. Many of the small Palmer booklets were printed there as well. The PSC Printery did not print the early Green Books.

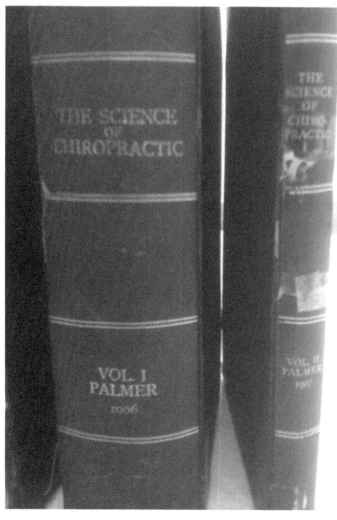

Leatherbound editions of Vol. 1 and Vol. 2

Chapter 17
Green Book Master List

A Green Book is any one of the books written by D.D. Palmer, B.J. Palmer or the faculty of the Palmer School of Chiropractic, for use in teaching chiropractic principles and methods. In addition, if a book was published with a volume number as part of the B.J. Palmer chiropractic series, all future editions are considered a Green Book even if the volume number was dropped.

There are some books published by B.J. Palmer and other PSC faculty that should not be considered Green Books such as *'Round the World with B.J.*, *Radio Salesmanship*, and Mabel Palmer's *Stepping Stones*. None of these or other books in their class meet the definition of a Green Book. Other books like Stephenson's *Art of Chiropractic* and Pharaoh's *Correlative Chiropractic Hygiene* are defined as Green Books.

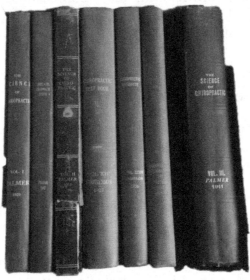

Green Books

Green Book Master List

We created the Green Book Master List (GBML) as a comprehensive designation system for the Green Books. This system is a way to distinguish between every edition of the Palmer Green Books. The GBML includes detailed identifying descriptions of originally printed Palmer Green Books. Each listing on the GBML is comprised of title, volume, edition, author, printing date, number of pages, city and publisher, physical characteristics, as well as ratings on rarity, value, and desirability. The list includes six reprints, which were printed between 1949 and 1979. It is important to be aware of the reprints so that they are not mistaken for original books because some were reprinted between 50-79 years ago.

Each book has been assigned a specific number or a Green Book Master Number (GBMN). The GBMN allows collectors to easily identify a specific Green Book. This master list number should be used when buying, selling, or trading books. It will ensure all parties know exactly what book is being discussed.

The GBML and the specific GBMNs were developed primarily for collectors. However, this designation system should also be adopted by historians and anyone interested in the development of ideas as they emerged from the Palmers and the original school of chiropractic over the course of the first half of the twentieth century.

The complete GBML with each individual GBMN is listed in Appendix 6 as a bibliographic list of Green Books with author, volume, title, and cover color information. More details about each book may be found below.

What is a "Set of Green Books?"

Chiropractors collect Green Books for a variety of reasons. Some seek the written knowledge contained within the texts. Others collect Green Books as a hobby, like collecting wine, stamps, or baseball cards. Green Book collectors have a deep emotional connection to the Palmers and the chiropractic profession. These individuals are passionate about their lives as chiropractors and collecting Green Books serves as a material connection to the profession they love.

Generally stated, collectors are trying to acquire each of the individual Green Book volume numbers and obtain what they would consider a complete set of Green Books published. While this sounds like a simple task, it is actually very complicated as some volume numbers were reused and many of the editions were significantly altered as B.J. revised his work over decades. Collectors consider some books with the same volume number to be different books. As an example, Vol. 1 1906 is a completely different book than the revised Vol. 1 1910, 1917 or 1920.

It is common for Green Book aficionados to say they have "a set of Green Books." However, that general statement does not reveal the specifics about their collection. Up until now a "set of Green Books" has never been defined.

Here are five classifications to describe various collections of Green Books:

Level 1 Set

A minimum of 20 books including any volume or non-volume numbered Green Books. This is essentially a beginner's collection of Green Books. A collection of less than 20 Green Books is not yet considered a set.

Level 2 Set

A set of one edition of all the unique volume and non-volume numbered Green Books. This would include one book of each of the reused volumes published as Vol. 3, Vol. 4, Vol. 14, Vol. 34, Vol. 37, plus *Correlative Chiropractic Hygiene* and *The Art of Chiropractic*. Collectors consider the 1906 Vol. 1 as a different book than the other revised editions. A Level 2 set only needs one copy of Vol. 1. This would be a total of 44 books (It does not have to include original copies of D.D. Palmer's two books, the signed and numbered or the supplements to editions, etc.)

Level 3 Set

A set of all first editions. This is the same as the Level 2 set, except all the volumes are first editions. The 1906 Vol. 1 would be needed. (Vol. 10 first edition is not required, as only two copies of this book are known to exist).

Level 4 Set

A set of all the volumes and all printings of the published volumes. D.D. Palmer's two books and the supplements are needed. Level 4 does not require the special leather bound editions, special editions, signed & numbered, although these may certainly count for a required book in the set.

Level 5 Set

Some collectors have taken collecting to extremes and sought a copy of each book ever printed. This level of collecting would essentially include every book on the GBML. It is a set of all volumes, all editions, all printings. This is also called a Green Book Master List collection.

Set Examples

Each of these levels may be collected as all signed editions. Example Level 2 set: all signed copies. Some will describe their collections as a Level X set minus four, indicating they need four books to have that level of set.

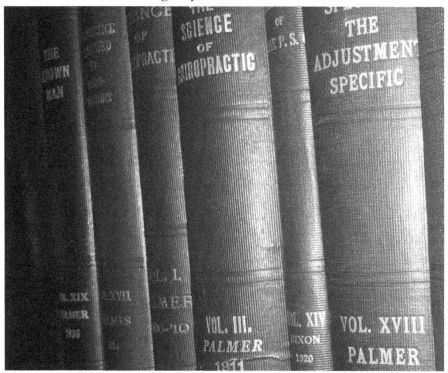

Green Book Master List

GBMN 1

Title: The Science, Art and Philosophy
of Chiropractic
"The Chiropractor's Adjuster"
Volume: None
Edition: First
Author: D.D. Palmer
Printing Date: 1910
Pages: 1007
Publisher: Portland Printing House Co.
City: Portland, Oregon
Rarity: 9.6
Value: 9.6
Desirability: 9.5
Physical Characteristics:

This book has green cloth boards with gold print, the spine reading "The Chiropractor's Adjuster by D.D. Palmer, 1910, Portland Printing House Co." The inside papers are dark green. This edition will have the thin red on white striped headband or binding threads. For specific detail about the physical characteristics used to differentiate the various printings of D.D. Palmer's 1910 book, consult Appendix 7.

Date Acquired:

Price:

Notes:

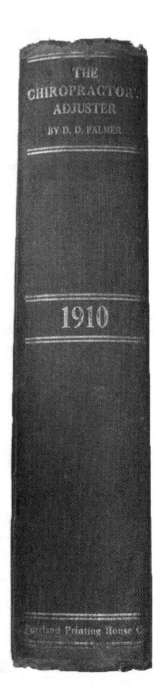

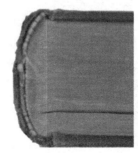

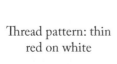

Thread pattern: thin
red on white

GBMN 2

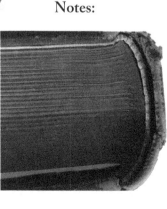

Title: The Science, Art and Philosophy
of Chiropractic
"The Chiropractor's Adjuster"

Volume: None

Edition: First

Author: D.D. Palmer

Printing Date: 1910

Pages: 1007

Publisher: Portland Printing House Co.

City: Portland, Oregon

Distinctive Marks: Red/maroon leather boards. Thread pattern: thin red on white.

Rarity: 10

Value: 10

Desirability: 10

Physical Characteristics:

This is a red leather covered presentation version of the original 1910 first edition (GBMN 1). It is common for an author to have a fancier covered printing done of their book to present to special supporters. It is unknown if there were more than one printed.

Date Acquired:

Price:

Notes:

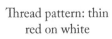

Thread pattern: thin
red on white

GBMN 3

Title: The Science, Art and Philosophy
of Chiropractic
"The Chiropractor's Adjuster"

Volume: None

Edition: First

Author: D.D. Palmer

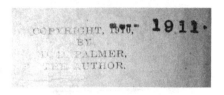

Printing Date: 1910 (1911 overstamp)

Pages: 1007

Publisher: Portland Printing House

City: Portland, Oregon

Distinctive Marks: Green board with purple 1911 overstamp. Thread pattern: thin red on white.

Rarity: 9.6

Value: 9.6

Desirability: 9.5

Physical Characteristics:

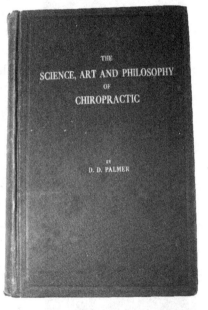

This book has the same characteristics as GBMN 1 with an additional small purple inked 1911 stamped over the printed 1910 on the copyright page of the book. For specific detail about the physical characteristics used to differentiate the various print-ings of D.D. Palmer's 1910 book, consult Appendix 7.

Date Acquired:

Price:

Notes:

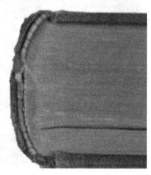

Thread pattern: thin
red on white

GBMN 4

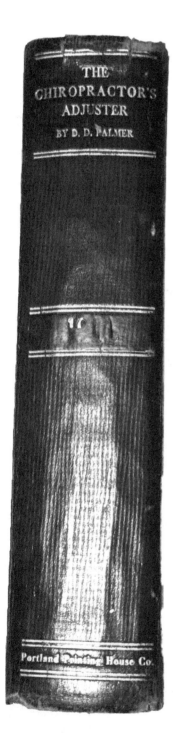

Title: The Science, Art and Philosophy
of Chiropractic
"The Chiropractor's Adjuster"

Volume: None

Edition: First

Author: D.D. Palmer

Printing Date: 1910 (1911 overstamp)

Pages: 1007

Publisher: Portland Printing House Co.

City: Portland, Oregon

Distinctive Marks: Red/maroon leather board with purple 1911 overstamp. Thread pattern: thin red on white.

Rarity: 10

Value: 10

Desirability: 10

Physical Characteristics:

This is a red leather covered presentation version of the original 1911 overstamped first edition (GBMN 3). It is the same as GBMN 2, with the additional 1911 purple overstamp on the 1910 copyright date. It is unknown if there were more than one printed.

Date Acquired:

Price:

Notes:

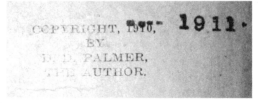

GBMN 5

Title: The Science, Art and Philosophy
          of Chiropractic
       "The Chiropractor's Adjuster"
Volume: None
Edition: Reprint of first edition
Author: D.D. Palmer
Printing Date: 1949
Pages: 1007
Publisher: Chiropractic Research Foundation
City: Webster City, Iowa
Rarity: 6
Value: 5
Desirability: 4
Physical Characteristics:

This 1940s reprint is almost exactly the same as the original 1910 book. The book's size, cover color, paper thickness and text font is all nearly identical to the original 1910 edition. The copyright page is identical to the 1910 original book with a 1910 copyright date. It is nearly impossible to tell them apart. The headband or binding threads of this 1940s printing is thick blue and white threads. There is a 1940s reprint with thick red and yellow binding threads (See GBMN 6). For specific detail about the physical characteristics used to differentiate the various printings of D.D. Palmer's 1910 book, consult Appendix 7.

Date Acquired:

Price:

Notes:

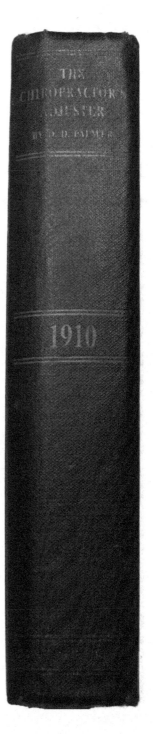

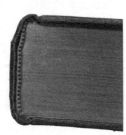

Thread pattern: thin
blue on white

GBMN 6

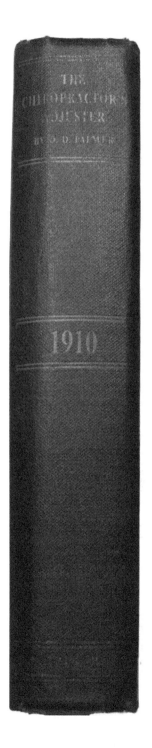

Title: The Science, Art and Philosophy
of Chiropractic
"The Chiropractor's Adjuster"

Volume: None

Edition: Reprint of first edition

Author: D.D. Palmer

Printing Date: 1949

Pages: 1007

Publisher: Chiropractic Research Foundation

City: Webster City, Iowa

Rarity: 9

Value: 6.5

Desirability: 4

Physical Characteristics:

Same as GBMN 5 except binding threads are thick red and yellow.

Date Acquired:

Price:

Notes:

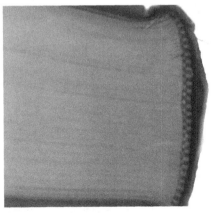

Thread pattern: thick red with yellow

GBMN 7

Title: The Science, Art and Philosophy
of Chiropractic
"The Chiropractor's Adjuster"
Volume: None
Edition: Reprint of first edition
Author: D.D. Palmer
Printing Date: 1966
Pages: 1007
Publisher: Palmer School of Chiropractic
City: Davenport, Iowa
Rarity: 1
Value: 2
Desirability: 3
Physical Characteristics:

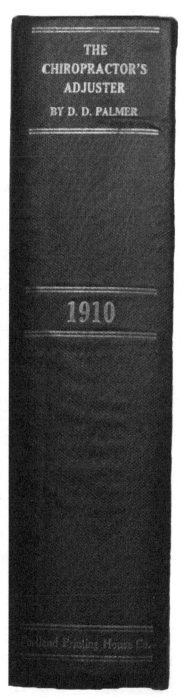

The grandson of D.D. Palmer, Daniel David Palmer II (Dr. Dave Palmer), reprinted the original 1910 book in 1966. This book does not identify itself as a reprint on the copyright page. It has the addition of a two-page foreword in the front of the book containing a message from Dr. Dave and a 1966 date at the end of that page. The 1966 reprint by Dr. Dave Palmer is what most of the profession has seen. This version was the first time the founder's book was readily available to the profession. The book has been printed numerous times over the 50 plus years since the 1966 printing. The headband in the spine in this book will have thick yellow and red stripes. Identifying a true 1966 printing of the book has not been established.

Date Acquired:

Price:

Notes:

GBMN 8

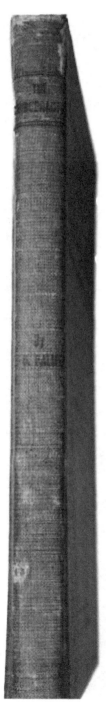

Title: The Chiropractor
Volume: None
Edition: First
Author: D.D. Palmer
Printing Date: 1914
Pages: 115
Publisher: Beacon Light Printing Co.
City: Los Angeles, California
Rarity: 10
Value: 10
Desirability: 10
Physical Characteristics:

This small (6x9) light green covered book had gold lettering of the title on the cover. It was produced by Mary Palmer just over three months after D.D. Palmer died in Los Angles. Palmer's widow, Mary Palmer, completed the publication using the newly revised and updated notes of the founder. For more information see Appendix 2. This book had a small print run with an estimated 50 books printed in 1914. An inside page has a transparent spider web pattern that goes over the D.D. Palmer image.

Date Acquired:

Price:

Notes:

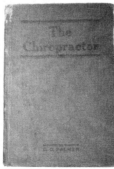

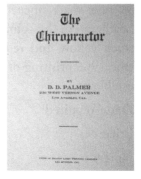

GBMN 9

Title: The Chiropractor
Volume: None
Edition: Reprint of first edition
Author: D.D. Palmer
Printing Date: 1969
Pages: 115
Publisher: Earl R. Bebout
City: Indianapolis, Indiana
Rarity: 4
Value: 4.5
Desirability: 5
Physical Characteristics:

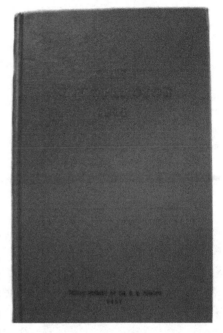

This edition of *The Chiropractor* was published with a red cover. Dr. Earl Bebout, the president of Bebout Chiropractic College, printed at least 200 and maybe more of this book. There two print runs. For more information see Appendix 2. Citing the desire to share with the profession D.D. Palmer's largely unknown second book, Bebout re-printed the original.

Date Acquired:

Price:

Notes:

GBMN 10

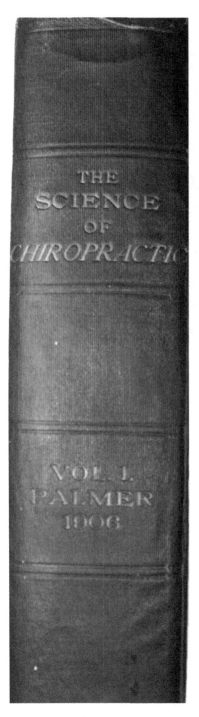

Title: The Science of Chiropractic
Volume: 1
Edition: First
Author: D.D. Palmer, B.J. Palmer
Printing Date: 1906
Pages: 420
Publisher: Palmer School of Chiropractic
City: Davenport, Iowa
Distinctive Marks: Green cover
Rarity: 9.7
Value: 9.8
Desirability: 10
Physical Characteristics:

This 1906 book was printed in the standard Green Book format. The title page lists it as a 1906 first edition. There is no oval image of D.D. Palmer pasted over his signature in front of the book.

Date Acquired:

Price:

Notes:

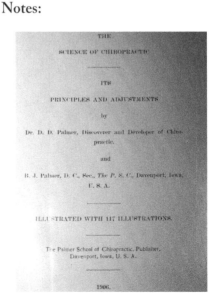

GBMN 11

Title: The Science of Chiropractic
Volume: 1
Edition: First
Author: D.D. Palmer, B.J. Palmer
Printing Date: 1906
Pages: 420
Publisher: Palmer School of Chiropractic
City: Davenport, Iowa
Distinctive Marks: Red and black leather with red tips
Rarity: 10
Value: 10
Desirability: 10
Physical Characteristics:

The book is a presentation copy of the 1906 first edition. It has a red leather spine and black covers with red triangle shaped tips. The spine reads Vol. 1. An oval picture of D.D. Palmer is pasted across from his signature on the front pages. The book was covered in Davenport by a company called Wunder Brothers (Bros). There is a distinctive stamp from this company in the back cover.

Date Acquired:

Price:

Notes:

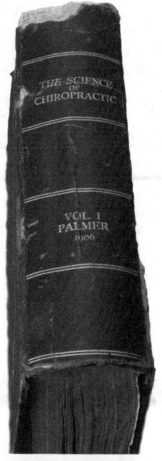

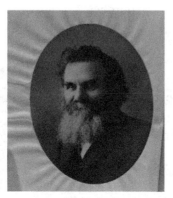

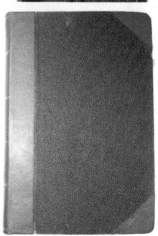

GBMN 12

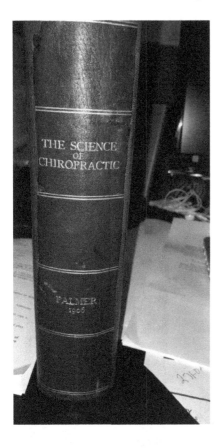

Title: The Science of Chiropractic
Volume: 1
Edition: First
Author: D.D. Palmer, B.J. Palmer
Printing Date: 1906
Pages: 420
Publisher: Palmer School of Chiropractic
City: Davenport, Iowa
Distinctive Marks: Red and black leather with no volume number on spine, no red tips (Numbered edition)
Rarity: 10
Value: 10
Desirability: 10
Physical Characteristics:

The book is a presentation copy of the 1906 first edition. It has a red leather spine and black covers. This 1906 edition has no Vol. 1 on the red spine and the covers are solid black with no red triangular shaped tips. These books seem to be the first books of the Palmer's very first book to come off the press. They are numbered editions. On an inside front page, dead center, is a printed number.

Date Acquired:

Price:

Notes:

42

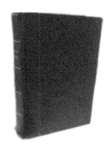

GBMN 13

Title: The Science of Chiropractic
Volume: 1
Edition: Second
Author: B.J. Palmer
Printing Date: 1910
Pages: 440
Publisher: Palmer School of Chiropractic
City: Davenport, Iowa:
Rarity: 8
Value: 7.5
Desirability: 7
Physical Characteristics:

This 1910 book was printed in the standard Green Book format. The title page lists it as a 1910 second edition. This edition contains significant revisions of the original 1906 first edition as well as new chapters. The book is smaller than the 1906 edition because most of the images have been removed.

Date Acquired:

Price:

Notes:

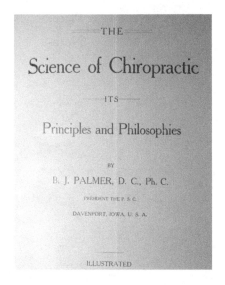

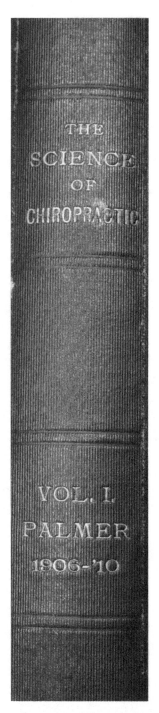

GBMN 14

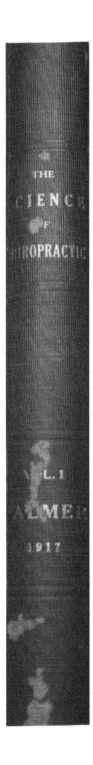

Title: The Science of Chiropractic
Volume: 1
Edition: Third
Author: B.J. Palmer
Printing Date: 1917
Pages: 332
Publisher: Palmer School of Chiropractic
City: Davenport, Iowa
Rarity: 6
Value: 6
Desirability: 6
Physical Characteristics:

This 1917 book was printed in the standard Green Book format except the cover was red. Some copies are faded to a tan color. The title page lists it as a 1917 third edition. This 1917 third edition has 90 pages less than the 1910 second edition. There are a few updates to the material and an updated image of B.J. appears on the front page.

Date Acquired:

Price:

Notes:

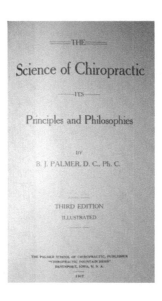

GBMN 15

Title: The Science of Chiropractic
Volume: 1
Edition: Fourth
Author: B.J. Palmer
Printing Date: 1920
Pages: 332
Publisher: Palmer School of Chiropractic
City: Davenport, Iowa
Rarity: 2
Value: 3
Desirability: 4
Physical Characteristics:

This 1920 book was printed in the standard Green Book format. The title page lists it as a 1920 fourth edition. This book is the same as the 1917 third edition with a 1920 printing date. Like many of the early volumes, more books were needed in the 1920s. This is one of the most common books as many were printed in 1920.

Date Acquired:

Price:

Notes:

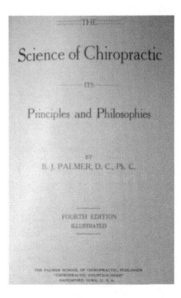

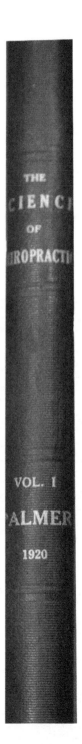

GBMN 16

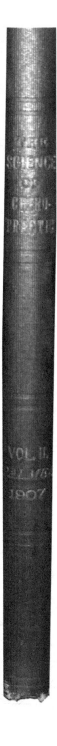

Title: The Science of Chiropractic
Volume: 2
Edition: First
Author: B.J. Palmer
Printing Date: 1907
Pages: 162
Publisher: Palmer School of Chiropractic
City: Davenport, Iowa
Rarity: 9.3
Value: 9.3
Desirability: 9.3
Physical Characteristics:

This 1907 book was printed in the standard Green Book format. The title page lists it as a 1907 first edition. This book was published in 1907 and is considered to be B.J. Palmer's first book.

Date Acquired:

Price:

Notes:

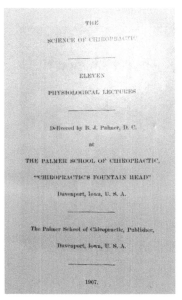

GBMN 17

Title: The Science of Chiropractic
Volume: 2
Edition: First
Author: B.J. Palmer
Printing Date: 1907
Pages: 162
Publisher: Palmer School of Chiropractic
City: Davenport, Iowa
Distinctive Marks: Red and black leather covers with red tips
Rarity: 10
Value: 10
Desirability: 10
Physical Characteristics:

This book is a presentation copy of the 1907 first edition. It has a red leather spine and black covers with red triangle shaped tips. Vol. 2 is printed on the spine. The book was covered in Davenport by a company called Wunder (Bros). There is a distinctive stamp from this company in the back cover.

Date Acquired:

Price:

Notes:

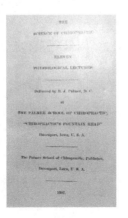

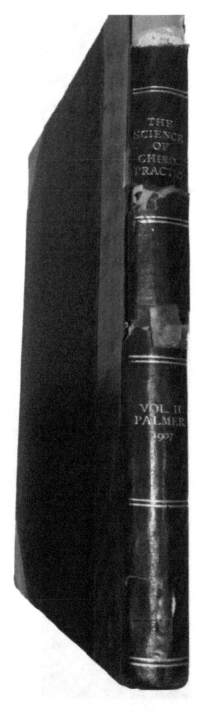

GBMN 18

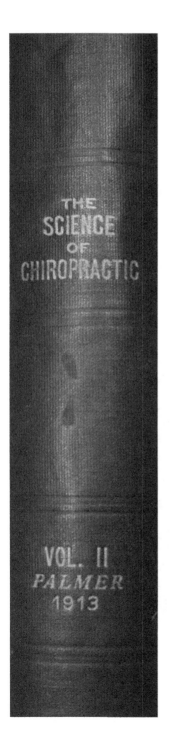

Title: The Science of Chiropractic
Volume: 2
Edition: Second
Author: B.J. Palmer
Printing Date: 1913
Pages: 677
Publisher: Palmer School of Chiropractic
City: Davenport, Iowa
Rarity: 8
Value: 7.5
Desirability: 7
Physical Characteristics:

This 1913 book was printed in the standard Green Book format. The title page lists it as a 1913 second edition. The second edition is a revised and updated edition of the book.

Date Acquired:

Price:

Notes:

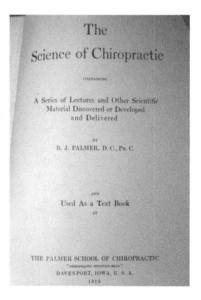

The

Science of Chiropractic

CONTAINING

A Series of Lectures and Other Scientific
Material Discovered or Developed
and Delivered

BY

B. J. PALMER, D. C., Ph. C.

AND

Used As a Text Book

AT

THE PALMER SCHOOL OF CHIROPRACTIC
"CHIROPRACTIC FOUNTAIN-HEAD"
DAVENPORT, IOWA, U. S. A.
1913

GBMN 19

Title: The Science of Chiropractic
Volume: 2
Edition: Third
Author: B.J. Palmer
Printing Date: 1917
Pages: 679
Publisher: Palmer School of Chiropractic
City: Davenport, Iowa
Rarity: 6
Value: 6.5
Desirability: 7
Physical Characteristics:

This 1917 book was printed in the standard Green Book format. The title page lists it as a 1917 third edition. The third edition is a revised and updated edition of the book

Date Acquired:

Price:

Notes:

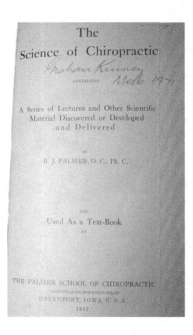

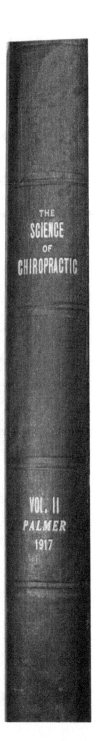

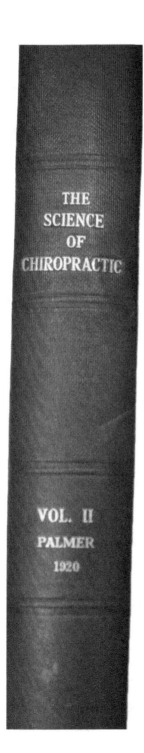

GBMN 20

Title: The Science of Chiropractic
Volume: 2
Edition: Fourth
Author: B.J. Palmer
Printing Date: 1920
Pages: 679
Publisher: Palmer School of Chiropractic
City: Davenport, Iowa
Rarity: 2
Value: 2.5
Desirability: 3
Physical Characteristics:

This 1920 book was printed in the standard Green Book format. The title page lists it as a 1920 fourth edition. This book is the same as the 1917 third edition with a 1920 printing date. Like many of the early volumes, more books were needed in the 1920s. This is one of the most common books as many were printed in 1920.

Date Acquired:

Price:

Notes:

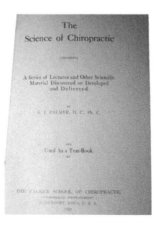

GBMN 21

Title: The Science of Chiropractic
Volume: 3
Edition: First
Author: B.J. Palmer
Printing Date: 1908
Pages: 360
Publisher: Palmer School of Chiropractic
City: Davenport, Iowa
Rarity: 9.1
Value: 9.1
Desirability: 9.1
Physical Characteristics:

This 1908 book was printed in the standard Green Book format. The title page lists it as a 1908 first edition.

Date Acquired:

Price:

Notes:

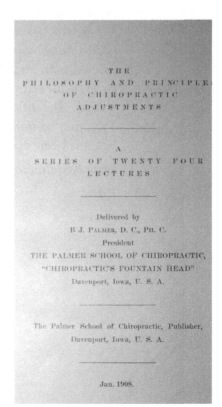

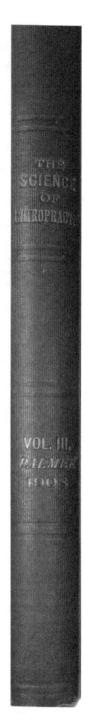

GBMN 22

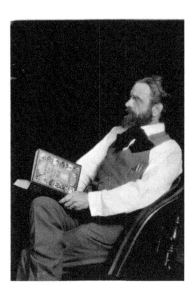

There are no known copies of this book.

Title: The Science of Chiropractic
Volume: 3
Edition: First
Author: B.J. Palmer
Printing Date: 1908
Pages: 360
Publisher: Palmer School of Chiropractic
City: Davenport, Iowa
Distinctive Marks: SUSPECTED - red & black leather cover
Rarity: 10
Value: 10
Desirability: 10
Physical Characteristics:

This book is suspected to exist as another first edition like Vol. 1, Vol. 2, and Vol. 6, which were printed as red and black presentation copies. This book would be printed with a red leather spine and black covers with red triangular tips as a special edition. The title page would list it as a 1908 first edition. To date a known copy has not been doc-umented.

Date Acquired:

Price:

Notes:

GBMN 23

Title: The Science of Chiropractic
Volume: 3
Edition: Second
Author: B.J. Palmer
Printing Date: 1911
Pages: 567
Publisher: Palmer School of Chiropractic
City: Davenport, Iowa
Rarity: 8
Value: 7.5
Desirability: 7
Physical Characteristics:

This 1911 book was printed in the standard Green Book format. The title page lists it as a 1911 second edition. B.J. continued his practice of going back and revising the material in his early books. The Vol. 3, 1908 first edition, was revised and expanded in 1911.

Date Acquired:

Price:

Notes:

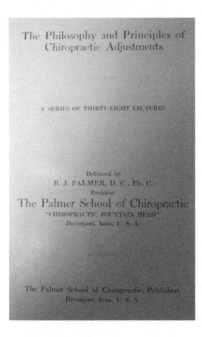

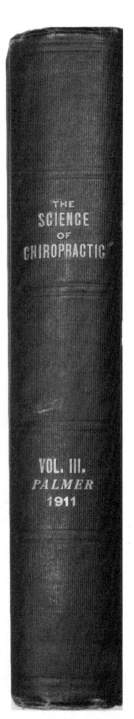

GBMN 24

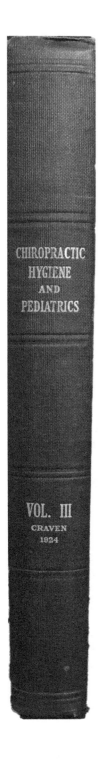

Title: A Textbook on Hygiene and Pediatrics from a Chiropractic Standpoint

Volume: 3 (reissued volume number)

Edition: First

Author: John H. Craven

Printing Date: 1924

Pages: 407

Publisher: John H. Craven

City: Davenport, Iowa

Rarity: 6

Value: 6

Desirability: 6

Physical Characteristics:

This 1924 book was printed in the standard Green Book format and had a single printing done by Palmer. B.J. Palmer published *Palmer Technique of Chiropractic* as Vol. 13 in 1920. This made the 1911 Vol. 3 *Science of Chiropractic* obsolete and unnecessary as it was the volume that covered technique.

Date Acquired:

Price:

Notes:

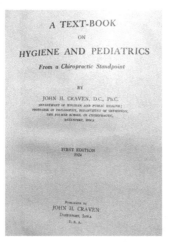

GBMN 25

Title: The Science of Chiropractic:
            Causes Localized
Volume: 4
Edition: First
Author: B.J. Palmer
Printing Date: 1908
Pages: 108
Publisher: Palmer School of Chiropractic
City: Davenport, Iowa
Rarity: 9
Value: 9.25
Desirability: 9.5
Physical Characteristics:

This 1908 book was printed in the standard Green Book format and had a single printing done by Palmer.

Date Acquired:

Price:

Notes:

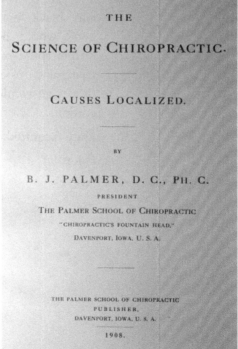

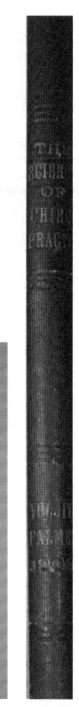

GBMN 26

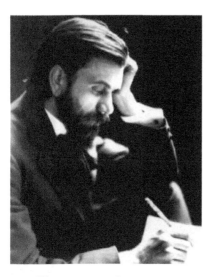

There are no known
copies of this book.

Title: The Science of Chiropractic:
Causes Localized
Volume: 4
Edition: First
Author: B.J. Palmer
Printing Date: 1908
Pages: 108
Publisher: Palmer School of Chiropractic
City: Davenport, Iowa
Distinctive Marks: SUSPECTED -
red & black leather cover
Rarity: 10
Value: 10
Desirability: 10
Physical Characteristics:

This book is suspected to exist as
another first edition like Vol. 1, Vol. 2,
and Vol. 6, which were printed as red
and black presentation copies. This
book would be printed with a red
leather spine and black covers with red
triangular tips as a special edition. The
title page would list it as a 1908 first
edition.

Date Acquired:

Price:

Notes:

GBMN 27

Title: The Chiropractic Adjuster
Volume: 4 (reissued volume number)
Edition: First
Author: D.D. Palmer, B.J. Palmer
Printing Date: 1921
Pages: 912
Publisher: Palmer School of Chiropractic
City: Davenport, Iowa
Rarity: 7
Value: 7.5
Desirability: 8
Physical Characteristics:

This 1921 book was printed in the standard Green Book format and had a single printing done by Palmer.

Date Acquired:

Price:

Notes:

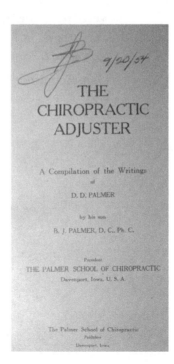

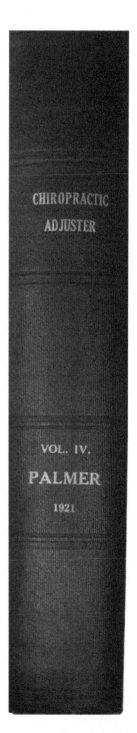

GBMN 28

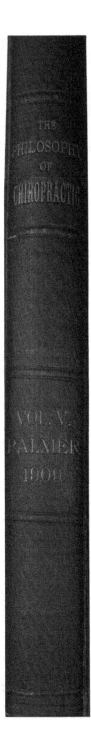

Title: The Philosophy of Chiropractic
Volume: 5
Edition: First
Author: B.J. Palmer
Printing Date: 1909
Pages: 579
Publisher: Palmer School of Chiropractic
City: Davenport, Iowa
Rarity: 8.8
Value: 8.4
Desirability: 8
Physical Characteristics:

This 1909 book was printed in the standard Green Book format. The title page lists it as a 1909 first edition. With this 1909 book, B.J. Palmer makes a subtle change to his chiropractic series. Previous volumes were titled the *Science of Chiropractic*. The title of Vol. 5 is *The Philosophy of Chiropractic* on the spine.

Date Acquired:

Price:

Notes:

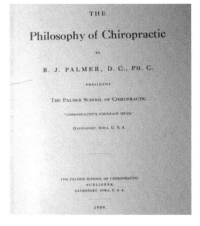

GBMN 29

Title: The Philosophy of Chiropractic
Volume: 5
Edition: First
Author: B.J. Palmer
Printing Date: 1909
Pages: 579
Publisher: Palmer School of Chiropractic
City: Davenport, Iowa
Distinctive Marks: SUSPECTED - red & black leather cover
Rarity: 10
Value: 10
Desirability: 10
Physical Characteristics:

This book is suspected to exist as another first edition like Vol. 1, Vol. 2, and Vol. 6, which were printed as red and black presentation copies. This book would be printed with a red leather spine and black covers with red triangular tips as a special edition. The title page would list it as a 1909 first edition.

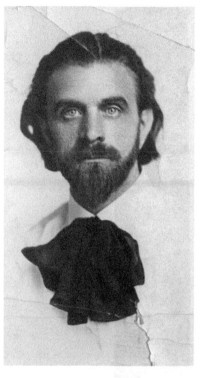

There are no known copies of this book.

Date Acquired:

Price:

Notes:

GBMN 30

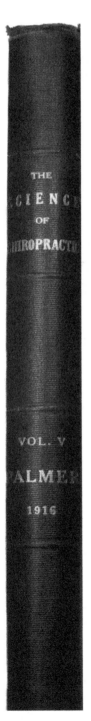

Title: The Philosophy of Chiropractic
Volume: 5
Edition: Second
Author: B.J. Palmer, J.H. Craven
Printing Date: 1916
Pages: 428
Publisher: Palmer School of Chiropractic
City: Davenport, Iowa
Rarity: 8
Value: 7
Desirability: 6
Physical Characteristics:

This 1916 book was printed in the standard Green Book format. The title page lists it as a 1916 second edition. John H. Craven is listed as collaborator to this updated second edition. The material was reduced by 130 pages. The spine of the book was been changed to *The Science of Chiropractic*, while the title page reads *The Philosophy of Chiropractic*.

Date Acquired:

Price:

Notes:

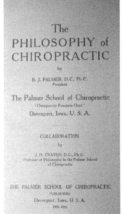

GBMN 31

Title: The Philosophy of Chiropractic
Volume: 5
Edition: Third
Author: B.J. Palmer, J.H. Craven
Printing Date: 1919 (1918 on spine)
Pages: 428
Publisher: Palmer School of Chiropractic
City: Davenport, Iowa
Rarity: 6
Value: 6.5
Desirability: 7
Physical Characteristics:

This 1919 book was printed in the standard Green Book format. The spine has a 1918 date and the title page lists it as a 1919 third edition. This book is the same as the 1916 second edition with a 1919 printing date. Many of the Vol. 5 books have different dates printed on the spine as compared to the title page. This is the first book in the series to have this confusing discrepancy.

Date Acquired:

Price:

Notes:

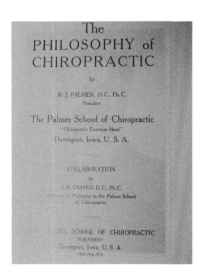

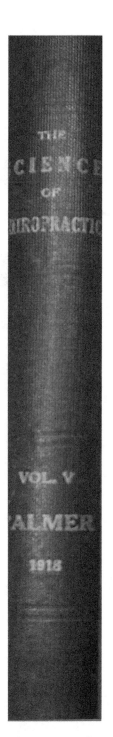

GBMN 32

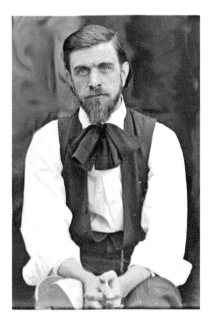

There are no known
copies of this book.

Title: The Philosophy of Chiropractic
Volume: 5
Edition: Third
Author: B.J. Palmer, J.H. Craven
Printing Date: 1919 (1918 on spine)
Pages: 428
Publisher: Palmer School of Chiropractic
City: Davenport, Iowa
Distinctive Marks: SUSPECTED -
brown leather cover
Rarity: 10
Value: 8.5
Desirability: 7
Physical Characteristics:
    This book is suspected to exist as
other Green Books printed in 1919 had
this special edition in brown leatherette.
This 1919 book would be printed with
brown leather covers as a special edition.
The title page would list it as a 1919
third edition.

Date Acquired:

Price:

Notes:

GBMN 33

Title: The Philosophy of Chiropractic
Volume: 5
Edition: Fourth
Author: B.J. Palmer, J.H. Craven
Printing Date: 1920 (1919 on Spine)
Pages: 428
Publisher: Palmer School of Chiropractic
City: Davenport, Iowa
Rarity: 6
Value: 6
Desirability: 6
Physical Characteristics:

This 1920 book was printed in the standard Green Book format. The spine has a 1919 date and the title page lists it as a 1920 fourth edition. This book is the same as the 1918 third edition with a 1920 printing date.

Date Acquired:

Price:

Notes:

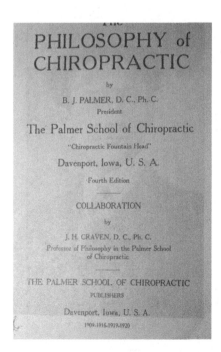

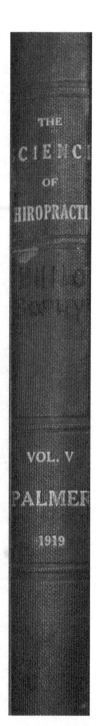

GBMN 34

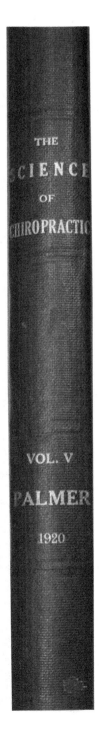

Title: The Philosophy of Chiropractic
Volume: 5
Edition: Fifth
Author: B.J. Palmer, J.H. Craven
Printing Date: 1920
Pages: 428
Publisher: Palmer School of Chiropractic
City: Davenport, Iowa
Rarity: 6
Value: 6
Desirability: 6
Physical Characteristics:

This 1920 book was printed in the standard Green Book format. The title page lists it as a 1920 fifth edition. This book is the same as the 1920 fourth edition with a 1920 printing date.

Date Acquired:

Price:

Notes:

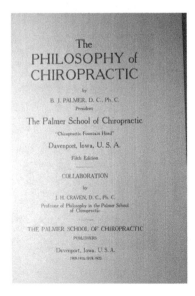

GBMN 35

Title: The Philosophy of Chiropractic
Volume: 5
Edition: Sixth
Author: B.J. Palmer, J.H. Craven
Printing Date: 1922 (1920 on title page)
Pages: 428
Publisher: Palmer School of Chiropractic
City: Davenport, Iowa
Rarity: 5
Value: 5
Desirability: 5
Physical Characteristics:

This 1922 book was printed in the standard Green Book format. The spine has a 1922 date and the title page lists it as a 1920 sixth edition. This book is the same as the 1920 fifth edition with a 1922 printing date.

Date Acquired:

Price:

Notes:

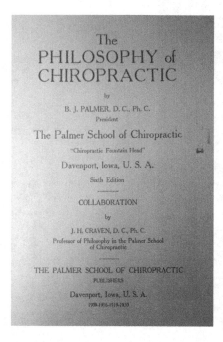

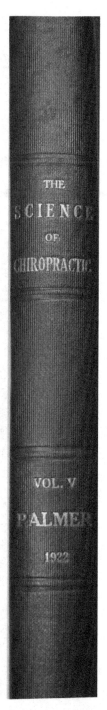

GBMN 36

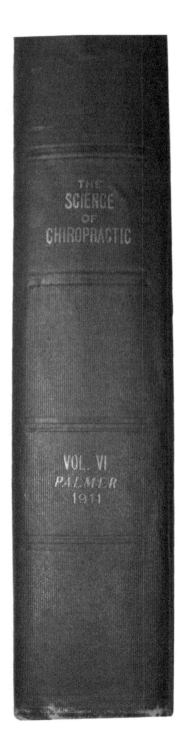

Title: The Philosophy Science and Art of Chiropractic Nerve Tracing
Volume: 6
Edition: First
Author: B.J. Palmer
Printing Date: 1911
Pages: 789
Publisher: Palmer School of Chiropractic
City: Davenport, Iowa
Rarity: 9.3
Value: 9.3
Desirability: 9.2
Physical Characteristics:

This 1911 book was printed with the standard Green Book format. It is a thick book at nearly 800 pages. The title page lists it as a 1911 first edition.

Date Acquired:

Price:

Notes:

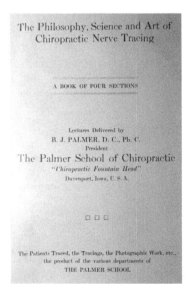

GBMN 37

Title: The Philosophy Science and Art of Chiropractic Nerve Tracing
Volume: 6
Edition: First
Author: B.J. Palmer
Printing Date: 1911
Pages: 789
Publisher: Palmer School of Chiropractic
City: Davenport, Iowa
Distinctive Marks: Red and black leather covers with red tips
Rarity: 10
Value: 10
Desirability: 10
Physical Characteristics:

This is a presentation copy of the 1911 first edition. The spine is red leather with black covers and red triangle tips. This book looks very similar to other red and black leather presentation copies of Vol. 1 and 2. A slight difference is a thin gold line along the red and black boarders. It is suspected this was covered by Wunder Bros. in Davenport. There is one known example, but there may be others.

Date Acquired:

Price:

Notes:

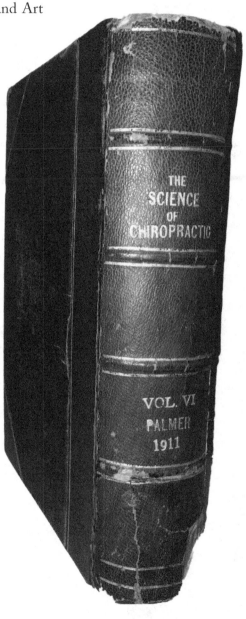

GBMN 38

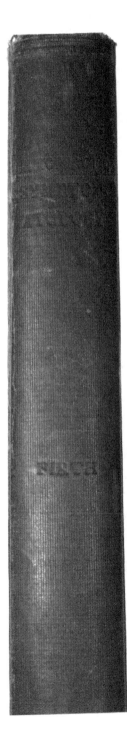

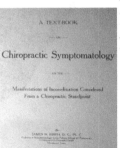

Title: A Text-book on Chiropractic Symptomatology

Volume: 7

Edition: First

Author: James N. Firth

Printing Date: 1914

Pages: 424

Publisher: James N. Firth

City: Davenport, Iowa

Rarity: 9

Value: 8

Desirability: 7

Physical Characteristics:

This dark blue covered book was written by PSC faculty member, James Firth. The book was intended to be used as a textbook for students at the PSC. The title page lists it as a 1914 first edition. The first edition did not have a volume number on the spine as it was not initially a part of B.J. Palmer's chiropractic series. This book received heavy use by PSC students and is usually found in poor condition.

Date Acquired:

Price:

Notes:

GBMN 39

Title: A Text-book on Chiropractic
Symptomatology
Volume: 7
Edition: Supplement to first edition
Author: James N. Firth
Printing Date: 1919
Pages: 100
Publisher: James N. Firth
City: Davenport, Iowa
Rarity: 9.3
Value: 7.2
Desirability: 5
Physical Characteristics:

This light green book was printed
in 1919 by Firth as a companion to
his 1914 first edition. The cover has
black lettering and the title page lists
it as a supplement to the first edition.
It does not have a volume number on
the spine.

Date Acquired:

Price:

Notes:

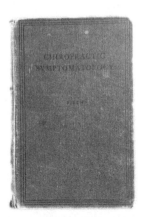
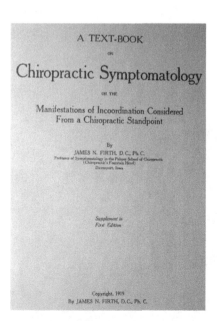

GBMN 40

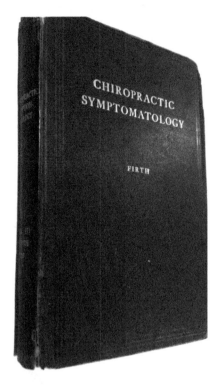

Title: A Text-book on Chiropractic Symptomatology

Volume: 7

Edition: Second

Author: James N. Firth

Printing Date: 1919

Pages: 424

Publisher: James N. Firth

City: Davenport, Iowa

Distinctive Marks: Soft brown leather cover

Rarity: 10

Value: 8

Desirability: 6

Physical Characteristics:

This is another printing of the 1919 second edition done in a soft brown leather cover. The title page lists it as a 1919 second edition. Firth's book is now officially part of the chiropractic series. Vol. 7 now appears on the spine.

Date Acquired:

Price:

Notes:

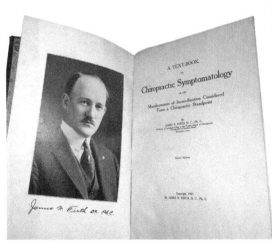

GBMN 41

Title: A Text-book on Chiropractic Symptomatology

Volume: 7

Edition: Second

Author: James N. Firth

Printing Date: 1919

Pages: 465

Publisher: James N. Firth

City: Davenport, Iowa

Rarity: 5

Value: 4

Desirability: 3

Physical Characteristics:

This 1919 book was printed in the standard Green Book format for the first time. The title page lists it as a 1919 second edition. Firth's book is now officially part of the chiropractic series. Vol. 7 now appears on the spine of this traditionally green bound book. Firth has combined his first edition with the supplement and updated the material. This book received heavy use by PSC students and is usually found in poor condition.

Date Acquired:

Price:

Notes:

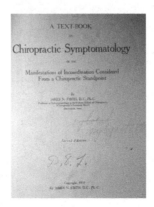

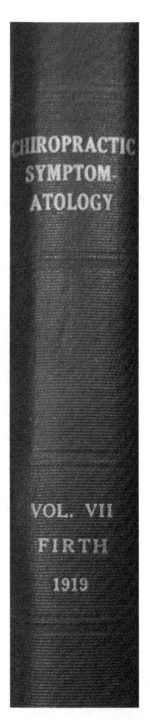

GBMN 42

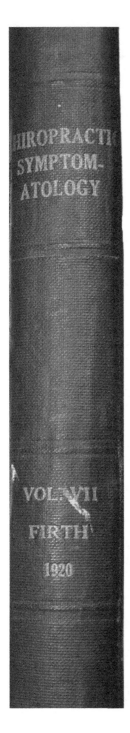

Title: A Text-book on Chiropractic Symptomatology

Volume: 7

Edition: Second

Author: James N. Firth

Printing Date: 1920

Pages: 465

Publisher: James N. Firth

City: Davenport, Iowa

Rarity: 5

Value: 4

Desirability: 3

Physical Characteristics:

This 1920 book was printed in the standard Green Book format. The title page lists it as a 1920 second edition. This book is the same as the 1919 second edition with a 1920 printing date. This book received heavy use by PSC students and is usually found in poor condition.

Date Acquired:

Price:

Notes:

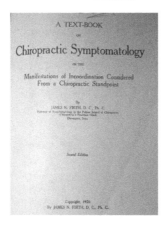

GBMN 43

Title: A Text-book on Chiropractic Symptomatology
Volume: 7
Edition: Second
Author: James N. Firth
Printing Date: 1921
Pages: 465
Publisher: James N. Firth
City: Davenport, Iowa
Rarity: 5
Value: 4
Desirability: 3
Physical Characteristics:

This 1921 book was printed in the standard Green Book format. The title page lists it as a 1921 second edition. This book is the same as the 1919 second edition with a 1921 printing date. This book received heavy use by PSC students and is usually found in poor condition.

Date Acquired:

Price:

Notes:

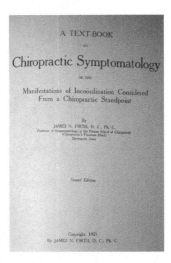

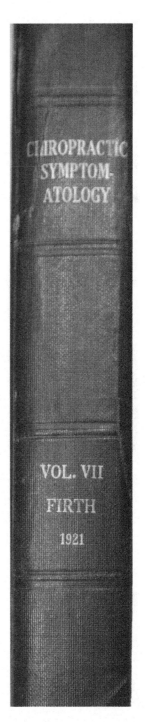

GBMN 44

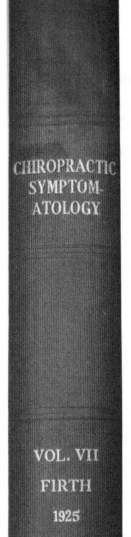

Title: A Text-book on Chiropractic
                Symptomatology
Volume: 7
Edition: Second
Author: James N. Firth
Printing Date: 1925
Pages: 465
Publisher: James N. Firth
City: Davenport, Iowa
Rarity: 5
Value: 4
Desirability: 3
Physical Characteristics:

This 1925 book was printed in the standard Green Book format. The title page lists it as a 1925 second edition. This book is the same as the 1919 second edition with a 1925 printing date.

Date Acquired:

Price:

Notes:

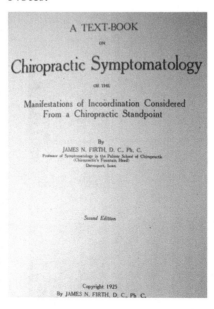

GBMN 45

Title: A Text-book on Chiropractic Diagnosis
Volume: 7
Edition: Third
Author: James N. Firth
Printing Date: 1929
Pages: 592
Publisher: Lincoln Chiropractic College
City: Indianapolis, Indiana
Rarity: 7
Value: 5.5
Desirability: 4
Physical Characteristics:

This 1929 book was printed with the standard Green Book format. The title page lists it as a 1929 third edition. Firth left the PSC faculty in 1925 and soon after joined the faculty at Lincoln Chiropractic College. While teaching at Lincoln Chiropractic College, Firth printed a third edition of his book which was revised and updated. The title changed to *Chiropractic Diagnosis* but it was still a green cloth cover with Vol. 7 on the spine.

Date Acquired:

Price:

Notes:

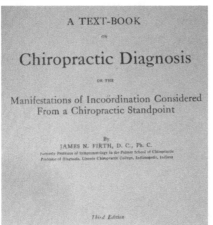

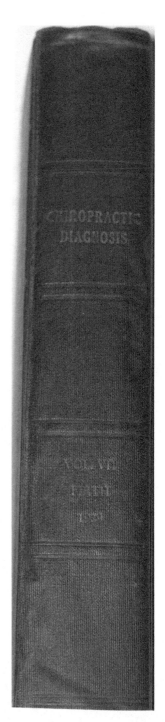

GBMN 46

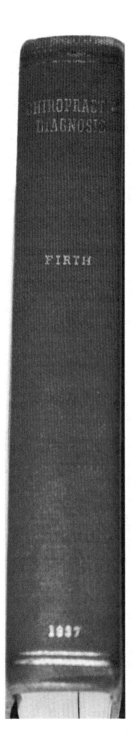

Title: A Text-book on Chiropractic Diagnosis
Volume: 7
Edition: Fourth
Author: James N. Firth
Printing Date: 1937
Pages: 576
Publisher: Lincoln Chiropractic College
City: Indianapolis, Indiana
Rarity: 5
Value: 4.5
Desirability: 4
Physical Characteristics:

The cover is red. While still at Lincoln Chiropractic College, Firth produced a fourth edition of his book. The title page lists it as a 1937 fourth edition. This edition continues with the *Chiropractic Diagnosis* title but the book was no longer green and did not have a volume number on the spine. This book is a later edition of an official numbered volume from the Palmer chiropractic series so it is still defined as a Green Book.

Date Acquired:

Price:

Notes:

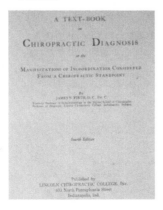

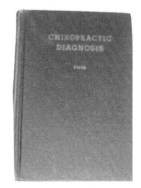

GBMN 47

Title: A Text-book on Chiropractic Diagnosis
Volume: 7
Edition: Fifth
Author: James N. Firth
Printing Date: 1948
Pages: 577
Publisher: Lincoln Chiropractic College
City: Indianapolis, Indiana
Rarity: 4
Value: 3.5
Desirability: 3
Physical Characteristics:

The cover is red. While still at Lincoln Chiropractic College, Firth produced a fifth edition of his book. The title page lists it as a 1948 fifth edition. This edition continues with the *Chiropractic Diagnosis* title without a volume number. A red (GBMN 47) and a blue (GBMN 48) covered printing are known. This book is a later edition of an official numbered volume from the Palmer chiropractic series so it is still defined as a Green Book.

Date Acquired:

Price:

Notes:

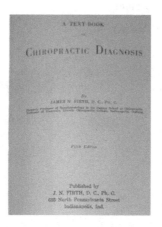

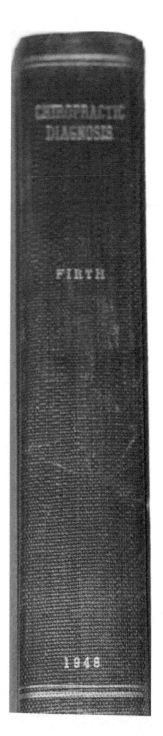

GBMN 48

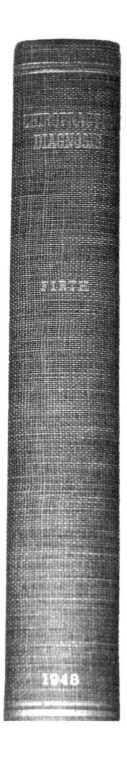

Title: A Text-book on Chiropractic Diagnosis
Volume: 7
Edition: Fifth
Author: James N. Firth
Printing Date: 1948
Pages: 577
Publisher: Lincoln Chiropractic College
City: Indianapolis, Indiana
Rarity: 6
Value: 4.5
Desirability: 3
Physical Characteristics:

The cover is blue. While still at Lincoln Chiropractic College, Firth produced a fifth edition of his book. The title page lists it as a 1948 fifth edition. This edition continues with the *Chiropractic Diagnosis* title without a volume number and a red (GBMN 47) and a blue (GBMN 48) covered printing are known. This book is a later edition of an official numbered volume from the Palmer chiropractic series so it is still defined as a Green Book.

Date Acquired:

Price:

Notes:

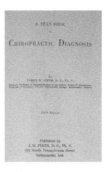
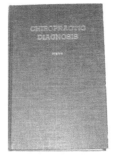

GBMN 49

Title: A Text Book on Chiropractic
Physiology
Volume: 8
Edition: First
Author: Harry E. Vedder
Printing Date: 1916
Pages: 414
Publisher: Harry E. Vedder
City: Davenport, Iowa
Rarity: 8.5
Value: 8.5
Desirability: 8.5
Physical Characteristics:

This 1916 book was printed with a brick red cover. The first edition did not have a volume number on the spine. The book color is often faded and the spine may look tan. PSC faculty member, Harry E. Vedder, published this book as a textbook for students.

Date Acquired:

Price:

Notes:

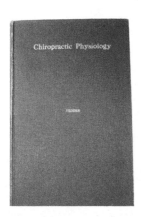

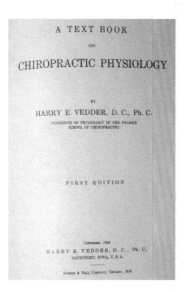

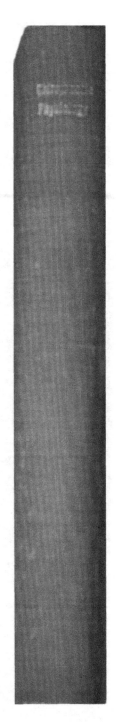

GBMN 50

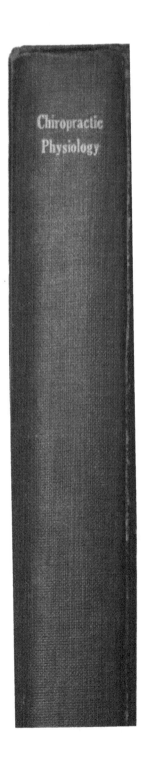

Title: A Text Book on Chiropractic Physiology
Volume: 8
Edition: Second
Author: Harry E. Vedder
Printing Date: 1918
Pages: 414
Publisher: Harry E. Vedder
City: Davenport, Iowa
Rarity: 7
Value: 7
Desirability: 7
Physical Characteristics:

This 1918 book was printed with the same brick red cover as the first edition. The title page lists it as a 1918 second edition. There was still no volume number on this edition. The book is often faded and the spine may look tan.

Date Acquired:

Price:

Notes:

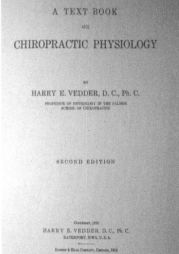

GBMN 51

Title: A Text Book on Chiropractic Physiology
Volume: 8
Edition: Third
Author: Harry E. Vedder
Printing Date: 1920 (1918 on title page)
Pages: 414
Publisher: Harry E. Vedder
City: Davenport, Iowa
Rarity: 6
Value: 5.5
Desirability: 5
Physical Characteristics:

This 1920 book was printed in the standard Green Book format for the first time. The title page lists it as a 1918 third edition but the spine has a 1920 date. The third edition is a 1920 printing of the original 1916 first edition. Chiropractic is misspelled on the front cover as, "Chiropractric Physiology."

Date Acquired:

Price:

Notes:

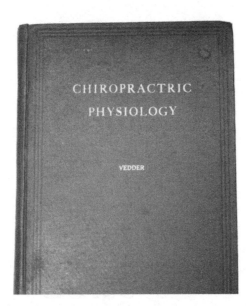
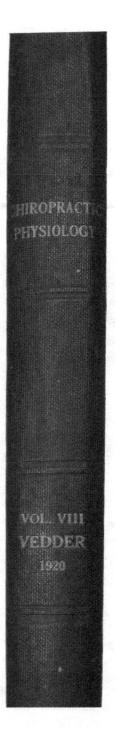

GBMN 52

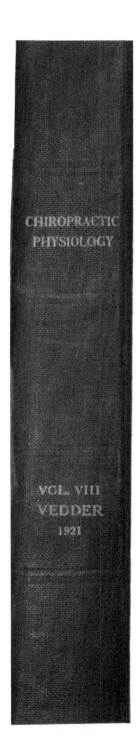

Title: A Text Book on Chiropractic Physiology
Volume: 8
Edition: Fourth
Author: Harry E. Vedder
Printing Date: 1921
Publisher: Harry E. Vedder
City: Davenport, Iowa
Pages: 414
Rarity: 4
Value: 3.5
Desirability: 3
Physical Characteristics:

This 1921 book was printed in the standard Green Book format. The title page lists it as a 1921 fourth edition. The fourth edition is a 1921 printing of the original 1916 first edition.

Date Acquired:

Price:

Notes:

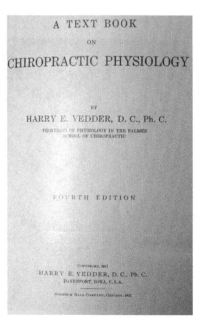

GBMN 53

Title: A Text Book on Chiropractic Physiology
Volume: 8
Edition: Fifth
Author: Harry E. Vedder
Printing Date: 1922
Pages: 414
Publisher: Harry E. Vedder
City: Davenport, Iowa
Rarity: 4
Value: 3.5
Desirability: 3
Physical Characteristics:

This 1922 book was printed in the standard Green Book format. The title page lists it as a 1922 fifth edition. The fifth edition is a 1922 printing of the original 1916 first edition.

Date Acquired:

Price:

Notes:

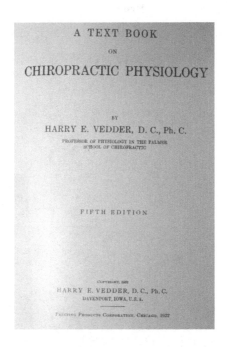

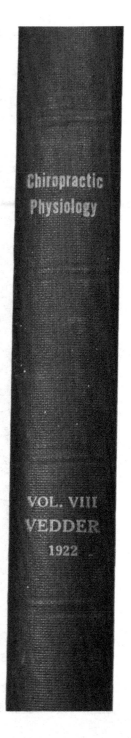

GBMN 54

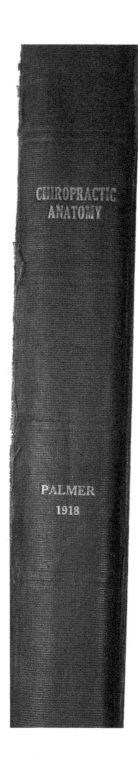

Title: Chiropractic Anatomy
Volume: 9
Edition: First
Author: Mabel H. Palmer
Printing Date: 1918
Pages: 487
Publisher: Mabel H. Palmer
City: Davenport, Iowa
Rarity: 8
Value: 8
Desirability: 8
Physical Characteristics:

This 1918 book was printed in the standard Green Book format except it did not list a volume number on the spine. The title page lists it as a 1918 first edition.

Date Acquired:

Price:

Notes:

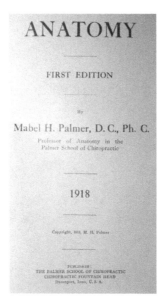

ANATOMY

FIRST EDITION

By

Mabel H. Palmer, D. C., Ph. C.

Professor of Anatomy in the
Palmer School of Chiropractic

1918

Copyright, 1918, M. H. Palmer

PUBLISHED
THE PALMER SCHOOL OF CHIROPRACTIC
CHIROPRACTIC FOUNTAIN HEAD
Davenport, Iowa, U. S. A.

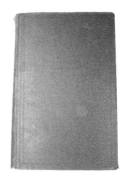

GBMN 55

Title: Chiropractic Anatomy
Volume: 9
Edition: Second
Author: Mabel H. Palmer
Printing Date: 1919
Pages: 569
Publisher: Mabel H. Palmer
City: Davenport, Iowa
Rarity: 6
Value: 5.5
Desirability: 5
Physical Characteristics:

This 1919 book was printed in the standard Green Book format. Vol. 9 appears on the spine for the first time. The title page lists it as a 1919 second edition. The second edition is a revised and updated edition of the book.

Date Acquired:

Price:

Notes:

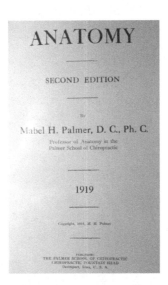

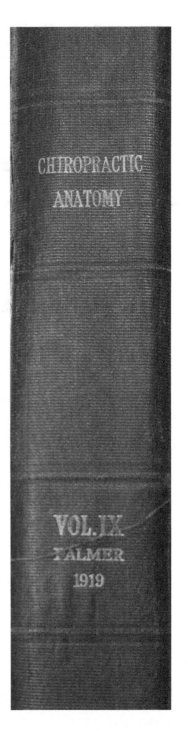

GBMN 56

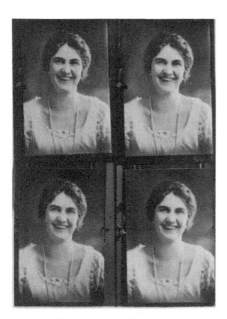

There are no known copies of this book.

Title: Chiropractic Anatomy
Volume: 9
Edition: Second
Author: Mable H. Palmer
Printing Date: 1919
Pages: 569
Publisher: Mabel H. Palmer
City: Davenport, Iowa
Distinctive Marks: SUSPECTED - soft brown leather cover
Rarity: 10
Variety: 8
Desirability: 6
Physical Characteristics:

This book is suspected to exist as other Green Books printed in 1919 had this special edition in brown leatherette. To date, a known copy has not been documented. This 1919 book would be printed with brown leather covers as a special edition. The title page would list it as a 1919 second edition.

Date Acquired:

Price:

Notes:

GBMN 57

Title: Chiropractic Anatomy
Volume: 9
Edition: Third
Author: Mable H. Palmer
Printing Date: 1922 (1920 on title page)
Pages: 569
Publisher: Mabel H. Palmer
City: Davenport, Iowa
Rarity: 5
Value: 5
Desirability: 5
Physical Characteristics:

This 1919 book was printed in the standard Green Book format. The title page lists it as a 1920 third edition, but the spine has a 1919 date. The third edition is a reprinting of the second edition.

Date Acquired:

Price:

Notes:

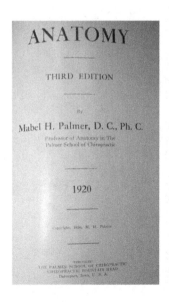

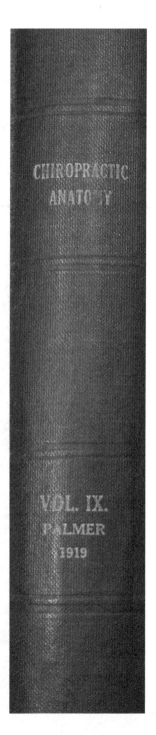

GBMN 58

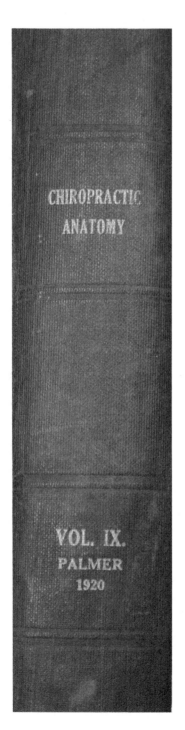

Title: Chiropractic Anatomy
Volume: 9
Edition: Fourth
Author: Mable H. Palmer
Printing Date: 1920
Pages: 569
Publisher: Mabel H. Palmer
City: Davenport, Iowa
Rarity: 4
Value: 4
Desirability: 4
Physical Characteristics:
    This 1920 book was printed in the standard Green Book format. The title page lists it as a 1920 fourth edition. The fourth edition is a reprinting of the second edition.

Date Acquired:

Price:

Notes:

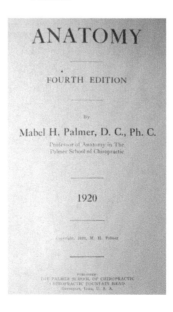

GBMN 59

Title: Chiropractic Anatomy
Volume: 9
Edition: Fourth
Author: Mable H. Palmer
Printing Date: 1922 (1920 on title page)
Pages: 569
Publisher: Mabel H. Palmer
City: Davenport, Iowa
Rarity: 4
Value: 4
Desirability: 4
Physical Characteristics:

This 1922 book was printed in the standard Green Book format. The title page lists it as a 1920 fourth edition but the spine has a 1922 date. The fourth edition is a reprinting of the second edition.

Date Acquired:

Price:

Notes:

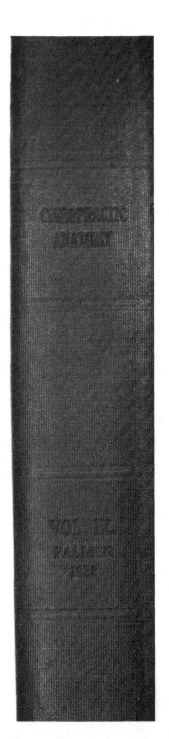

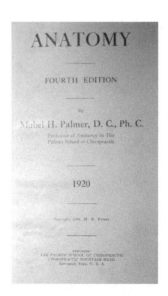

GBMN 60

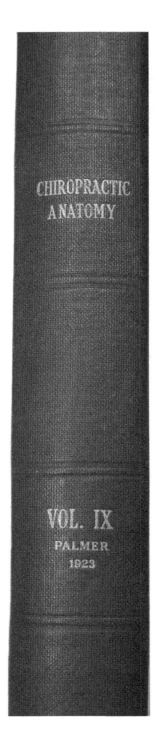

Title: Chiropractic Anatomy
Volume: 9
Edition: Fifth
Author: Mable H. Palmer
Printing Date: 1923
Pages: 573
Publisher: Mabel H. Palmer
City: Davenport, Iowa
Rarity: 4
Value: 4
Desirability: 4
Physical Characteristics:

This 1923 book was printed in the standard Green Book format. The title page lists it as a 1923 fifth edition. The fifth edition is a revised and updated edition of the book.

Date Acquired:

Price:

Notes:

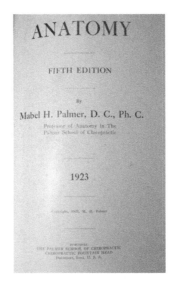

GBMN 61

Title: Text on Spinography
Volume: 10
Edition: First
Author: Earnest A. Thompson
Printing Date: 1918
Pages: 31
Publisher: Earnest A. Thompson
City: Davenport, Iowa
Rarity: 10
Value: 10
Desirability: 10
Physical Characteristics:

Earnest Thompson was a PSC faculty member in charge of the Spinography (X-ray) Department. The first edition in this series started as a soft covered booklet. It was titled *Text on Spinography* and had no volume number. Printed in 1918, it is a small booklet (6x9) and has only 31 pages.

Date Acquired:

Price:

Notes:

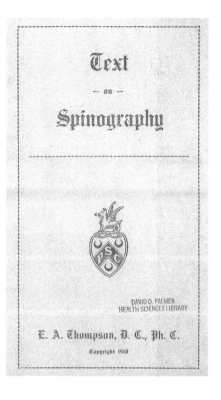

GBMN 62

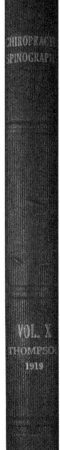

Title: Text on Chiropractic Spinography
Volume: 10
Edition: Second
Author: Earnest A. Thompson
Printing Date: 1919
Pages: 194
Publisher: Earnest A. Thompson
City: Davenport, Iowa
Rarity: 6
Value: 6
Desirability: 6
Physical Characteristics:

This 1919 book was printed in the standard Green Book format for the first time. The title page lists it as a 1919 second edition. The second edition is a revised and updated book compared to the first edition.

Date Acquired:

Price:

Notes:

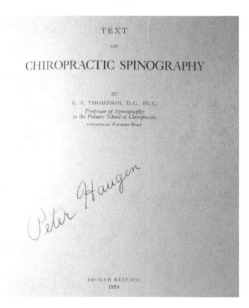

GBMN 63

Title: Text on Chiropractic Spinography
Volume: 10
Edition: Second
Author: Earnest A. Thompson
Printing Date: 1919
Pages: 194
Publisher: Earnest A. Thompson
City: Davenport, Iowa
Distinctive Marks: Soft brown leather cover
Rarity: 10
Value: 8
Desirability: 6
Physical Characteristics:

This is another printing of the 1919 second edition done in a soft brown leather cover.

Date Acquired:

Price:

Notes:

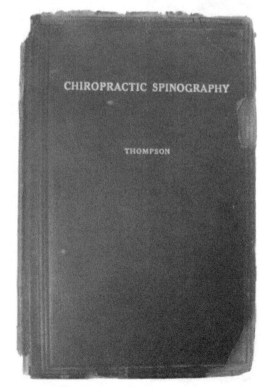

GBMN 64

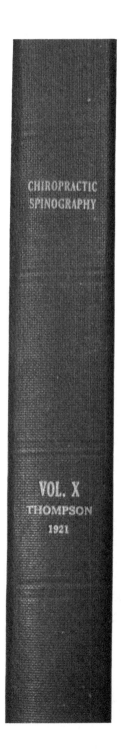

Title: Text on Chiropractic Spinography
Volume: 10
Edition: Third
Author: Earnest A. Thompson
Printing Date: 1921
Pages: 346
Publisher: Earnest A. Thompson
City: Davenport, Iowa
Rarity: 4
Value: 3.5
Desirability: 3
Physical Characteristics:

This 1921 book was printed in the standard Green Book format. The title page lists it as a 1921 third edition. The third edition is a revised and updated book compared to the second edition.

Date Acquired:

Price:

Notes:

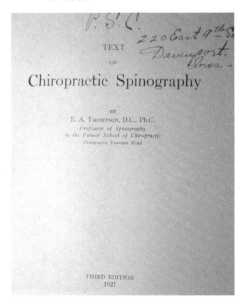

GBMN 65

Title: Text on Chiropractic Spinography
Volume: 10
Edition: Fourth
Author: Earnest A. Thompson
Printing Date: 1923
Pages: 426
Publisher: Earnest A. Thompson
City: Davenport, Iowa
Rarity: 4
Value: 3.5
Desirability: 3
Physical Characteristics:

This 1923 book was printed in the standard Green Book format. The title page lists it as a 1923 fourth edition. The fourth edition is a revised and updated book compared to the third edition

Date Acquired:

Price:

Notes:

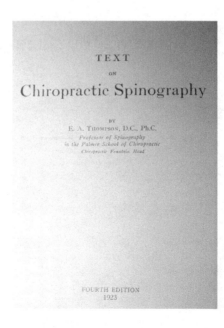

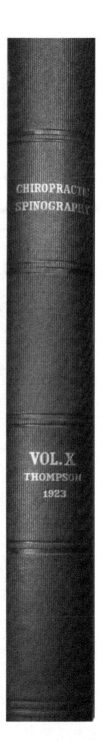

GBMN 66

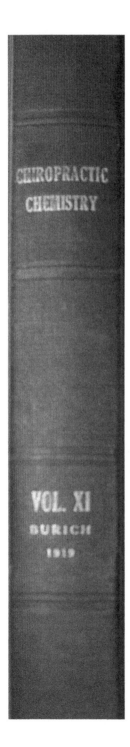

Title: A Text Book on Chiropractic Chemistry
Volume: 11
Edition: First
Author: Stephen J. Burich
Printing Date: 1919
Pages: 430
Publisher: Stephen J. Burich
City: Davenport, Iowa
Rarity: 4
Value: 4
Desirability: 4
Physical Characteristics:

This 1919 book was printed in the standard Green Book format. The title page lists it as a 1919 first edition.

Date Acquired:

Price:

Notes:

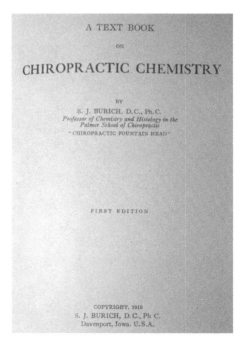

GBMN 67

Title: A Text Book on Chiropractic
Chemistry
Volume: 11
Edition: First
Author: Stephen J. Burich
Printing Date: 1919
Pages: 430
Publisher: Stephen J. Burich
City: Davenport, Iowa
Distinctive Marks: Soft brown leather cover
Rarity: 10
Value: 8
Desirability: 6
Physical Characteristics:

This is another printing of the 1919 first edition done in a soft brown leather cover.

Date Acquired:

Price:

Notes:

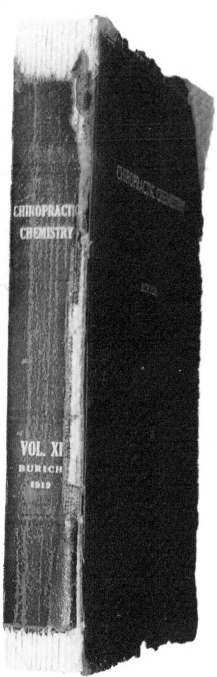

GBMN 68

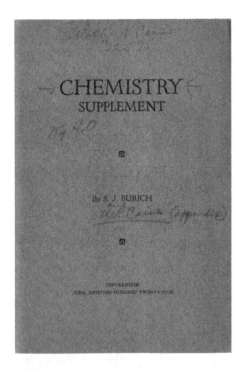

Title: Chemistry Supplement
Volume: 11
Edition: Supplement
Author: Stephen J. Burich
Printing Date: 1925
Pages: 43
Publisher: Stephen J. Burich
City: Davenport, Iowa
Rarity: 10
Value: 6
Desirability: 2
Physical Characteristics:

This small (6x9) soft covered booklet is from June 1925. It was to be used in connection with *Chiropractic Chemistry* as a guide to study and as a supplement to that text. It is exceptionally rare and very few are known to have survived.

Date Acquired:

Price:

Notes:

GBMN 69

Title: A Text Book on Chiropractic Chemistry
Volume: 11
Edition: Second
Author: Stephen J. Burich
Printing Date: 1920
Pages: 430
Publisher: Stephen J. Burich
City: Davenport, Iowa
Rarity: 3
Value: 2.5
Desirability: 2
Physical Characteristics:

This 1920 book was printed in the standard Green Book format. The title page lists it as a 1920 second edition. The second edition is a 1920 reprinting of the first edition.

Date Acquired:

Price:

Notes:

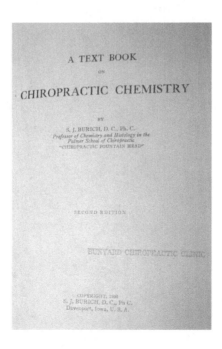

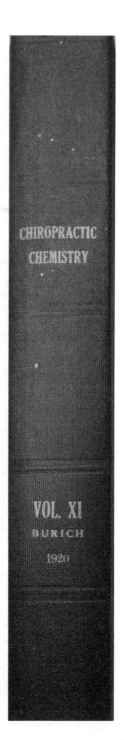

GBMN 70

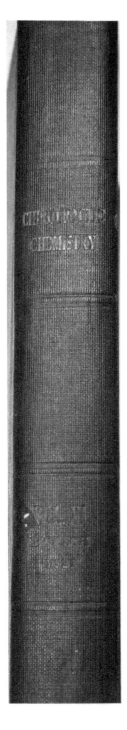

Title: A Text Book on Chiropractic Chemistry
Volume: 11
Edition: Third
Author: Stephen J. Burich
Printing Date: 1921 (1920 on title page)
Pages: 432
Publisher: Stephen J. Burich
City: Davenport, Iowa
Rarity: 3
Value: 2.5
Desirability: 2
Physical Characteristics:

This 1921 book was printed in the standard Green Book format. The spine has a 1921 date. The title page lists it as a 1920 third edition. The third edition is a 1921 reprinting of the 1919 first edition.

Date Acquired:

Price:

Notes:

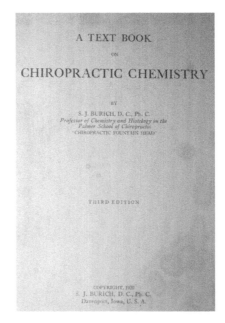

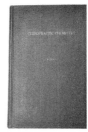

GBMN 71

Title: A Text Book on Chiropractic Gynecology
Volume: 12
Edition: First
Author: Harry E. Vedder
Printing Date: 1919
Pages: 407
Publisher: Harry E. Vedder
City: Davenport, Iowa
Rarity: 5
Value: 4
Desirability: 3
Physical Characteristics:

This 1919 book was printed in the standard Green Book format. The title page lists it as a 1919 first edition.

Date Acquired:

Price:

Notes:

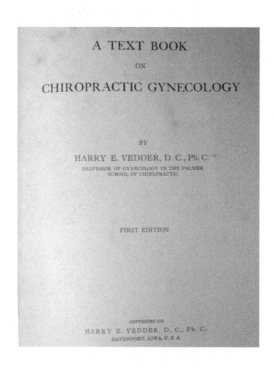

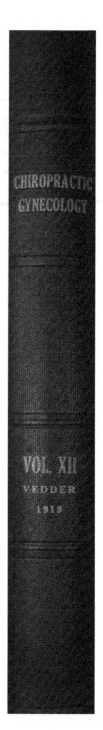

GBMN 72

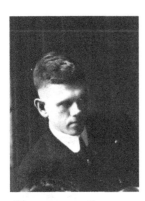

There are no known copies of this book.

Title: A Text Book on Chiropractic Gynecology
Volume: 12
Edition: First
Author: Harry E. Vedder
Printing Date: 1919
Pages: 407
Publisher: Harry E. Vedder
City: Davenport, Iowa
Distinctive Marks: SUSPECTED - soft brown leather cover
Rarity: 10
Value: 8
Desirability: 6
Physical Characteristics:

This book is suspected to exist as other Green Books printed in 1919 had this special edition in brown leatherette. To date a known copy has not been documented. This 1919 book would be printed with brown leather covers as a special edition. The title page would list it as a 1919 first edition.

Date Acquired:

Price:

Notes:

GBMN 73

Title: A Text Book on Chiropractic Gynecology
Volume: 12
Edition: Second
Author: Harry E. Vedder
Printing Date: 1920
Pages: 407
Publisher: Harry E. Vedder
City: Davenport, Iowa
Rarity: 3
Value: 2
Desirability: 2.5
Physical Characteristics:

This 1920 book was printed in the standard Green Book format. The title page lists it as a 1920 second edition. This second edition is a 1920 printing of the 1919 first edition.

Date Acquired:

Price:

Notes:

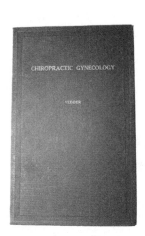
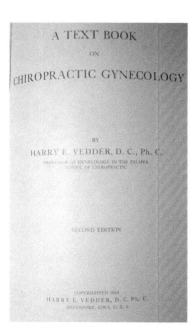
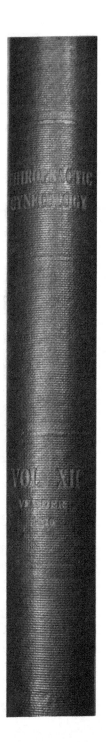

GBMN 74

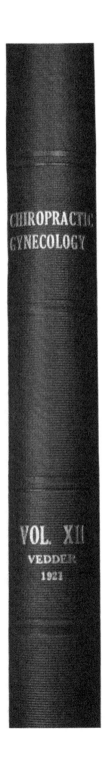

Title: A Text Book on Chiropractic Gynecology
Volume: 12
Edition: Third
Author: Harry E. Vedder
Printing Date: 1921
Pages: 407
Publisher: Harry E. Vedder
City: Davenport, Iowa
Rarity: 3
Value: 2
Desirability: 2.5
Physical Characteristics:

This 1921 book was printed in the standard Green Book format. The title page lists it as a 1921 third edition. This third edition is a 1921 printing of the 1919 first edition.

Date Acquired:

Price:

Notes:

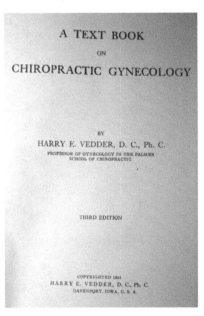

GBMN 75

Title: A Text Book on Chiropractic Gynecology
Volume: 12
Edition: Fourth
Author: Harry E. Vedder
Printing Date: 1923
Pages: 474
Publisher: Harry E. Vedder
City: Davenport, Iowa
Rarity: 3
Value: 2.5
Desirability: 2
Physical Characteristics:

This 1923 book was printed in the standard Green Book format. The title page lists it as a 1923 fourth edition. This fourth edition is a revised and updated edition.

Date Acquired:

Price:

Notes:

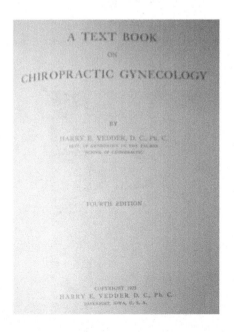

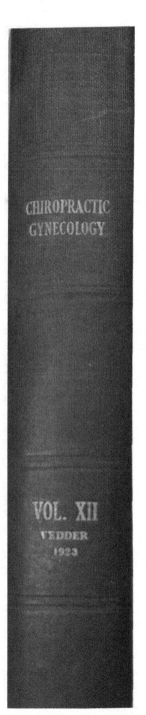

GBMN 76

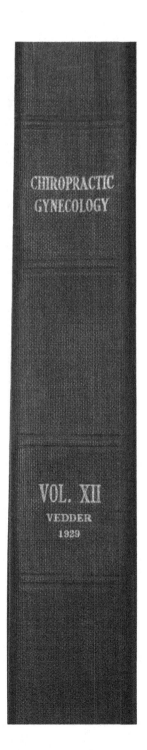

Title: A Text Book on Chiropractic Gynecology
Volume: 12
Edition: Fifth
Author: Harry E. Vedder
Printing Date: 1929
Pages: 474
Publisher: Harry E. Vedder
City: Indianapolis, Indiana
Rarity: 7
Value: 4.5
Desirability: 2
Physical Characteristics:

This 1929 book was printed in the standard Green Book format. The title page lists it as a 1929 fifth edition. Harry Vedder left the PSC faculty in 1926 and soon after joined the faculty at Lincoln Chiropractic College. While teaching at Lincoln Chiropractic College, Vedder printed the fifth edition which was a 1929 printing of the 1923 fourth edition.

Date Acquired:

Price:

Notes:

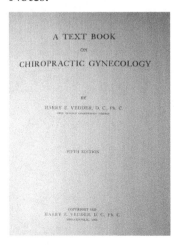

GBMN 77

Title: A Text Book on Palmer Technique
of Chiropractic
Volume: 13
Edition: First
Author: B.J. Palmer
Printing Date: 1920
Pages: 531
Publisher: Palmer School of Chiropractic
City: Davenport, Iowa
Rarity: 6
Value: 6
Desirability: 6
Physical Characteristics:

This 1920 book was printed in the standard Green Book format and had a single printing.

Date Acquired:

Price:

Notes:

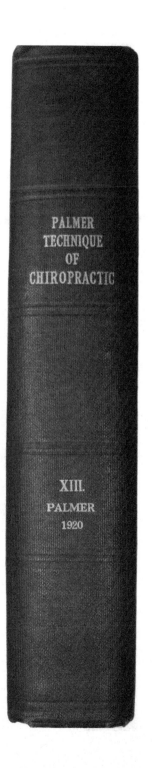

GBMN 78

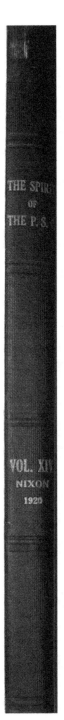

Title: The Spirit of the P.S.C.

Volume: 14

Edition: First

Author: James L. Nixon

Printing Date: 1920

Pages: 199

Publisher: Palmer School of Chiropractic

City: Davenport, Iowa

Rarity: 8

Value: 7.5

Desirability : 7

Physical Characteristics:

This 1920 book was printed in the standard Green Book format and had a single printing.

Date Acquired:

Price:

Notes:

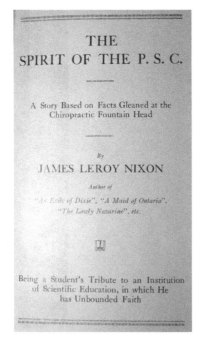

THE
SPIRIT OF THE P. S. C.

A Story Based on Facts Gleaned at the
Chiropractic Fountain Head

By
JAMES LEROY NIXON

Author of
"An Exile of Dixie", "A Maid of Ontario",
"The Lowly Nazarine", etc.

Being a Student's Tribute to an Institution
of Scientific Education, in which He
has Unbounded Faith

GBMN 79

Title: Chiropractic Textbook
Volume: 14 (reissued volume number)
Edition: First
Author: Ralph W. Stephenson
Printing Date: 1927
Pages: 396
Publisher: Ralph W. Stephenson
City: Davenport, Iowa
Rarity: 8
Value: 8
Desirability: 8
Physical Characteristics:

This 1927 book was printed in the standard Green Book format. This first edition can be easily identified from the second edition as it has 396 pages.

Date Acquired:

Price:

Notes:

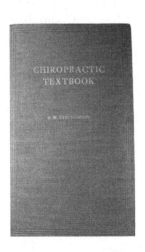

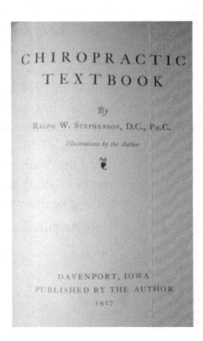

CHIROPRACTIC
TEXTBOOK

By

RALPH W. STEPHENSON, D.C., PH.C.

Illustrations by the Author

DAVENPORT, IOWA
PUBLISHED BY THE AUTHOR
1927

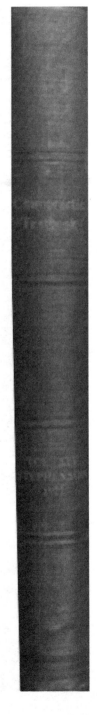

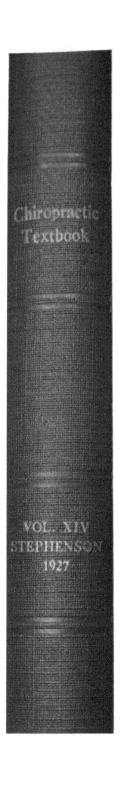

GBMN 80

Title: Chiropractic Textbook
Volume: 14 (reissued volume number)
Edition: Second
Author: Ralph W. Stephenson, Galen Price
Printing Date: 1940 (1927 on spine)
Pages: 414
Publisher: Palmer School of Chiropractic
City: Davenport, Iowa
Rarity: 7
Value: 7
Desirability: 7
Physical Characteristics:

This 1940 book was printed in the standard Green Book format. The spine and title page list a 1927 date. This book was mistakenly thought to have been printed in 1927. The second edition of this book was produced in 1940 with the addition of material on upper cervical adjusting by Galen Price (PSC 1936). This revised edition kept the 1927 copyright and gave no indication of the 1940 printing date. The book has 414 pages while the first edition in 1927 has 396 pages. Stephenson was planning to revise the first edition to include the new upper cervical material at the time of his accidental death in 1936. With the death of Stephenson, Galen Price was tasked with adding this new material to the text of this revised second edition.

Date Acquired:

Price:

Notes:

GBMN 81

Title: Chiropractic Textbook
Volume: 14 (reissued volume number)
Edition: Third
Author: Ralph W. Stephenson, Galen Price
Printing Date: 1946 (1927 on spine)
Pages: 414
Publisher: Palmer School of Chiropractic
City: Davenport, Iowa
Rarity: 5
Value: 4
Desirability: 3
Physical Characteristics:

This 1946 book was printed in the standard Green Book format. The spine reads 1927, but the inside lists a 1946 date. The third edition is another printing of the 1940 second edition.

Date Acquired:

Price:

Notes:

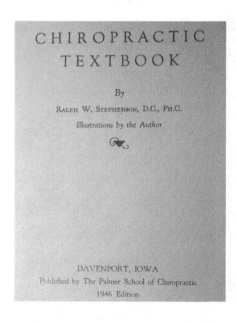

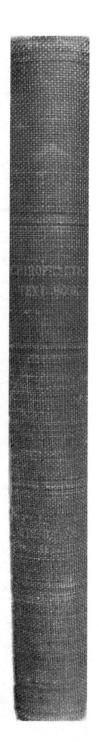

GBMN 82

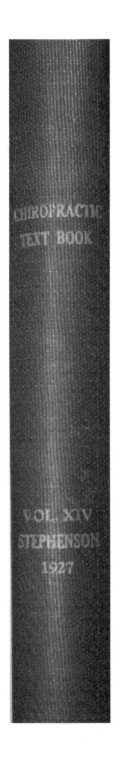

Title: Chiropractic Textbook
Volume: 14 (reissued volume number)
Edition: Fourth
Author: Ralph W. Stephenson, Galen Price
Printing Date: 1948 (1927 on spine)
Pages: 414
Publisher: Palmer School of Chiropractic
City: Davenport, Iowa
Rarity: 4
Value: 3.5
Desirability: 3
Physical Characteristics:

This 1948 book was printed in the standard Green Book format. The spine reads 1927, but the inside lists a 1948 date. The fourth edition is another printing of the 1940 second edition.

Date Acquired:

Price:

Notes:

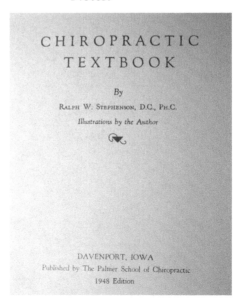

CHIROPRACTIC
TEXTBOOK

By
RALPH W. STEPHENSON, D.C., PH.C.
Illustrations by the Author

DAVENPORT, IOWA
Published by The Palmer School of Chiropractic
1948 Edition

GBMN 83

Title: A Text-Book on Chiropractic Orthopedy
Volume: 15
Edition: First
Author: John H. Craven
Printing Date: 1921
Pages: 399
Publisher: John H. Craven
City: Davenport, Iowa
Rarity: 3
Value: 2.5
Desirability: 2
Physical Characteristics:

This 1921 first edition book was printed in the standard Green Book format. The spine reads "Vol. XV." The title page reads, "First Edition."

Date Acquired:

Price:

Notes:

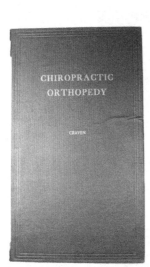
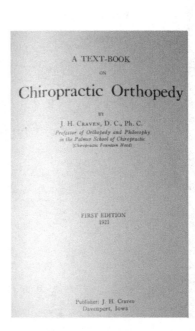
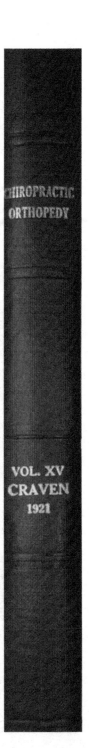

GBMN 84

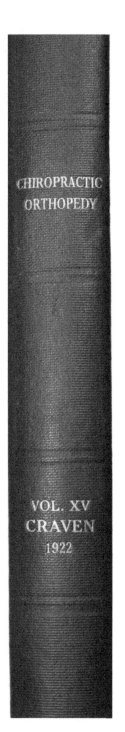

Title: A Text-Book on Chiropractic Orthopedy
Volume: 15
Edition: Second
Author: John H. Craven
Printing Date: 1922
Pages: 399
Publisher: John H. Craven
City: Davenport, Iowa
Rarity: 2
Value: 2
Desirability: 2
Physical Characteristics:

This 1922 book was printed in the standard Green Book format. This has a dark green cover. The title page lists it as a 1922 second edition. There are both a dark green (GBMN 84) and light green (GBMN 85) covered printings of this book.

Date Acquired:

Price:

Notes:

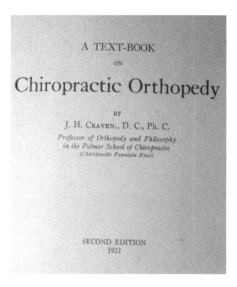

GBMN 85

Title: A Text-Book on Chiropractic Orthopedy

Volume: 15
Edition: Second
Author: John H. Craven
Printing Date: 1922
Pages: 399
Publisher: John H. Craven
City: Davenport, Iowa
Rarity: 6
Value: 1.5
Desirability: 5
Physical Characteristics:

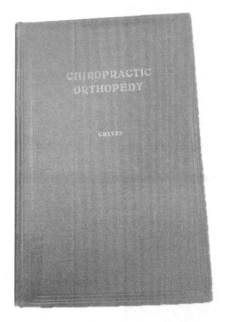

This second edition book was printed in the standard Green Book format with a slightly lighter green cover. The cover font is different than the dark green covered second edition. It is missing the dedication page and the image of Craven with the printed signature. It is likely a later printing but that has not been confirmed. The title page lists it as a 1922 second edition. There are both a dark green (GBMN 84) and light green (GBMN 85) covered printings of this book.

Date Acquired:

Price:

Notes:

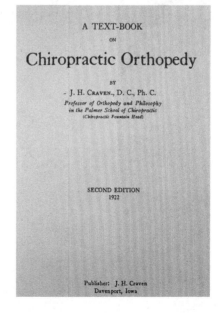

A TEXT-BOOK
ON
Chiropractic Orthopedy
BY
- J. H. CRAVEN., D. C., Ph. C.
Professor of Orthopedy and Philosophy
in the Palmer School of Chiropractic
(Chiropractic Fountain Head)

SECOND EDITION
1922

Publisher: J. H. Craven
Davenport, Iowa

GBMN 86

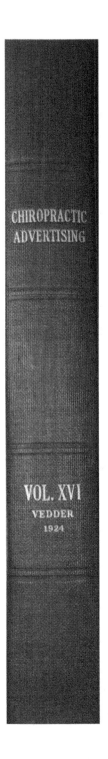

Title: Chiropractic Advertising
Volume: 16
Edition: First
Author: Harry E. Vedder
Printing Date: 1924
Pages: 244
Publisher: Harry E. Vedder
City: Davenport, Iowa
Rarity: 9
Value: 8.5
Desirability: 8
Physical Characteristics:

This 1924 book was printed in the standard Green Book format and had a single printing.

Date Acquired:

Price:

Notes:

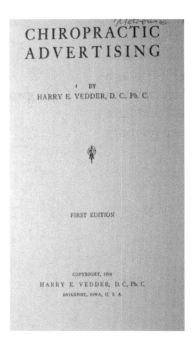

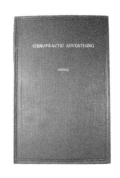

GBMN 87

Title: Malpractice As Applied to Chiropractors
Volume: 17
Edition: First
Author: Arthur T. Holmes LLB esquire
Printing Date: 1924
Pages: 253
Publisher: Arthur T. Holmes
City: Chicago, Illinois
Rarity: 8
Value: 8
Desirability: 8
Physical Characteristics:

This 1924 book was printed in the standard Green Book format and had a single printing.

Date Acquired:

Price:

Notes:

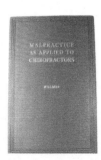

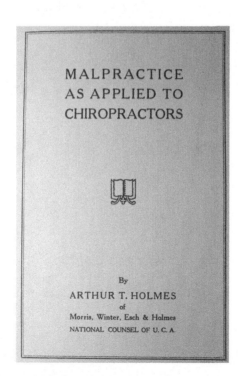

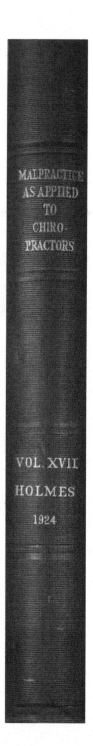

GBMN 88

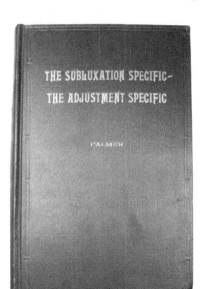

Title: The Subluxation Specific; the Adjustment Specific; and Exposition of the Cause of All Dis-ease
Volume: 18
Edition: First
Author: B.J. Palmer
Printing Date: 1934
Pages: 870
Publisher: Palmer School of Chiropractic
City: Davenport, Iowa
Rarity: 7.5
Value: 8.5
Desirability: 9.5
Physical Characteristics:

This 1934 book was printed in the standard Green Book format. The spine reads "Vol. XVIII." The title page reads, "First Edition."

Date Acquired:

Price:

Notes:

GBMN 89

Title: The Subluxation Specific; the Adjustment Specific; and Exposition of the Cause of All Dis-ease
Volume: 18
Edition: First
Author: B.J. Palmer
Printing Date: 1934
Pages: 870
Publisher: Palmer School of Chiropractic
City: Davenport, Iowa
Distinctive Marks: Signed and numbered edition
Rarity: 9
Value: 9.3
Desirability: 9.5
Physical Characteristics:

This is a special edition printing of the 1934 edition. It has an additional page in the front with a printed number and a printed script inscription. The B.J. initials are done with a live hand. It appears that 400 were printed; earlier numbers have some minor added value.

Date Acquired:

Price:

Notes:

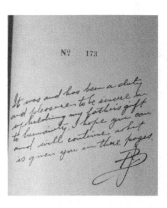

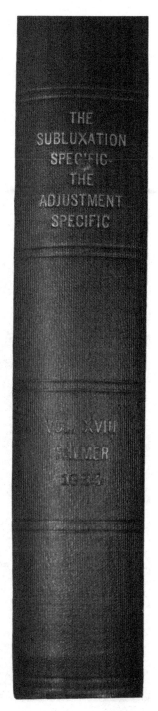

GBMN 90

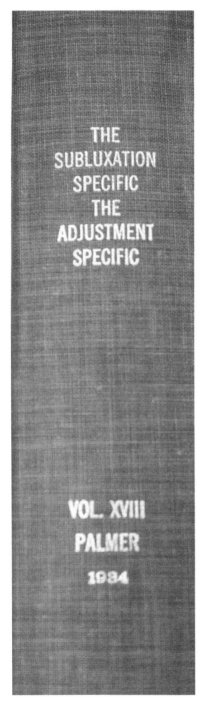

Title: The Subluxation Specific; the Adjustment Specific; and Exposition of the Cause of All Dis-ease
Volume: 18
Edition: First (reprint)
Author: B.J. Palmer
Printing Date: 1977
Pages: 870
Publisher: Chiropractic Publishers
City: Davenport, Iowa
Rarity: 5
Value: 4
Desirability: 3
Physical Characteristics:

This is a 1977 printing of the 1934 edition. There are no obvious indications that it is a modern reprint except for the cover being noticeably lighter in color and the cloth cover material is courser fibers. The book is slightly thicker and more square than the original.

Date Acquired:

Price:

Notes:

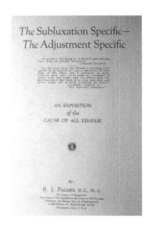

GBMN 91

Title: The Known Man
Volume: 19
Edition: First
Author: B.J. Palmer
Printing Date: 1936
Pages: 342
Publisher: Palmer School of Chiropractic
City: Davenport, Iowa
Rarity: 9.5
Value: 9.3
Desirability: 9
Physical Characteristics:

This 1936 book was printed in the standard Green Book format and had a single printing done by Palmer. The spine reads "Vol. XIX."

Date Acquired:

Price:

Notes:

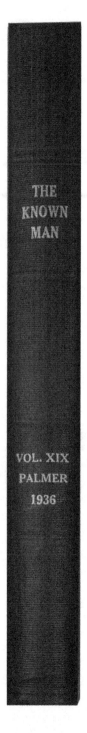

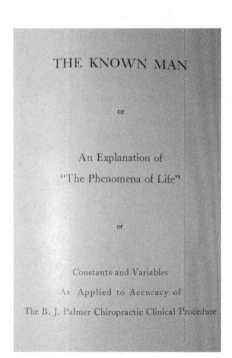

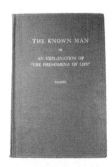

GBMN 92

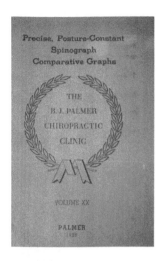

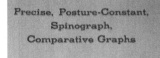

Title: Precise, Posture-Constant, Spinograph, Comparative Graphs; An Exposition of Innate Natural Adaptation Following HIO Adjustment Proving Measurement Correction of Vertebral Subluxations
Volume: 20
Edition: First
Author: B.J. Palmer
Printing Date: 1938
Pages: 207
Publisher: Palmer School of Chiropractic
City: Davenport, Iowa
Rarity: 7
Value: 7
Desirability: 7
Physical Characteristics:

This is a large (11x16) oversized gold spiral bound book. It does have volume 20 on the front cover. B.J. Palmer had at least one copy bound in black leather and it was labeled Property of the B.J. Palmer Chiropractic Clinic.

Date Acquired:

Price:

Notes:

GBMN 93

Title: Modern X-ray Practice and Chiropractic
Spinography

Volume: 21

Edition: First

Author: Percy A. Remier

Printing Date: 1938

Pages: 474

Publisher: Palmer School of Chiropractic

City: Davenport, Iowa

Rarity: 5

Value: 4

Desirability: 3

Physical Characteristics:

This 1938 book was printed in the standard Green Book format. The title page lists it as a 1938 first edition. The first edition of this book is individually numbered.

Date Acquired:

Price:

Notes:

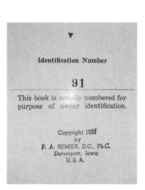

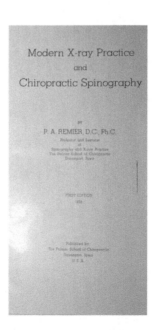

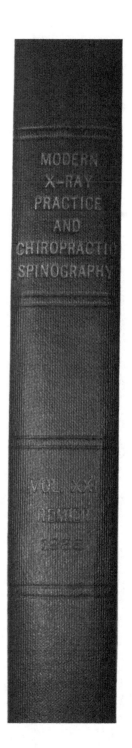

GBMN 94

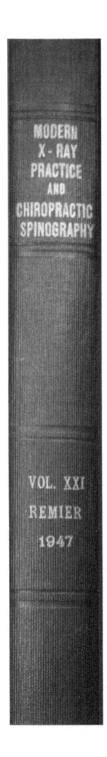

Title: Modern X-ray Practice and Chiropractic Spinography

Volume: 21

Edition: Second

Author: Percy A. Remier

Printing Date: 1947

Pages: 479

Publisher: Palmer School of Chiropractic

City: Davenport, Iowa

Rarity: 3

Value: 2.5

Desirability: 2

Physical Characteristics:

This 1947 book was printed in the standard Green Book format. The title page lists it as a 1947 second edition. The second edition has been revised and updated compared to the first edition

Date Acquired:

Price:

Notes:

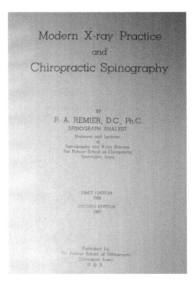

GBMN 95

Title: Modern X-ray Practice and Chiropractic Spinography

Volume: 21

Edition: Third

Author: Percy A. Remier

Printing Date: 1957

Pages: 422

Publisher: Palmer School of Chiropractic

City: Davenport, Iowa

Rarity: 1.5

Value: 1.5

Desirability: 1.5

Physical Characteristics:

This 1957 book was printed in the standard Green Book format. The title page lists it as a 1957 third edition. The third edition has been revised and updated compared to the second edition.

Date Acquired:

Price:

Notes:

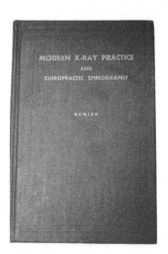

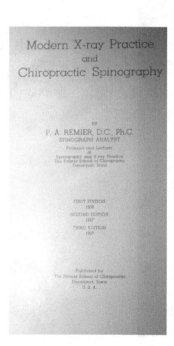

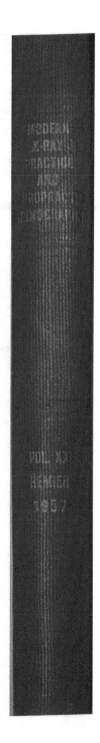

GBMN 96

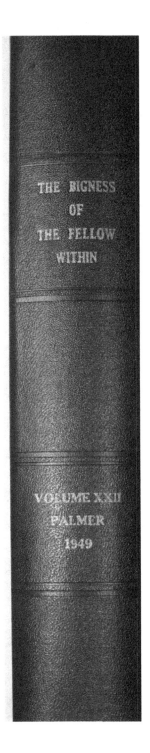

Title: The Bigness of the Fellow Within
Volume: 22
Edition: First
Author: B.J. Palmer
Printing Date: 1949
Pages: 943
Publisher: Palmer School of Chiropractic
City: Davenport, Iowa
Rarity: 7
Value: 8
Desirability: 9
Physical Characteristics:

This 1949 book was printed in the standard Green Book format and had a single printing done by Palmer.

Date Acquired:

Price:

Notes:

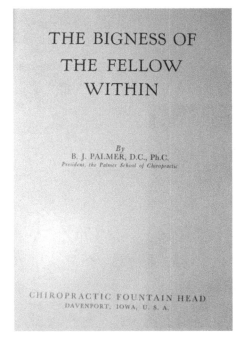

THE BIGNESS OF
THE FELLOW
WITHIN

By
B. J. PALMER, D.C., Ph.C.
President, the Palmer School of Chiropractic

CHIROPRACTIC FOUNTAIN HEAD
DAVENPORT, IOWA, U. S. A.

GBMN 97

Title: The Bigness of the Fellow Within
Volume: 22
Edition: Second
Author: B.J. Palmer
Printing Date: 1978
Pages: 943
Publisher: Sherman College of Straight Chiropractic
City: Spartanburg, South Carolina
Rarity: 5
Value: 4
Desirability: 3
Physical Characteristics:

This is a 1978 printing of the 1949 edition produced in a very small print run by Sherman College of Straight Chiropractic. It is in the standard Green Book format but the book is thicker and has slightly different lettering on the spine. The front page identifies the book as printed by Sherman and the title page reads "Second Edition."

Date Acquired:

Price:

Notes:

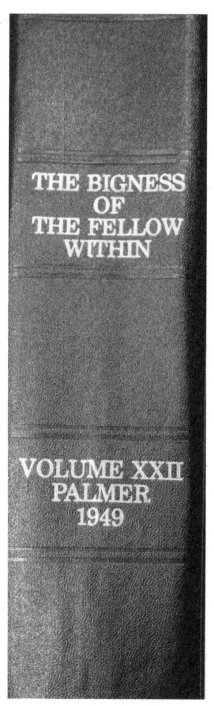

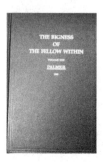

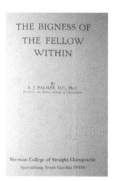

GBMN 98

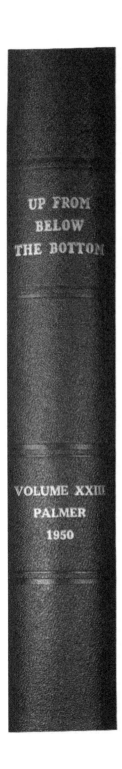

Title: Up From Below the Bottom
Volume: 23
Edition: First
Author: B.J. Palmer
Printing Date: 1950
Pages: 865
Publisher: Palmer School of Chiropractic
City: Davenport, Iowa
Rarity: 6
Value: 6
Desirability: 6
Physical Characteristics:

This 1950 book was printed in the standard Green Book format and had a single printing done by Palmer.

Date Acquired:

Price:

Notes:

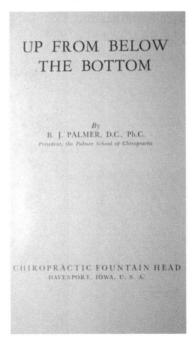

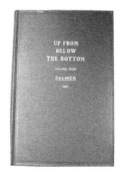

GBMN 99

Title: Up From Below the Bottom
Volume: 23
Edition: Second
Author: B.J. Palmer
Printing Date: 1979
Pages: 865
Publisher: Sherman College of Straight Chiropractic
City: Spartanburg, South Carolina
Rarity: 5
Value: 4
Desirability: 3
Physical Characteristics:

This is a 1979 printing of the 1950 edition produced in a very small print run by Sherman College of Straight Chiropractic. It is in the standard Green Book format but the book is thicker. It is square and has slightly different lettering on the spine. The front page identifies the book as printed by Sherman and title page reads a second edition in 1979.

Date Acquired:

Price:

Notes:

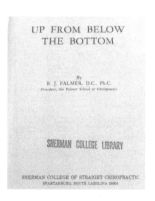

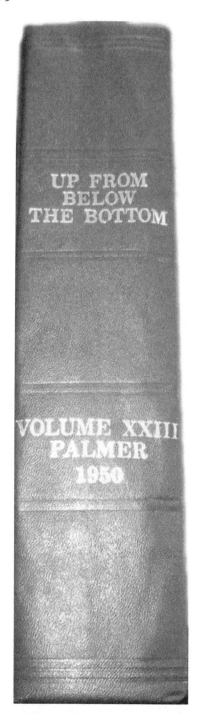

GBMN 100

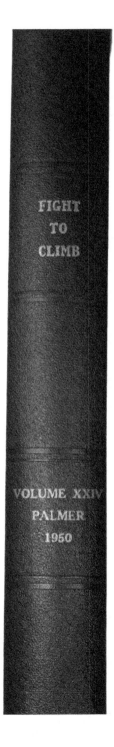

Title: Fight to Climb
Volume: 24
Edition: First
Author: B.J. Palmer
Printing Date: 1950
Pages: 715
Publisher: Palmer School of Chiropractic
City: Davenport, Iowa
Rarity: 6
Value: 6
Desirability: 6
Physical Characteristics:

This 1950 book was printed in the standard Green Book format and had a single printing done by Palmer.

Date Acquired:

Price:

Notes:

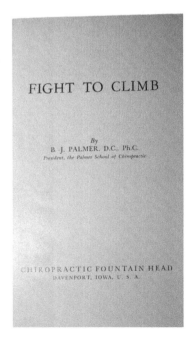

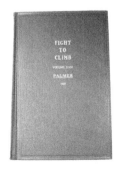

GBMN 101

Title: Chiropractic Clinical Controlled Research
Volume: 25
Edition: First
Author: B.J. Palmer
Printing Date: 1951
Pages: 744
Publisher: Palmer School of Chiropractic
City: Davenport, Iowa
Rarity: 6
Value: 6
Desirability: 6
Physical Characteristics:

    This 1951 book was printed in the standard Green Book format and had a single printing done by Palmer.

Date Acquired:

Price:

Notes:

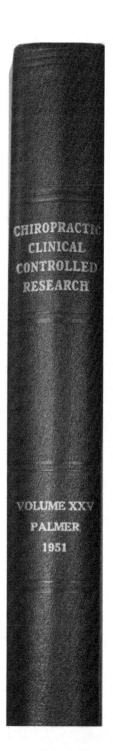

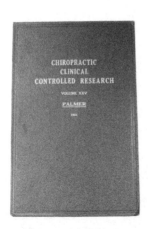

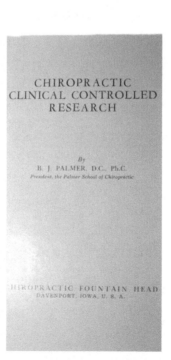

GBMN 102

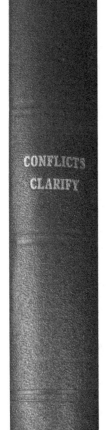

Title: Conflicts Clarify
Volume: 26
Edition: First
Author: B.J. Palmer
Printing Date: 1951
Pages: 747
Publisher: Palmer School of Chiropractic
City: Davenport, Iowa
Rarity: 6
Value: 6
Desirability: 6
Physical Characteristics:
    This 1951 book was printed in the standard Green Book format and had a single printing done by Palmer.

Date Acquired:

Price:

Notes:

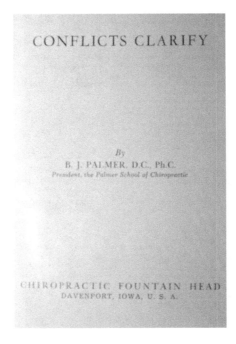

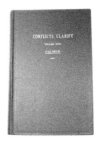

GBMN 103

Title: History Repeats
Volume: 27
Edition: First
Author: B.J. Palmer
Printing Date: 1951
Pages: 778
Publisher: Palmer School of Chiropractic
City: Davenport, Iowa
Rarity: 6
Value: 6
Desirability: 6
Physical Characteristics:

This 1951 book was printed in the standard Green Book format and had a single printing done by Palmer.

Date Acquired:

Price:

Notes:

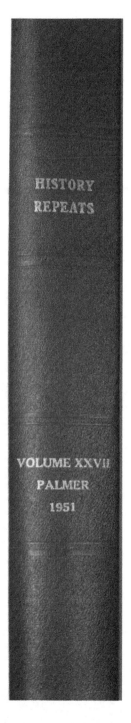

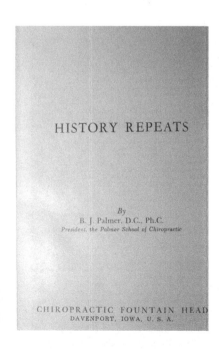

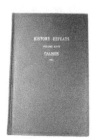

GBMN 104

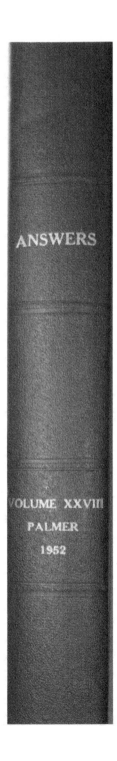

Title: Answers
Volume: 28
Edition: First
Author: B.J. Palmer
Printing Date: 1952
Pages: 840
Publisher: Palmer School of Chiropractic
City: Davenport, Iowa
Rarity: 6
Value: 6
Desirability: 6
Physical Characteristics:

This 1952 book was printed in the standard Green Book format and had a single printing done by Palmer. It was likely first offered at the PSC Lyceum August 1952.

Date Acquired:

Price:

Notes:

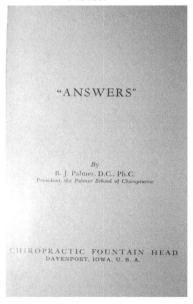

"ANSWERS"

By
B. J. Palmer, D.C., Ph.C.
President, the Palmer School of Chiropractic

CHIROPRACTIC FOUNTAIN HEAD
DAVENPORT, IOWA, U. S. A.

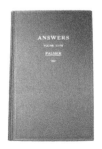

GBMN 105

Title: Upside Down and Right
          Side Up with B.J.
Volume: 29
Edition: First
Author: B.J. Palmer
Printing Date: 1953
Pages: 1036
Publisher: Palmer School of Chiropractic
City: Davenport, Iowa
Rarity: 6
Value: 6
Desirability: 6
Physical Characteristics:

This 1953 book was printed in the standard Green Book format and had a single printing done by Palmer. It was likely first offered at the PSC Lyceum, August 1953.

Date Acquired:

Price:

Notes:

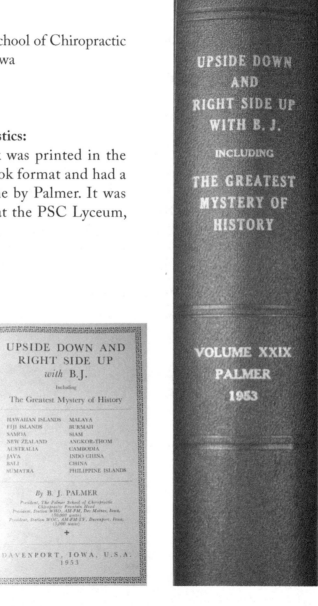

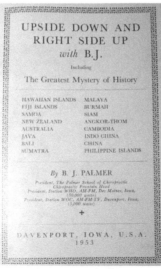

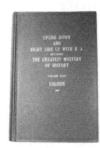

GBMN 106

Title: Chiropractic Philosophy, Science and Art: What it does, How it does, and Why It Does It
Volume: 32
Edition: First
Author: B.J. Palmer
Printing Date: 1955
Pages: 260
Publisher: Palmer School of Chiropractic
City: Davenport, Iowa
Rarity: 6
Value: 6
Desirability: 6
Physical Characteristics:

This 1955 book was printed in the standard Green Book format and had a single printing done by Palmer. This volume was reprinted in 1980 by ADIO. This modern printing looks very similar to the original 1955 printing except the green covers have a textured pattern and the book has details of the ADIO printing on the inside pages.

Date Acquired:

Price:

Notes:

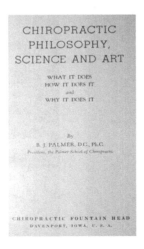

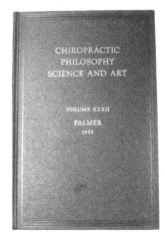

GBMN 107

Title: Fame and Fortune and the Know-how
and Show-how to Attain it
Volume: 33
Edition: First
Author: B.J. Palmer
Printing Date: 1955
Pages: 130
Publisher: Palmer School of Chiropractic
City: Davenport, Iowa
Rarity: 6
Value: 6
Desirability: 6
Physical Characteristics:

This 1953 book was printed in the standard
Green Book format and had a single printing
done by Palmer.

Date Acquired:

Price:

Notes:

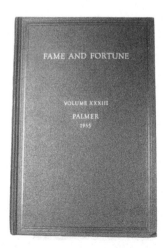

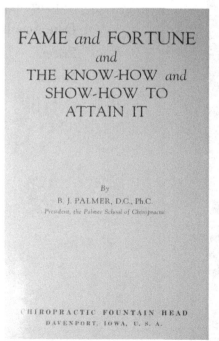

FAME *and* FORTUNE
and
THE KNOW-HOW *and*
SHOW-HOW TO
ATTAIN IT

By
B. J. PALMER, D.C., Ph.C.
President, the Palmer School of Chiropractic

CHIROPRACTIC FOUNTAIN HEAD
DAVENPORT, IOWA, U. S. A.

GBMN 108

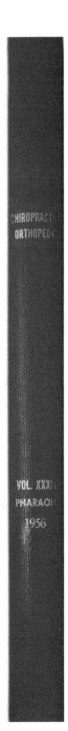

Title: Chiropractic Orthopedy
Volume: 34
Edition: First
Author: Donald Pharaoh
Printing Date: 1956
Pages: 311
Publisher: Palmer School of Chiropractic
City: Davenport, Iowa
Rarity: 3
Value: 2.5
Desirability: 2
Physical Characteristics:

    PSC faculty member Donald Pharaoh published this book in 1956 as a textbook for students. This 1956 book was printed in the standard Green Book format except it had a red cover. There was a single printing done by Palmer. There was a softcover reprint in 1975.

Date Acquired:

Price:

Notes:

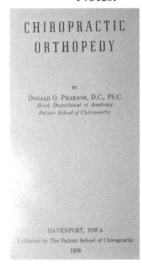

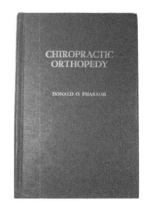

GBMN 109

Title: Evolution or Revolution
Volume: 34 (reissued volume number)
Edition: First
Author: B.J. Palmer
Printing Date: 1957
Pages: 126
Publisher: Palmer School of Chiropractic
City: Davenport, Iowa
Rarity: 5
Value: 5.5
Desirability: 6
Physical Characteristics:

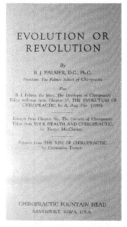

This 1957 book was printed in the standard Green Book format and had a single printing done by Palmer. During the PSC Lyceum in August of 1956, many in the profession honored B.J. Palmer's 75th birthday. The celebration was called "Operation 75." During the planning process donations had been collected from individual doctors across the world. Among other gifts, B.J. was presented with a check. B.J. used these funds to produce his next book. B.J. wrote Vol. 34 while in Sarasota over the winter 1956-57. The book was sent free of charge to those who had donated to B.J.'s birthday fund. Each edition had a printed form letter from B.J. Some had his script initials handwritten and some had personal handwritten inscriptions. Books with the original letter have more value ($20-$40). B.J. received many personal thank you notes from those doctors that received their complimentary Vol. 34. In 1958 B.J. produced a compilation of these as a small booklet titled "What They Say."

Date Acquired:

Price:

Notes:

GBMN 110

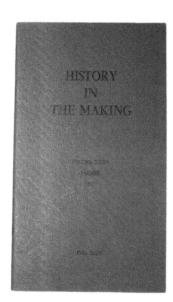

Title: History in the Making
Volume: 35
Edition: First
Author: B.J. Palmer
Printing Date: 1957
Pages: 72
Publisher: Palmer School of Chiropractic
City: Davenport, Iowa
Rarity: 5
Value: 5
Desirability: 5
Physical Characteristics:

A small (6x9) red soft covered book-let. The cover reads "Volume XXXV" and it had a single printing done by Palmer. The book is a bit of an oddity. B.J. Palmer had already produced Vol. 34 in 1957. It is unclear why he completely broke from his tradition and produced this red soft covered edition also in 1957. It is very small with only 72 pages, which could have easily been incorporated into *Palmer's Law of Life,* published in 1958. It is possible B.J. thought he needed something for sale at the 1957 PSC Lyceum as *Evolution or Revolution* was mailed to donors of his Operation 75. A modern reprint looks identical, but it does list a modern printing date on the inside title page.

Date Acquired:

Price:

Notes:

GBMN 111

Title: Palmer's Law of Life
Volume: 36
Edition: First
Author: B.J. Palmer
Printing Date: 1958
Pages: 150
Publisher: Palmer School of Chiropractic
City: Davenport, Iowa
Rarity: 5
Value: 5
Desirability: 5
Physical Characteristics:

This 1958 book was printed in the standard Green Book format and had a single printing done by Palmer.

Date Acquired:

Price:

Notes:

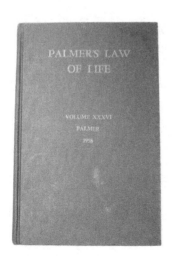

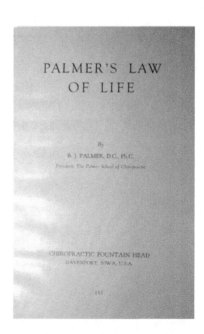

GBMN 112

Title: The Glory of Going On
Volume: 37 (reissued volume number)
Edition: First
Author: B.J. Palmer
Printing Date: 1961
Pages: 255
Publisher: Palmer School of Chiropractic
City: Davenport, Iowa
Rarity: 5
Value: 5
Desirability: 5
Physical Characteristics:

This was the last book B.J. wrote and had printed while he was alive. This 1961 book was printed in the standard Green Book format and had a single printing done by Palmer.

Date Acquired:

Price:

Notes:

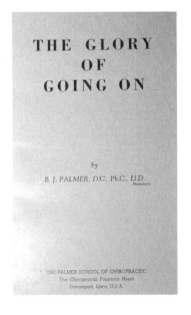

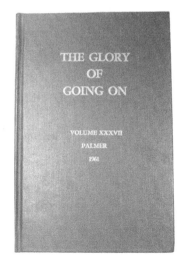

GBMN 113

Title: Healing Hands
Volume: 37
Edition: First
Author: Joseph Edward Maynard
Printing Date: 1959
Pages: 365
Publisher: Jonorm Publishing Company,
City: Freeport, New York
Rarity: 5
Value: 4
Desirability: 3
Physical Characteristics:

Dr. Joe Maynard was a 1949 PSC graduate. Maynard compiled many of the personal stories B.J. told over the years into a history of the Palmer family. Maynard wrote the stories as B.J. told them and may have added some of his own embellishments. The book was released during the PSC Lyceum in 1959 with an apparent endorsement from B.J. The book was printed with the standard Green Book format with a green cover and Vol. 37 on the spine. The original book had a purple dust cover.

Date Acquired:

Price:

Notes:

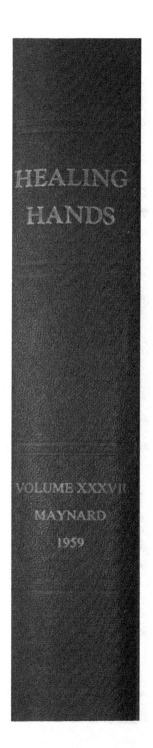

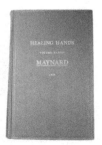

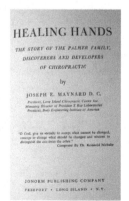

HEALING HANDS

THE STORY OF THE PALMER FAMILY,
DISCOVERERS AND DEVELOPERS
OF CHIROPRACTIC

by

JOSEPH E. MAYNARD D. C.

President, Long Island Chiropractic Center Inc.
Managing Director of Precision X Ray Laboratories
President, Body Engineering Institute of America

"O God, give us serenity to accept what cannot be changed,
courage to change what should be changed and wisdom to
distinguish the one from the other."
Composed By Dr. Reinhold Niebuhr

JONORM PUBLISHING COMPANY
FREEPORT · LONG ISLAND · N.Y.

GBMN 114

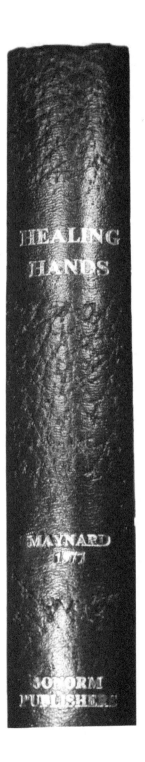

Title: Healing Hands
Volume: 37
Edition: Second
Author: Joseph Edward Maynard
Printing Date: 1977
Pages: 407
Publisher: Jonorm Publishers, 1977
City: Mobile, Alabama
Rarity: 3
Value: 3
Desirability: 3
Physical Characteristics:

Dr. Maynard revised his book and printed the second edition in 1977. This printing was a special limited autographed edition. The book has a brown cover and it no longer reads Vol. 37 on the spine. This book had a green dust cover.

Date Acquired:

Price:

Notes:

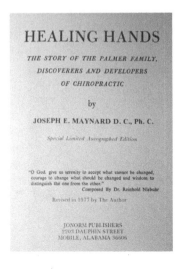

HEALING HANDS

THE STORY OF THE PALMER FAMILY,
DISCOVERERS AND DEVELOPERS
OF CHIROPRACTIC

by

JOSEPH E. MAYNARD D. C., Ph. C.

Special Limited Autographed Edition

"O God, give us serenity to accept what cannot be changed,
courage to change what should be changed and wisdom to
distinguish the one from the other."
Composed By Dr. Reinhold Niebuhr

Revised in 1977 by The Author

JONORM PUBLISHERS
2205 DAUPHIN STREET
MOBILE, ALABAMA 36606

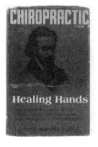

GBMN 115

Title: Healing Hands
Volume: 37
Edition: Third
Author: Joseph Edward Maynard
Printing Date: 1982
Pages: 407
Publisher: Jonorm Publishers
City: Mobile, Alabama
Rarity: 3
Value: 2.5
Desirability: 2
Physical Characteristics:

Blue hard cover with title and author on cover. This edition does have personalized copies with the ownder's name on the cover.

Date Acquired:

Price:

Notes:

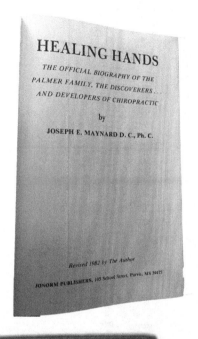

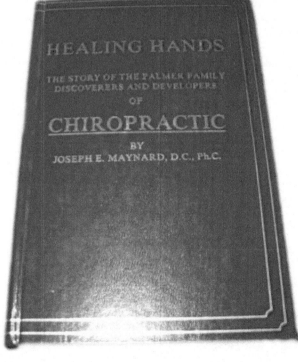

GBMN 116

Title: Healing Hands
Volume: 37
Edition: Fourth
Author: Joseph Edward Maynard
Printing Date: 1991
Pages: 408
Publisher: Jonorm Publishers
City: Woodstock, Georgia
Rarity: 3
Value: 2.5
Desirability: 2
Physical Characteristics:

The fourth edition is listed as a revised edition and the title page reads a 1991 copyright. The cover is again green with no volume number on the spine. This book had a white dust cover.

Date Acquired:

Price:

Notes:

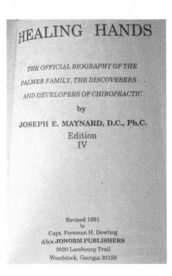

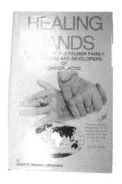

GBMN 117

Title: The Great Divide
Volume: 38
Edition: First
Author: B.J. Palmer
Printing Date: 1966
Pages: 163
Publisher: Palmer School of Chiropractic
City: Davenport, Iowa
Rarity: 5
Value: 4.5
Desirability: 4
Physical Characteristics:

The last two Palmer Green books Vols. 38 and 39 were published after B.J. Palmer's death. The books were printed in 1966, but the spine and title page reads 1961, the year B.J. died. The books are dark green covered, with the title and volume number on the spine. While the color is similar to the standard Green Book format the cloth cover is a courser material and the gold lettering is different. The cover is not indented near the border like the standard Green Book format. The book could easily be mistaken for a modern reprint. All the reprints known do state a modern printing date on the title page.

Date Acquired:

Price:

Notes:

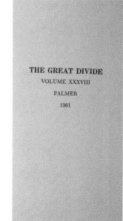

GBMN 118

Title: Our Masterpiece
Volume: 39
Edition: First
Author: B.J. Palmer
Printing Date: 1966
Pages: 156
Publisher: Palmer School of Chiropractic
City: Davenport, Iowa
Rarity: 5
Value: 4.5
Desirability: 4
Physical Characteristics:

The last two Palmer Green books Vols. 38 and 39 were published after B.J. Palmer's death. The books were printed in 1966, but the spine and title page lists 1961, the year B.J. died. The books are dark green covered with the title and volume number on the spine. While the color is similar to the standard green book format the cloth cover is a courser material and the gold lettering is different. The cover is not indented near the border like the standard Green Book format. The book could easily be mistaken for a modern reprint. All the reprints known do state a modern printing date on the title page.

Date Acquired:

Price:

Notes:

"OUR MASTERPIECE"
VOLUME XXXIX
PALMER
1961

GBMN 119

Title: Correlative Chiropractic Hygiene
Volume: None
Edition: First
Author: Donald Otis Pharaoh
Printing Date: 1946
Pages: 223
Publisher: Palmer School of Chiropractic
City: Davenport, Iowa
Distinctive Marks: Dark green cover
Rarity: 3
Value: 3
Desirability: 3
Physical Characteristics:

This book is in the standard Green Book format except there is no volume number on the spine. The spine reads Pharoah 1947 and the title page reads 1946. There are dark green (GBMN 119) and light green (GBMN 120) covered printings of this book.

Date Acquired:

Price:

Notes:

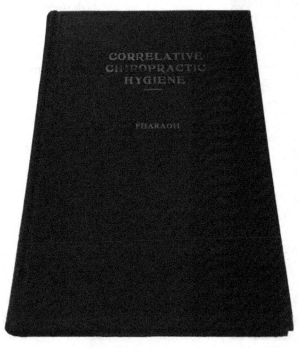

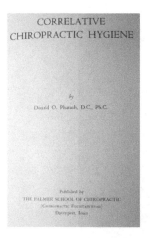

GBMN 120

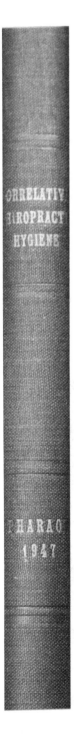

Title: Correlative Chiropractic Hygiene
Volume: None
Edition: First
Author: Donald Otis Pharaoh
Printing Date: 1946
Pages: 223
Publisher: Palmer School of Chiropractic
City: Davenport, Iowa
Distinctive Marks: Light green cover
Rarity: 3
Value: 3
Desirability: 3
Physical Characteristics:
This book is in the standard Green Book format except the cover is a lighter lime green and there is no volume number on the spine. The spine reads Pharaoh 1947 and the title page reads 1946. There are dark green (GBMN 119) and light green (GBMN 120) covered printings of this book.

Date Acquired:

Price:

Notes:

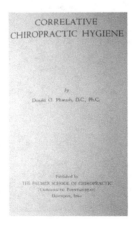

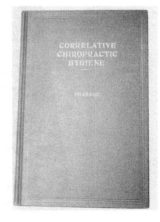

GBMN 121

Title: The Art of Chiropractic
Volume: None
Edition: First
Author: R.W. Stephenson
Printing Date: 1927
Pages: 88
Publisher: R.W. Stephenson
City: Davenport, Iowa
Rarity: 6
Value: 5
Desirability: 4
Physical Characteristics:

Small (6x9 inch) gray covered book with *The Art of Chiropractic* by R. W. Stephenson on the cover. Nothing on the spine. The title page lists 1927 edition.

Date Acquired:

Price:

Notes:

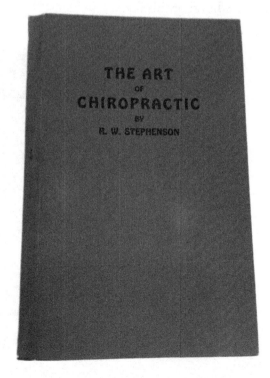

GBMN 122

Title: The Art of Chiropractic
Volume: None
Edition: Second
Author: R.W. Stephenson, W.H. Quigley
Printing Date: 1947
Pages: 72
Publisher: Palmer School of Chiropractic
City: Davenport, Iowa
Rarity: 5
Value: 4.5
Desirability: 4
Physical Characteristics:

Small (6x9 inch) lime green covered book with *The Art of Chiropractic* by R. W. Stephenson and (revised edition) on the cover. This edition was published by Quigley and the faculty of the Technique Department. There is nothing on the spine. The title page lists it as a 1947 revised edition. There are both a light green (GBMN 122) and copper (GBMN 123) covered revised edition of this book.

Date Acquired:

Price:

Notes:

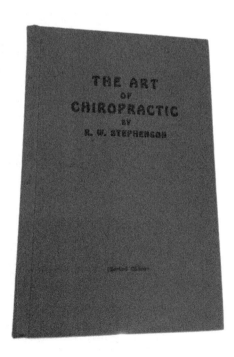

GBMN 123

Title: The Art of Chiropractic
Volume: None
Edition: Second
Author: R.W. Stephenson, W.H. Quigley
Printing Date: 1947
Pages: 72
Publisher: Palmer School of Chiropractic
City: Davenport, Iowa
Rarity: 5
Value: 4.5
Desirability: 4
Physical Characteristics:

Small (6x9 inch) copper covered book with *The Art of Chiropractic* by R. W. Stephenson and (revised edition) on the cover. This edition was produced by Quigley and the Technique Department. There is nothing on the spine. The title page lists it as a 1947 revised edition. There are both a light green (GBMN 122) and copper (GBMN 123) covered revised edition of this book.

Date Acquired:

Price:

Notes:

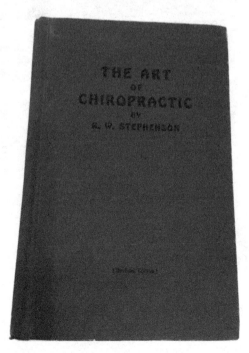

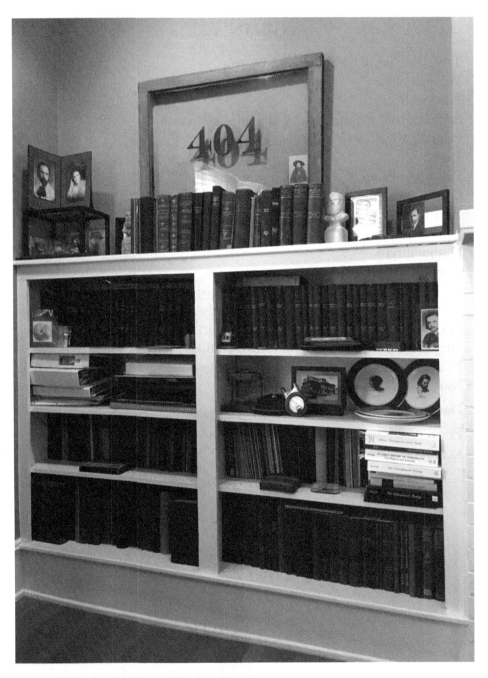

Private Collection
(including Room 404 door transom from D.D. Palmer's 4th floor Ryan Block offices)

Chapter 18
How To Value a Green Book

Collecting and studying Green Books is an enjoyable way to deepen your philosophical, scientific, and clinical roots while owning a part of history. Being a Green Book collector allows you to enjoy a rare type of camaraderie with colleagues. It is our hope that this guide will open up new pathways to fair exchange, enriching conversations, and a newfound passion for all things chiropractic.

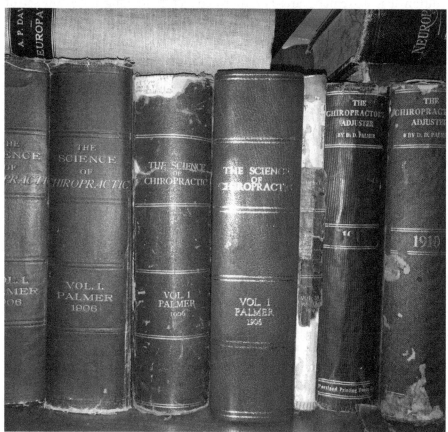

Green Book Value

As a general statement, the rarer a book is the more value it holds. However, it is more complicated than that. Just because something is rare does not make it valuable. The desirability of a book plays a significant role in its value.

Books written by D.D. or B.J Palmer are more desirable to collectors than books authored by PSC faculty. This is evident in the value of the non-Palmer authored Green Books. For example, a B.J. Palmer authored Green Book with a similar rarity to a John Craven authored Green Book, will have significantly different value.

However, a few faculty authored Green Books do have a very high value. For example, Vol. 16 or *Chiropractic Advertising* was written by Harry Vedder. If this book followed the trend of other faculty volumes it would hold a lower value than it does. Since Vol. 16 was only printed as a single edition it is extremely rare. For those collectors looking for a full set of books, Vol. 16 is hard to locate. Without it the collector does not have a full set of Green Books. Thus, the book is both rare and desirable, so its value is correspondingly higher than most other faculty written Green Books.

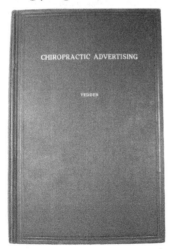 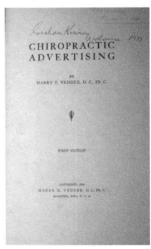

Chiropractic Advertising (Vo. 16)

The value of Green Books continually changes. Fluctuations in value have many factors such as the success of the chiropractic profession and the state of the economy in general. If doctors of chiropractic are profitable as a profession there will be doctors looking for Green Books to collect. Disposable income is an important factor when collecting.

Rarity and Desirability Scale

In this guide, we rated both the rarity and the desirability using a 1 to 10 scale of each book as a way to determine the value of a Green Book. The average score of rarity and desirability, is the value. By showing the rarity and desirability the collector gains more information about collecting books. The collector may find a book they need for their collection and the price may be more than they want to spend. Some books that are above an 8 on the rarity scale may not have another book available for sale in years or once in a decade. Knowing if the book is very rare or is more common will help the collector make a decision to buy the book now or wait for another book to be found for sale.

Rarity Scale

- **1-3** Very common books that are easy to find
- **4-6** Less common books to find, but with patience they can be found
- **7-8** More rare books, they do not come up for sale very often
- **9-10** Very rare books, no copies may come for sale for years to a decade

Desirability Scale

- **1-3** These books have limited interest or excitement
- **4-6** Moderate interest due to author, date, or subject
- **7-8** Higher desirability, these are usually early or high interest B.J. Palmer books
- **9-10** These are the showpiece of collections. Very early B.J or any of the D.D. books

Valuing Green Books

Because of future price fluctuations, we have chosen not to set specific prices for individual books. To say a specific book is worth $100 today makes the price fixed. We wanted a system that can be adaptive to the future market.

In today's market, a $60 Green Book is a 3 on the value scale. It is worth more than a 2 on the scale and not as much as a 4 on the scale. This same scale will be used for future pricing regardless of whether a 3 on the value scale is worth $50 or $200 one day.

To use this guide, a Green Book with similar value rating can be used to determine the current pricing of another Green Book that has the same value rating. We may not be able to say what a book is worth in the future, however, we developed this system so that collectors can tell the value based on other books sold with the same value rating.

The value scale is not linear, it is exponential. At the lower end of the scale, the price difference between a 3 and a 4 may only be $60. As the value numbers increase, the price goes up exponentially. The difference in value between a 9 and a 9.5 may be $1,500. This exponential increase is because around 20% of the books command significant prices. The other 80% of the books range from 0 to $500 in current price. The last 20% ranges from $500 to $7,000. A linear scale did not account for the massive jump in value of the top 20%.

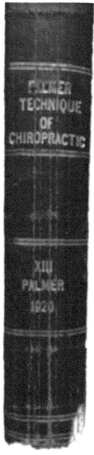

Vol. 13 (1920)

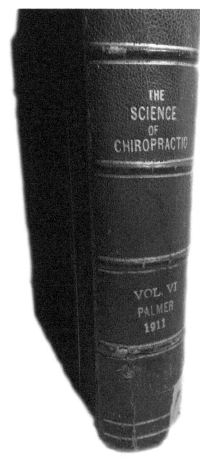

Vol. 6 (1911)

Wheeling and Dealing

Ultimately, the value of a Green Book is what someone is willing to pay for it. Buyers and sellers have other factors in play that may determine the book's ultimate sale price. A collector that is looking for a specific book to complete a collection may value a book higher than what our chart determines. Buyers may "over pay" because they need a specific book, or a seller may offer a bargain price because they need the money.

Some buyers or sellers may desire the sale of a group of books as a package deal, as opposed to "picking" an individual book out of a collection. The sale of 10 books as a lot, in a single transaction, has both advantages and disadvantages. You may over pay for nine books and under pay for one to get the book you need for your collection.

As previously mentioned, condition plays a significant role in value. Our chart assumes a complete book is in good condition with a solid binding and no obvious damage besides appropriate wear for its age. A book in mint condition may bring a higher price, just as a book in poor condition will have a lower price.

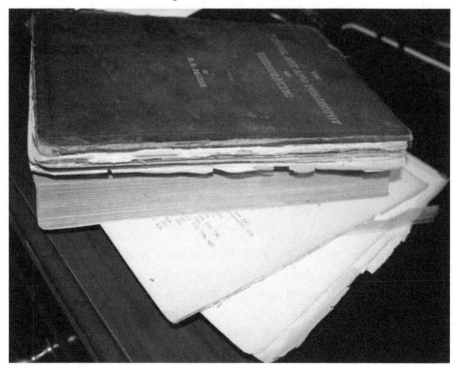

Damaged copy of *The Science, Art, and Philosophy of Chiropractic* (1910)

Assessing Green Book Condition

When considering the purchase of a Green Book for your collection, the book's condition is one of the most important factors affecting the value. There are many more factors to be considered. The bottom line is to make sure you know what you are getting. A picture of the book is the best way for you to see the book's condition. Make sure you look at the book and check the components listed in the assessment guide for Green Book condition in Appendix 5.

Can You Repair or Restore Your Green Book?

Damaged books can absolutely be fixed. There are a few things to consider before initiating a book repair. The first thing is the value of the book. Is it in original good condition? To determine whether to restore or repair a book you need to evaluate the cost. Compare the value of doing nothing to the value of the completed, restored book. For example, if it would cost $150 to fix a book but it is only worth $100 in original good condition, a collector should just spend the $100 and buy a book that is in good condition. Also, it is easier to decide to restore a book worth $1,000 than a book worth $200. Since most Palmer Green Books are less than $200 in value, it is hard to justify spending more than that on a minor repair. Simply stated, fixing a damaged book should be considered only if it makes financial sense. For some of the rare and highly valued Green Books, a full restoration is a reasonable and advisable solution.

Other questions require more complex answers. What is the overall condition of the book? Also, what issues are going to be addressed by fixing it? For this discussion two terms are needed: repair and restoration. A repair is fixing minor damage and a restoration is addressing more significant damage.

A book that can be repaired may only have minor damage, a detached page, or a cracked or loose binding. If the original parts are used and done by a professional, the repair will stabilize the book from further damage, and improve its value compared to leaving the book in its damaged condition. Repairs should always be done by professionals (not by a book owner with a hot glue gun). Signs of use like a torn page, faded cover, water stains, and edge wear cannot generally be repaired.

Restoration is when the damage cannot be repaired by using the original parts. Restoration is also required when parts are missing such as if the cover or spine is torn off, no longer attached and not complete. To restore the book to presentable condition, some material that was not original to the book must be added to it. Value will be lost from a restoration as compared to a book in good condition or one that has been repaired. The loss in value is determined by how much original material has been lost. In most cases a book that has been professionally restored is still more valuable than a book with major damage and/or parts missing.

Some books are "special" and have sentimental or other intangible value. If you love the book or it is a treasure for other reasons, spend the money and fix the issues.

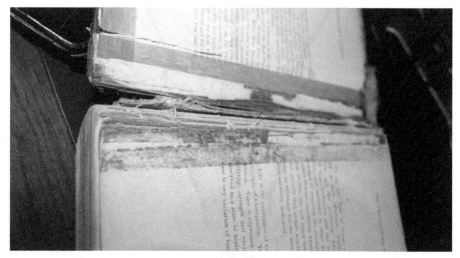

Damaged copy of *The Science, Art, and Philosophy of Chiropractic* (1910)

Trading Books With Other Collectors

Many Green Book collectors like to trade with other collectors. This is a great way for collectors to share their collecting activity. Oftentimes a collector will have duplicate books or they may be looking for a specific book and be willing to part with other books in their collection. If you know a collector has a duplicate of a book you need, find out what they need. Helping them find a book will likely result in them helping you. This hobby should be FUN. Trading is a very reasonable activity and keeps collectors from just buying and selling. The value rating will assist collectors in trading books with a similar value.

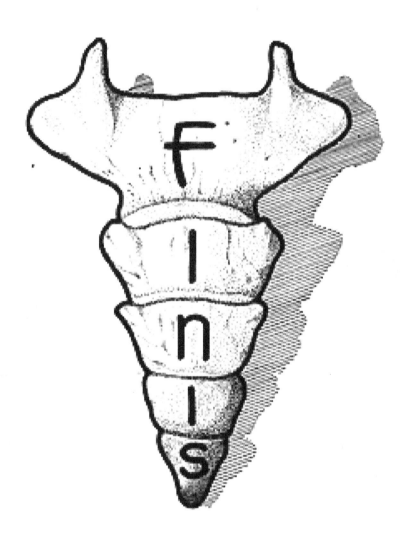

From Vol. 18

Appendix 1
D.D. Palmer's First Published Writing from 1872

D.D. Palmer's testimonial to Abba Lord, his first wife, was published as a letter to the editor of the *Religio-Philosophical Journal*. It is his first known published writing. The passage includes his earliest autobiographical account and his first use of "intelligence" to mean "spirit." He writes:

> I was raised a member of the Advent Church or Soul-Sleepers, for which I devoted the study hours of five years, to become a minister, but in spite of a threatening damnation and a kind father's council—"My son use your judgment in all religious matters, except when it conflicts with God's word, then allow His reason to be correct,"—I studied too much, thought too deeply, and finally my reason, or God's unmistakable word had to be laid aside. After spending many hours twisting my reason and the Bible and failing to make them harmonize, and many more discords arising, I chose to become, what the church called an Infidel and soon an Atheist. I then felt free and enjoyed a liberty which I never knew while fettered by the prejudices of the church and the Bible's narrow concocted plan of the future.
>
> For five years I attended Spiritual lectures and circles, for there I was allowed full liberty of thought and speech but found nothing to convince me of a future life but a tendency to make me more skeptical and Atheistical. When in that condition of mind I made the acquaintance of Miss Abba Lord, a very sensitive medium, who in time became my equal half and partner for life. Two weeks after we were pledged to each other, we conformed to the law and were publicly married at the residence of Wm. Drury, Esq. We married ourselves, using the following language: "Before God, men and angels I

take this man (or woman) to be my lawful wedded husband (or wife) to love and cherish till death do us part."

Here was more than I felt like saying—men I knew, but God and angels were myths to me. I was a disbeliever in psychometry, clairvoyance and all mediumistic phenomena, and I had satisfied myself it was a delusive humbug, and fancied that I should have no trouble to convince my equal partner that such was the case; for she was so purely honest that I knew she would not practice a knowing deception. Knowing the easiest way was the best, I patiently waited to inform her of the failures to guess correctly. During the first week she diagnosed ten cases of disease without a single failure, all of which were unknown to her previously. This was too good for guessing and I was compelled to acknowledge one humbug as truth. I soon found I could put her in mesmeric sleep— willing her to awake at any time desired by me, whether present or absent, and send her (spirit or intelligence) to any place however distant, leaving it with her when to return, which was usually about five minutes,—then her apparently lifeless body would be reanimated, telling me more or less of what she had seen and heard while absent. These experiments have satisfied me that the spirit can and does leave the body and return. The following facts I have daily evidence of, and not only believe, but know them to be positive facts, viz.: We live after the so-called death. Spirits can and do return. They give us any information that they have and desire to impart. The medium when under control can see without using the natural sight, speak a language of which she is not familiar, answer sealed or mental questions.

Yours for all truths, especially new truths,

D.D. Palmer

July 6, 1872

Appendix 2
D.D. Palmer's Second Book
The Chiropractor 1914 - Revealed
Abridged

Introduction

The Chiropractor by D.D. Palmer was printed by his widow, Mary Hudler Palmer, in 1914, a few months after the founder's death. It was largely unread within the chiropractic profession until 1969 when Dr. Earl Bebout of the Bebout Chiropractic College in Indianapolis, Indiana, first reprinted the book. Until this Bebout reprint, so few copies of the original book existed that it was essentially unknown to the profession that the founder had written a second book. Like the first D.D. Palmer book, it was a very small print run. The 1914 second book likely had even fewer books printed than the 1910 Palmer book. Dr. Dave Palmer had his grandfather's 1910 book reprinted in 1966, so it would be available to the profession.

Dr. Bebout had a unique distribution system for his reprinted Palmer book. He mailed 200 of them to chiropractors with the following letter:

> Dear Doctor: June 16, 1969
> This is a most unusual letter, with a most unusual offer. Read it carefully: then... it's up to you.
> Daniel David Palmer, father and founder of the science of Chiropractic, passed away in 1913. At this time he was preparing for publication his second book for Chiropractors on the subject of chiropractic. The manuscripts already prepared at the time were in 1914 published and copyrighted by Mary Palmer. It has been a little-known book; most Chiropractors, by far, during the past fifty years have never known of this book until a few weeks ago when we offered the first reprint of this book to chiropractors.

Republished with permission from the Association for the History of Chiropractic. Cite as: Foley, J. D.D. (2016). *Palmer's Second Book The Chiropractor 1914 - Revealed*. Chiropractic History, Vol. 36, No. 1, pp. 72-86.

A few years ago we became the owner of two of the originals. About five years ago a chiropractor wrote us pertaining to purchase of one of them. We offered it for $200. He immediately sent us his check.

About three years ago at Lyceum, we met the gentleman for the first time and, "how did you like the book?" His reply, "If I could not get another, I wouldn't take a thousand dollars for it." So, several months ago after a lot of thinking, we had the "Chiropractor" by D.D., 1914 reprinted, word for word by photocopy process. Nearly one-half of these have been disposed of already.

We have felt and still feel that every Chiropractor who practices chiropractic, who calls himself a Chiropractor should have this book. As he reads the chapters, 20 of them and a little more than one hundred pages, he will appreciate, we believe more than never the bigness of the science of Chiropractic and the bigness of the man who gave us Chiropractic: a thinker, a student, a philosopher, a scientist Daniel David Palmer.

Our first reprint edition is of deluxe type paper and binding, a very beautiful book to behold and to possess in one's library. One most of you will pick up and read parts many times. We indeed honor the memory of D.D. and appreciate what he has done for chiropractors and suffering mankind.

Our regular price has been and is $8. You may pay cash with order or charge same. Yes, if you don't want to or can't pay $8 then make us a contribution or pay nothing and keep the book if you desire or return it to us if you desire. Postage enclosed herewith.

The above is our way of making sure that all who desire may have as their very own, this book, as a proud memento to the honor and memory of Daniel David Palmer.

This letter and copy of the Chiropractor is being mailed out to 200 Chiropractors as a trial balloon. We are not so much interested in making a nice profit on a few hundred books as we are in placing the books in the hands of great numbers of chiropractors. The book comes to you with no strings attached. The book is yours, now. We would like to hear from as many of you as possible, and we will do our best to answer each letter.

Thanks to each of you and Sincerely

E.R. Bebout, DC

P.S. This letter above has just now been written on our 54th wedding anniversary.

The Chiropractor is a small book at just 115 pages. The binding of the original book had a hand done component consistent with a small run book printed at this time. (Morrison, Tony. R.R. Donnelley & Sons Printing Co., interview with author, December 7, 2012). A few added features of the book, when combined with this binding, makes the book's production costs at the higher end of what would have been available. If the sole purpose of printing the book was to make financial gain, the book could have easily been printed at less cost to make a larger profit per book sold. Based on the book's production quality, profit was not the sole purpose of publishing the book by the Palmer widow. In 1921, B.J. Palmer published volume four of his Green Book series titled *The Chiropractic Adjuster*. The book was D.D. Palmer's writings that had been sanitized by B.J. to remove what B.J. considered the unpleasant distractions of his father's writings. This book included articles from *The Chiropractor* (1914) along with the founder's *The Science Art and Philosophy of Chiropractic* (1910). Vol. 4 is presented as "A Compilation of the Writings of D.D. Palmer by his son B.J. Palmer." B.J. says, "My father only wrote two books. Each of these consisted of writings he compiled. The one was printed before his death, the other Mrs. Mary Palmer published immediately after his death." The reason given by B.J. for the production of this book was that "No library should be without D.D. Palmer's books in it. There has been a call for them. This book is the effort to meet that demand." Both of D.D. Palmer's books had limited print runs, making them extremely scarce. B.J.'s Vol. 4 was an effort to make his father's writings more available to the profession through this edited version. The author emphasizes that B.J. says D.D.'s widow published the second book immediately after his death. D.D. Palmer died on 20 October 1913 and *The Chiropractor* was copyrighted on 22 January 1914. This would leave three months from the founder's passing for the book's manuscript to be completed and ready to print. This seems like a short, but reasonable period of time for Mary Palmer to complete this task.

The Summer of 1913

D.D. Palmer moved to Los Angeles, Calif., in 1911, soon after publishing his 1910 tome, *The Science, Art and Philosophy of Chiropractic* (also known as *The Chiropractors Adjuster* or merely *The Adjuster*).

Palmer was no longer affiliated with the Portland-based D.D. Palmer Chiropractic College after yet another falling out with a school partner, Dr. John LaValley, in the fall of 1910. While living in Los Angeles, Palmer taught at the Ratledge Chiropractic College which was a short distance away from his residence. Dr. Ratledge opened his school in 1911 and he was able to convince D.D. Palmer to teach there in 1912.

Palmer and his fifth wife, Mary (Molly), traveled and lectured during the summer of 1913. They left southern California on 17 May and returned 8 September. During the first part of this trip, he was in Oklahoma City and gave four or five lectures over a period of two weeks at the Carver Chiropractic College. The president, Dr. Willard Carver, was both an attorney and chiropractor who had known the Palmer family from before chiropractic was founded. Dr. Carver reports that D.D. Palmer approached two prospective students of his school and offered them a set of 20 written lectures and a diploma for $50. Dr. Carver confronted D.D. Palmer and ended his teaching at the Carver school. Carver reports that D.D. soon left Oklahoma and headed to Davenport.

Longtime D.D. Palmer acquaintance, C. Sterling Cooley, recounts a similar story in an affidavit dated 14 August 1914. Dr. Cooley reported that while in Medford, Okla., in June 1913, he visited all day with D.D. and Mary Palmer. This visit with Cooley was just a few days before Palmer went to Oklahoma City to teach at Carver. Palmer told Cooley of his plan to sell his book, a set of lecture notes, and a diploma as a way to undermine B.J. and the P.S.C. These two sources corroborate each other's stories that D.D. Palmer had a set of lecture notes prepared for both his lectures at various schools, but also for sale with a diploma.

After leaving Oklahoma, D.D. and Mary visited Davenport for several months. During the summer of 1913 there was a minor reconciliation in the Palmer family as the three generations of Palmers shared some family time. The prior time D.D. was reported to have visited Davenport was in 1911. During this 1913 time in Davenport, it has been reported that D.D. Palmer lectured at the Palmer School of Chiropractic (P.S.C.), but was critical of his son, B.J., during those lectures. D.D. also lectured at the

Universal Chiropractic College (U.C.C.) and possibly at the Davenport Chiropractic College. Those schools were in direct competition for chiropractic students with the B.J. Palmer-operated P.S.C. This certainly did not help the father-son relationship that had been strained for many years. Unfortunately the truce did not last long as D.D. and B.J. got into a disagreement during a chiropractic parade that was to start on top of the hill at the P.S.C. and travel down Brady Street. D.D. and his wife left Davenport and returned to Los Angeles. Within two months the founder was dead of typhoid fever. D.D. Palmer died in Los Angeles on 20 October 1913 after a reported six week illness.

D.D. Palmer Lecture Notes

In the archives of Palmer College's Davenport campus are a set of D.D. Palmer lecture notes. The notes contain 20 lectures that are typed using a period typewriter that appears consistent with D.D. Palmer material. While studying these typed notes, the author recognized the lectures. The lecture titles were the same as articles in the 1914 D.D. Palmer book *The Chiropractor*. These typed lecture titles matched 20 of the 24 articles in *The Chiropractor*. There were four articles in *The Chiropractor* that were not in these typed notes. It is not known how this specific set of typed notes ended up in the Palmer archives. These 100-year-old typed notes are there and no other details are known about who owned them or how they got to Palmer.

As this author compared the actual lectures from the typed notes to the articles printed in *The Chiropractor*, it was obvious that the notes were the basis for the book. The typed notes were written by Palmer after he published his 1910 book. Palmer mentions repeatedly in the notes to refer to specific pages in *The Adjuster* (his 1910 book) for more information on a topic. Other dates listed in the typed notes confirm they were written after *The Adjuster* was published. It is apparent that Palmer was still adding material to these typed notes even into the late summer of 1912. In the article titled "Inflammation," Palmer mentions a 17 August 1912 Los Angeles Times newspaper article. At the end of the lecture titled "Nerve Vibrations" is a single line saying, "Notes from one of the lectures of the four weeks course by D.D. Palmer, Los Angeles, California." This line does not appear at the end of this same article printed in *The Chiropractor*. Dr. D.D. Palmer most certainly had a set of lecture notes developed after he published his 1910 book. He was lecturing at the Ratledge Chiropractic College in Los Angeles in 1912 before he left L.A. during the summer of 1913 and he taught short courses at other locations during that trip. It is likely he was even selling a set of notes in 1913 as reported by Carver and Cooley.

Further comparison of the individual lectures from the typed notes to the articles in *The Chiropractor* revealed various levels of revisions. Some articles like "Fever" were completely rewritten from the version in these typed notes. Others, like "Neuritis," "Arteritis," and "Rheumatism" are nearly identical in the typed notes and in the book.

The "Nerve Vibration" article in the book made reference to a newspaper article about Helen Keller hearing the vibration of a violin while visiting Petoskey, Michigan. A newspaper article about this Keller experience appeared in the Santa Ana Register and other newspapers on 13 August 1913. The addition of this detail into the article would indicate that the "Nerve Vibration" article from the typed notes was updated sometime after 13 August 1913, about two months before D.D. Palmer died.

Overall, nearly every article from the typed notes had noticeable additions in material and ideas when compared to the article written in *The Chiropractor*. There was only a small amount of content removed from the typed notes before being printed in the book. To this author, it is without question that the typed notes were added to and refined by D.D. Palmer. The fact that the typed notes were revised before being printed in *The Chiropractor* would imply these were typed by D.D. Palmer earlier, possibly in the fall of 1912 for use while teaching at the Ratledge school, rather than later in 1913 for his summer tour.

D.D. Palmer had been back in L.A. for over a week when he wrote to J.B. Olsen on 17 September 1913:

> Los Angeles, Cal., 420 W Vernon Ave
> J.B. Olson, D.C.--
> Yours of 4/19/13 came duly to hand, was taken with us East. We left here on May 17th and returned on Sep 8th. We made the trip one of sight seeing, one of seeing friends and relatives, one of chiropractic lectures and one of extreme hot weather for the three months out of the 3 and 1/2 we were gone in Oklahoma, Kansas, Nebraska and Iowa.

We were pleased to learn that Jacob is doing well. We frequently hear from Armstrong, but never from Marie or Graham. If you know their address, please give it in your next.

We are having it extremely hot here today, 107 in the shade, but <u>we do not have to work in the shade.</u>

I gave 22 lectures at the U.C.C. while in Davenport, for $220. I nearly made expenses while I was gone. The last trip out was on an excursion to Keokuk to see the Great Dam. On the return I cured a man of sun stroke by one thrust on the 5th dorsal. That is what I call definite, specific, scientific chiropractic, which is unknown to 99 out of a 100 chiropractors. My lectures have been increased, the last one is on "The Normal and Abnormal Movements of the Vertebral Column." I show therein that displacements increase the size of the foramina.

Look to the first two lines of your card and correct. Chiropractic is the Science (knowledge) of the principles which compose the scientific portion of chiropractic. Chiropractic is divided into three grand divisions, the Science, the Art, and the Philosophy. The Art is subdivided in Palpation, nerve-tracing and adjusting. Sixth and 7th lines. Nerves are stretched -- tension my boy causes 99 per cent of all diseases. Otherwise your card is up to date, abreast of the times. Some day I am going to get up a card for practitioners, also a booklet.

I have quite a lengthy lecture, in fact it will take two evenings to give it.

Truly, D.D. Palmer

P.S. At Davenport I offered an adjuster to the one who would give the greatest number of chiropractic principles. 221 were given.

This letter to Olsen was written after D.D. Palmer had returned to L.A. from his summer of 1913 travels. There are several bits of information contained in this letter that are relevant to this topic. D.D. added another lecture to his notes, "The Normal and Abnormal Movements of the Vertebral Column." This lecture was one of the four lectures printed in the book, but not contained in the typed notes found at Palmer College. D.D.'s addition of this new lecture supports the author's premise that the typed notes found at Palmer were early versions of the lectures, likely created before this summer 1913 tour. We can now document that twenty-one of the 24 articles contained in *The Chiropractor* were the up-to-date works of D.D. Palmer. Only three articles in the book are not documented in some manner. In this letter, Palmer also states he gave 22 lectures at the U.C.C. in Davenport. D.D. Palmer was in Davenport for an extended period if he delivered 22 lectures at the U.C.C. We do not know which 22 lectures he presented. In the last line of the letter, D.D. mentions giving away an *Adjuster* during his lecture at the U.C.C. During the summer of 1913, D.D. Palmer still had copies of his 1910 book available. This supports the 1914 affidavit by Cooley that D.D. was selling his book, a set of notes and a diploma in Oklahoma prior to going on to Davenport.

The three articles that are in the book and are not accounted for are "Constipation and Costiveness," "Pyorrea Alveolaris," and "The Moral and Religious Duty of the Chiropractor." Only one of these articles, "The Moral and Religious Duty of the Chiropractor," is controversial. This single article is the most provocative of all the Palmer writings.

Based on the typed notes in the Palmer archives and the collaborating information present, it is obvious that 22 of the 24 articles were revised and updated by D.D. Palmer to be published as his second book. The two other noncontroversial articles in the book also fit the work of D.D. Palmer, as there is no compelling reason for anyone to misrepresent them. The material in *The Chiropractor* did not consist of old notes or ideas that D.D. Palmer had discarded. What the author has revealed during his investigation indicates just the opposite. The articles were either newly written or recently revised from previous versions. It is entirely plausible that D.D. had begun the process.

Appendix 3
A Brief Review by D.D. Palmer

Biology is the science of life. Life is intelligent action, movements guided by intelligence. Life exists because of renitency and elasticity of tissue; these conditions not only permit, make it possible to receive, but actually create a response to an impulse. Impulses are thoughts in transmission over the nervous system. In telepathy thoughts are transmitted by the vibrations of ether; in spoken language they are transferred by the vibrations of the air.

The soul is intelligent life; it is the product from uniting intelligence and material, spirit and body; the result of a combination of the immaterial with the material. Vital makes possible organic functions, the power of motion and feeling.

The amount of tension depends upon the relative position of the osseous frame, the neuroskeleton, the skeleton of the vertebrates.

Health is a condition wherein all the functions are performed with a normal amount of force. Disease is an existence in which the action of an organ or organs are improperly performed. Death is a situation wherein action has ceased to be controlled by intelligence. The state of dissolution, or the act of a rolling stone, is not that of intelligence. Inflammation is a condition in which some local portion exhibits a higher temperature than any other, including the blood. Do not forget, in order to disturb functions, there must be in-ordinate nerve tension, also, a change in heat production. Fever is a state in which the whole body is above normal in temperature. Fever is diffused inflammation. Inflammation is associated with corns; the heat of which may be diffused if so, the patient has fever.

The neuroskeleton, when in normal position, is a protector of the nervous system, but, a nerve disturber when not properly placed. PRESSURE. There are three kinds of pressure, impingement, pinch and stricture; two forms of injury, contusion and concussion; each are lesional.

Pressure on any portion of the nervous system (the encephalon, spinal cord, the ganglionic chains, ganglia or nerves) increases or impairs its carrying capacity of impulses (motor or sensory), causing too much or not enough functionating: heat is one of those functions.

To impinge is to press on one side. Impinging and impinge are verbs, they denote action, something to be done, are always followed by on, upon or against. A nerve may be impinged on, upon or against. Impingement is a noun, denotes the act or condition of being impinged on, upon or against.

Pinching or squeezing is an act done by pressure on two sides, a material placed between two harder substances.

Spinal Adjustment displays two cuts on pages 146 and 147; the former is designed to "show the normal condition of the intervertebral discs."

In anatomy a disc is a circular organ or body which is plate-like. The epiphyseal plates of bone are situated on the upper and under surfaces of the body of the vertebra and the intervertebral fibrocartilage are known as discs, because they are like a plate, flat and round.

The cut on page 147 is "Showing compressed intervertebral discs and an impinged nerve from narrowing of the foramina."

The term foramina should be foramen, as nerve is referred to in the singular number.

To compress is to press or squeeze together, to reduce in volume by pressure, to make more compact.

The intervertebral cartilage is a connective tissue, nonvascular, contains no nerves. It is surrounded by a fibrovascular membrane, in which blood vessels and nerves are freely distributed, by which it receives nutrition. It contains a fibrous element, its base being of chrondin, a viscous, jelly-like substance which may be separated from the fibrous portion by boiling.

In the living subject it may be destroyed, necrosed, by excessive heat. Inflammation of the surrounding membrane liquifies, liberates the gelatin and very often destroys the fibrous portion. Its size is not and cannot be reduced by compression as shown in the cut.

A displaced vertebra, one whose articular surfaces are separated, en-larges the foramina, therefore, does not occlude the opening, does not pinch, compress or squeeze the outgoing nerves as they pass through the intervertebral foramina. The spinal nerves and their branches may be impinged upon or against, or stretched because of displaced vertebra, but not pinched.

"Impinged nerves from narrowing of the foramina."

The author here refers to nerves being pinched, not impinged.

Constriction is a condition of being narrowed by a binding force applied around a tubular orifice. A morbid contraction of a passageway, any hollow tube of the body. Constriction and stricture mean one and the same.

Illustrate stricture on board, contracture of nerve tissue, inflammation because of increased combustion of oxygen.

Compression is to press together, to make more compact, to reduce in volume, to make narrower in one direction.

A concussion is a shaking, a jarring, an agitation, or a shock caused by a collision.

The real and direct cause of disease is more or less nerve tension than normal. Displaced bones because of their pressure against, or non resistance of nerves, or that of stretching, cause an extra or a lessened amount of tension.

An abnormal performance of function of the body is denominated disease, the kind depends upon the tissue affected and the function disturbed.

The subtle and nicely discriminating transmission of physiological impulses, in health, whether of cells, the elementary structure of which organic substances are formed, individual organs, or the body as an organism, is directed by an intelligence known as spirit.

Sensory nerves are those nerve-fibers which carry sensory impulses from the exterior inward, to a nerve-center, resulting in sensation. Sensation is the recognizance of nerve vibration. Sensory nerve centers is where nerve vibration is identified. A sensory nerve is an afferent nerve, one which transfers peripheral impressions to the sensoria, sense-centers. Sensory ganglia are those masses of nervous substance which are thought to serve as a center of nervous influence. The most prominent of the sensory nerves are those of the olfactory, optic, auditory, gustatory, tactile and thermal. To these should be added that of cenesthesia, conscious existence, painful or pleasurable, depression or exaltation, the general sense of bodily, or self-existence, the subconscious sensation by the functioning of the internal organs. Sensory impressions are the effects of external agents or bodies upon the organs of sense. These external agents or bodies are always the same, impulses as originated are always perfect, if the nervous system is in a normal condition, the impressions, afferent impulses, can not be otherwise than normal.

We have the spiritual and physical impulses, those from the creator and the mind. All efferent impulses are motor. All motor impulses, whether of the spirit or the mind, are normal, providing the nerves of transmission are of normal tension.

All thoughts, orders, commands, directions of the mind, known as impulses, are normal if voluntary, the lines of communication are normal.

All thoughts, orders, commands, directions of the spirit, a segment of the Universal Intelligence, contains in miniature all intelligence and qualities of the All-Wise Spirit, just as one drop of the ocean contains all the qualities of the briny deep.

All spiritual impulses, those which cause intelligent organic action, life, are perfect when originated, as much so as their creator, as manifested in the new-born babe which has not been injured, whose impulses are carried over nerves of normal tension; but, if the tension-frame is displaced, luxuated ever so little, nerves stretched, vibration modified innervation increased or decreased, we have conditions known as disease.

The body when diseased manifests no new functions, develops no new forms of energy, adds no new space or accommodation.

While the larger share of diseases, abnormal functionating, are because of trauma, toxine and autosuggestion, there are minor causes such as inhalation of gas, smoke or flame, lack of food, water or air, decompression of the atmosphere in tunnels and caissons, an excess or a deficiency of heat, local exposure to the extremes of heat or cold which induces necroses, and exposure to X-rays may lead to caries.

Appendix 4
The Green Light Speech

This *Policy Talk* was delivered by Herbert M. Himes, D.C., Ph.C., head of the Technic Department, to the P.S.C. student body on January 4, 1956. It is known as "The Green Light Speech." The speech explains the new program described in Chapter 14 and detailed in Vol. 35.

The talk was recorded and shipped to B.J. Palmer in Sarasota, Florida. After listening to the talk, on January 7, 1956, B.J. writes to Himes,

> We are pleased beyond measure to KNOW YOU are behind this program 100%. It means that our life's work will come into its own. Our part of the work has been espoused and presented. NOW it is up to the profession to adopt or reject, all within the limitations of their horizons to understand. If OUR STUDENT BODY follows through, they will reach the concepts WE KNOW are true, and in this way spread THEIR influence TO the field, and in THIS WAY will evolve the profession EVENTUALLY into a solid phalanx from which MORE sick people over the world will profit.

Policy Talk by Marshall Himes:

I have something important to say this morning, but first, all of us here at P S.C. want to welcome all of you back from the holidays. We all are very happy that you-all have returned safely, and sincerely want to wish you the happiest of new years.

As I said, this is an important talk, and you are asked to pay close attention. It was decided to present this talk today because some ill-timed and ill-advised remarks have started a series of rumors. Rumors are vicious things, and rumor-mongers are unintentionally vicious. They suffer from a form of hoof-and-mouth disease. They hear something and cannot wait to hoof it to the first waiting ear, and there mouth what they heard, adding their own opinions and statements, thereby creating a situation that gets entirely out of hand.

We, and when I say we, I do not mean it in the sense that B.J. uses it. I refer to the entire faculty, the Dean's office and the business office.

We come to you today with a cards-on-the-table attitude, stating some conclusions and a series of propositions as clearly and as concisely as possible. Even so, there will be room for misunderstanding and mis-interpretation. I again ask you to pay close attention reserving remarks, opinions, and questions until we are finished.

The following is an extract from B.J.'s book "The Fight to Climb," page 507:

> "In 1895, D.D. Palmer brought forth a NEW principle with a NEW practice, which attained a NEW result. On the NATURAL, NORMAL SIDE it was:
>
> -if there are no concussion of forces, accidentally applied;
>
> -if there were no vertebral subluxation;
>
> -if all vertebral and spinal foramina were normally open to full size;
>
> -if there were no pressure upon nerves;
>
> -if there were no interference to any normal quantity flow of mental impulse supply between brain and body;
>
> -if there were no resistance to any transmission of nerve force flow;
>
> Then
>
> - there would be normal quantity of and/or normal speed of action of all tissue cell structure;
>
> -there would be normal function;
>
> -there would be chemical balance;
>
> -there would be functional, physiological, chemical health.
>
> On the ABNORMAL side, it further was:
>
> -a concussion of forces accidentally applied produced a vertebral subluxation.
>
> -a vertebral subluxation occluded a vertebral or spinal foramen.
>
> -the occluded foramen produced a pressure upon nerves.
>
> -Pressure upon nerves interfered with normal quantity flow of mental impulse supply between brain and body.
>
> -Pressure produced resistance to transmission.

-Resistance to transmission offered interference to transmission of mental impulse supply.

-This reduction in quantity flow created the beginning of ALL dis-ease, either functional, chemical, or pathological. In verity, he further said:

-a concussion of forces intentionally applied reduced a vertebral subluxation.

-A reduced vertebral subluxation opened the vertebral or spinal occlusion.

-Opened occlusion released pressure upon nerves.

-Released pressure upon nerves restored normal quantity flow of mental impulse supply between brain and body.

-Released pressure reduced resistance.

-Reduced resistance reduced interference.

-Increased quantity flow recreated restoration of health to ALL dis-ease - functional, chemical, or pathological. Diseases, as entities, were multiple; disease, as a condition, was single. As entities, each had its own cure; as a condition, there was but one cure. This is the 1895 PHILOSOPHY of D. D. Palmer's Chiropractic. That principle and practice was either right or wrong."

Our present day text book on philosophy states in Principle #30, and again in articles #122 and #123 that,

"the cause of dis-ease is interference with transmission of mental impulses; and, interference with transmission causes disease by preventing Innate Intelligence from producing adaptation in the tissue cell; hence it becomes unsound and not at ease."

Chiropractors the world over, who are worthy of the name, confining their practices to adjustment of the segments of the spinal column by hand only, are in whole-hearted agreement with the above principles. It is upon these principles, therefore, that we state the following conclusions and propositions:

Conclusion I. The first thirty-five years of our history was a period for evolving technics. Many were used, most were discarded. This was the period during which the very buildings housing you now were built. This was made possible because our graduates were REMOVING INTERFERENCE, gradually increasing their effectiveness, getting an ever increasing number of sick people well. The new science had caught on, and the very principles with which the profession worked were responsible.

Conclusion II. In 1930, the Hole-In-One or H-I-O or, as it is now called, Upper Cervical specific was introduced; B.J. produced his book on the subject in 1934 and the B.J.P.C.C. began to prove it in 1935. It was developed by one man; its purity is understood by some, and is practiced *exclusively* by relatively few. For sixteen years, the argument pro and con went on, comparing strict Upper Cervical Technic and results against the Meric system and general full-spine adjusting technics and results. Meanwhile, the B.J.P.C.C. and certain field men who were practicing strict upper cervical work were accumulating sufficient evidence to prove its effectiveness. Today, we are safe in stating that the majority of good Chiropractors recognize upper cervical work as the most effective SINGLE technic in Chiropractic.

Conclusion III. At Lyceum 1946, Dr. Hender was empowered to make the statement changing the name H-I-O to "Upper Cervical Specific" and adding that the PSC would stand behind any Chiropractor who adjusted the spinal column for the REMOVAL OF INTERFERENCE, when and where he found it.

Conclusion IV. Since 1946, many new graduates entered the field, and immediately entered the argument as stated above, no one advancing a satis-factory solution. Therefore, for twenty-five years, we have had a division in our Chiropractic ranks.

Conclusion V. Obviously the Member Schools of the NAACSC using various technics of adjusting the segments of the spinal column, have their percentage of successful and failure graduates even as we.

Conclusion VI. Leadership from the PSC has always been expected, and therefore, is now logical and imperative.

Conclusion VII. Until such time as the Chiropractor becomes the PRIN-CIPLE HEALER, legally and legislatively, we must have a circumscribed area of practice, and that area must be the ENTIRE spine.

Conclusion VIII. The consensus of opinion of the most staunch supporters of the PSC in the field, with the exception of few, was to the effect that occasionally some lower spine adjusting was necessary, should be thoroughly taught at school, and not discredited by the school causing a man to feel guilty or defensive when he used it .

Conclusion IX. It is time life be given to the 1946 announcement, and the so-called controversy between lower spine and upper cervical be given its death blow.

Therefore, we of the PSC propose to teach the Chiropractor of the future in the following manner:

Proposition I. Upper Cervical Specific will remain the main area of interest. Overwhelming evidence commands this attitude.

Proposition II. Investigate the lower spine in a practical research manner, assisting and encouraging the student to do likewise, for the purpose of eliminating any variables relative to the problem of interference.

In this connection, the program begins as a senior class project this quarter, known as a "Clinic Evaluation" or Pit Class. The pit class will be a two-hour class demonstration in the technics of: Taking a case history, physical examination, NCGH analysis., palpation, spinography, and adjustment. It will include the ENTIRE SPINE, and will be the foundation block for the eventual establishment of proper, standardized patient handling. These technics, so learned, will, when proper facilities have been provided, extend over into the student clinics, so the student may "learn by doing."

If you know of any person who is sick, ambulatory, available at 9:00 a.m. and is willing to appear before the class as an objective patient, we can assure them that the finest in Chiropractic care that the PSC has to offer will be theirs for the next three months.

Proposition III. We will demonstrate and insist upon sincerity of purpose and HONEST evaluation of all findings. This program will not lend itself to prove or disprove anything, merely to find and record FACTS surrounding the problems of interference, and its COMPLETE removal.

We make the following observations:

Observation I. This program will point up the high philosophical and artistic achievement of those men who can and do practice upper cervical work exclusively.

Observation II. It must be thoroughly understood that this program is not being adopted as an expedient, nor to meet any supposed competition, but instead, to render improved service to the patient, to the Chiropractor, and to the Chiropractic profession in general, removing the stigma of dogmatic pronouncements, by opening the spine to objective research.

Observation III. Some of you and some in the field will react as screaming alarmists, the "Chicken Little" type, who will think the sky is falling and we are going back to the dark ages of Chiropractic. Some others, both here and in the field, will hail this move as a return to the "Good Old Days" when "hit 'em high, hit 'em low, get all 26 and collect the dough" was the order of the day in most practices. You are both wrong, as the above statements indicate.

Observation IV. The theme of the program shall be, "To adjust where and when we find provable pressure, and how it shall be done most effectively."

Let it be made clear, here and now, that this will not be the practice of Meric Chiropractic as it was practiced in the '20's. I repeat, our theme is to adjust WHERE and WHEN we find PROVABLE PRESSURE developing and using the methods to do so most effectively.

If the dignity of Chiropractic is to ever reach its scientific achievements, and its recognizable value elevated to the level of the service it renders, then it must come from YOU, and educated out of the hands of those who are massaging, patting, rolling, rubbing, and jerking, eliminating all of the thoughtless, needless, and sometimes damaging adjusting that is done in the field today. Until that is done, we are worthy of being called glorified masseurs for which we receive three dollars a treatment.

Observation V. There are many points that have to be decided upon and researched. There are curricular changes that have to be made. This takes time and will require patience on your part. I ask you now, will you make a contribution to the success of Chiropractic and your own success by going along with us.

Observation VI. I plead, I beseech, I beg, I implore you; in short, I'm telling you, do not misrepresent this to your home town Chiropractor. To every writer of an indignant letter, demanding to know what is going on, I shall send a printed copy of this talk as a reply, and, as the saying goes, you shall be "hoist by your own petard."

Observation VII. In case you have any ideas that we are sneaking this into school while B.J. is in Florida, let me close this talk by reading two quotations from recent correspondence with him.

FIRST QUOTE:

> "In granting this program, as outlined, with exceptions noted, we do so knowing that if it is RIGHT, it will live and grow in the minds of more people. If it is WRONG, it will die and anything we might stubbornly refuse to yield on would be a dogmatic attitude in dealing with this problem."

SECOND QUOTE:

> "I do fully and most heartily concur in getting on top of this program, the sooner the better. We DO give YOU the greenest light we know, to go ahead."

Appendix 5
Book Condition

When considering the purchase of a Green Book for your collection, the books condition is one of the most important factors affecting the value. There are many factors to be considered. The bottom line is to make sure you know what you are getting. Besides viewing the book in person, detailed images of the book are the best way to see the book's condition for yourself. Make sure you look at the book and check these components:

Cover and spine - Any damage to cover, stains, color fading?

Binding – Is the binding tight and solid? Is it cracked, loose or even detached?

Pages – Are the pages attached? Any pages missing? Is there writing or highlighting? Any torn, discolored or damaged pages?

Grading Scale

Here is a list of terms so that you may more easily communicate about a particular book's condition. There are many different terms that can be used to describe a book's condition. Not all are mentioned here.

Mint or As New: The book is in the same immaculate condition as when it was published. This could be the description for a book that has been lost in a warehouse for years, never shelved, or even opened, yet it may still be an old book.

Fine or Excellent: The book approaches the condition of *Mint or As New* but without being as crisp. The book may have been opened and read but shows no wear. There are no defects to the book cover, binding or pages.

Very Good: Describes a book that shows some small signs of wear but has no significant damage. It has no tears or stains on either binding or paper. Any specific defects should be noted.

Good: Describes the average used worn book that has all pages present. There are more obvious signs of wear and has acceptable minor damage. The binding may be loose or cracked but not detached. Any defects should be noted.

Fair: A worn book with obvious heavy use that has complete text pages. The binding is very loose and beginning to be detached. Pages may be written on. There are stains and tears. All defects should be noted.

Poor: Describes a book that is excessively worn. There is obvious significant damage to cover, binding, and pages. Pages may be missing. The copy may be soiled, scuffed, stained or spotted and may have detached bindings and pages, etc.

Binding Copy: Describes a book in which the pages are in good to above condition but the binding is badly damaged, detached, or even nonexistent.

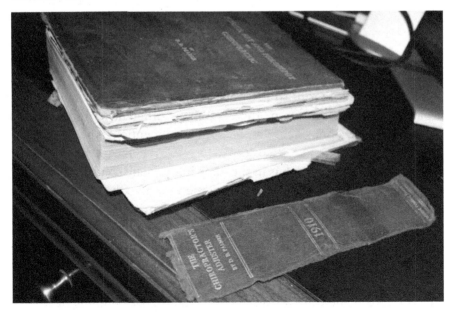

The Chiropractor's Adjuster with detached spine (1910)

Reading Copy: A copy usually in fair to poor condition but all the text is presented in a legible condition. The copy is okay to read but nothing more.

Working Copy: Even more damaged than the condition of a reading copy. The working copy will have numerous significant defects. It may be used to understand the basic structure of the book only.

Other Descriptors

Bowed or Warped: A condition of the covers or boards of a hard cover book. Bowed covers may turn inward toward the leaves or outward away from the leaves. This generally indicates some moisture issues at some point in the life of the book.

Chipped: Used to describe where small pieces are missing from the edges of the boards or where fraying has occurred on a dust jacket or the edge of a paperback.

Damp-stained: A light stain on the cover or on the leaves of a book caused by moisture such as a piece of food or perspiration. Generally not as severe as water stains.

Darkening or Fading: When book covers are exposed to light, the color darkens or it may fade and become lighter.

Edge-worn: Wear along the edges of hardback book covers.

Ex-library: The book was once in circulation at a library. This book could be in any of the above general conditions but more often than not has been well used. May have library stickers, stamps, or markings. Any former library book should be marked ex-library and have multiple stamps indicating it was officially withdrawn from circulation by the library.

Loose: The binding of a new book is very tight; that is, the book will not open easily and generally does not remain open to any given page. As the book is used, the binding becomes looser until a well-used book may lay flat and remain open to any page in the book.

Made-up Copy: A copy of a book whose parts have been assembled from one or more defective copies.

Moldy or Musty: Books stored in damp locations can get a musty smell to them and may have mold. Be very cautious of books in this condition. They can be dried out but a water damaged book will never be the same. The book may swell and be permanently altered.

Re-backed: A book that has been repaired by replacing the spine and mending the hinges.

Re-cased: A book that has been glued back into its covers after having been shaken loose.

Re-jointed: The book has been repaired preserving the original covers, including the spine.

Shaken: An adjective describing a book whose pages are beginning to come loose from the binding.

Shelf Wear: The wear that occurs as a book is placed onto and removed from a shelf. It may be to the tail (bottom) edge of the covers as they rub against the shelf, to the dust jacket or exterior of the covers (when no dust jacket is present) as the book rubs against its neighbors, or to the head of the spine due to being repeatedly pulled from the shelf.

Sunned: Faded from exposure to light or direct sunlight.

Tight: The book will not open easily and generally does not want to remain open to any given page.

Unopened: The leaves of the book are still joined at the folds, not slit apart.

Worming, Wormholes: Small holes resulting from bookworms (the larvae of various beetles).

Appendix 6
Bibliographic List of Green Books sorted by GBMN

The following Green Book Master List was designed to assist Green Book collectors to keep track of their books. The list includes cover-color information. No color indicates the book is Green. The books are listed according to Green Book Master Number and sorted by volume.

As you add a Green Book to your collection, first record the information on the individual GBMN listing of Chapter 17. List the date, price paid and make notes of its condition, uniqueness, damage, and any other purchasing information such as a history of previous owners.

The next step is to locate the Green Books in your collection on the following list. Check off the books you have.

Green Book Master List

☐ 1. *The Science, Art, and Philosophy of Chiropractic* (1910) - D.D. Palmer.

☐ 2. *The Science, Art, and Philosophy of Chiropractic* (1910) - D.D. Palmer. [red leather].

☐ 3. *The Science, Art, and Philosophy of Chiropractic* (1911) - D.D. Palmer.

☐ 4. *The Science, Art, and Philosophy of Chiropractic* (1911) - D.D. Palmer [red leather].

☐ 5. *The Science, Art, and Philosophy of Chiropractic* (1949) - D.D. Palmer [reprint, blue threads].

☐ 6. *The Science, Art, and Philosophy of Chiropractic* (1949) - D.D. Palmer [reprint, red threads].

☐ 7. *The Science, Art, and Philosophy of Chiropractic* (1966) - D.D. Palmer [Dr. Dave Palmer reprint].

☐ 8. *The Chiropractor* (1914) First edition - D.D. Palmer.

☐ 9. *The Chiropractor* (1969) - D.D. Palmer [Bebout reprint].

☐ 10. Vol. 1 *The Science of Chiropractic* (1906) First edition - Palmer.

☐ 11. Vol. 1 *The Science of Chiropractic* (1906) First edition - Palmer [red & black cover].

☐ 12. Vol. 1 *The Science of Chiropractic* (1906) First edition - Palmer [red & black cover, no red tips, no volume number on spine].

☐ 13. Vol. 1 *The Science of Chiropractic* (1906) and (1910) Second edition - Palmer.

☐ 14. Vol. 1 *The Science of Chiropractic* (1917) Third edition - Palmer.

☐ 15. Vol. 1 *The Science of Chiropractic* (1920) Fourth edition - Palmer.

☐ 16. Vol. 2 *The Science of Chiropractic* (1907) First edition - Palmer.

☐ 17. Vol. 2 *The Science of Chiropractic* (1907) First edition - Palmer [red & black cover].

☐ 18. Vol. 2 *The Science of Chiropractic* (1913) Second edition - Palmer.

☐ 19. Vol. 2 *The Science of Chiropractic* (1917) Third edition - Palmer.

☐ 20. Vol. 2 *The Science of Chiropractic* (1920) Fourth edition - Palmer.

☐ 21. Vol. 3 *The Science of Chiropractic* (1908) First edition - Palmer.

☐ 22. Vol. 3 *The Science of Chiropractic* (1908) First edition - Palmer [red & black cover] *suspected.

☐ 23. Vol. 3 *The Science of Chiropractic* (1908-1911) Second edition - Palmer.

☐ 24. Vol. 3 *Chiropractic Hygiene and Pediatrics* (1924) First edition - Craven.

☐ 25. Vol. 4 *The Science of Chiropractic: Causes Localized* (1908) First edition - Palmer.

☐ 26. Vol. 4 *The Science of Chiropractic: Causes Localized* (1908) First edition - Palmer [red & black cover] *suspected.

☐ 27. Vol. 4 *The Chiropractor Adjuster* (1921) First edition - Palmer.

☐ 28. Vol. 5 *The Philosophy of Chiropractic* (1909) First edition - Palmer.

☐ 29. Vol. 5 *The Philosophy of Chiropractic* (1909) First edition - Palmer [red & black cover] *suspected.

☐ 30. Vol. 5 *The Philosophy of Chiropractic* (1916) Second edition - Palmer.

☐ 31. Vol. 5 *The Philosophy of Chiropractic* (1919) Third edition - Palmer [1918 on spine].

☐ 32. Vol. 5 *The Philosophy of Chiropractic* (1919) - Palmer [soft brown cover] *suspected.

☐ 33. Vol. 5 *The Philosophy of Chiropractic* (1920) Fourth edition - Palmer [1919 on spine].

☐ 34. Vol. 5 *The Philosophy of Chiropractic* (1920) Fifth edition - Palmer [1920 on spine].

☐ 35. Vol. 5 *The Philosophy of Chiropractic* (1920) Sixth edition - Palmer [1922 on spine].

☐ 36. Vol. 6 *The Philosophy, Science, and Art of Chiropractic Nerve Tracing* (1911) First edition - Palmer.

☐ 37. Vol. 6 *The Philosophy Science and Art of Chiropractic Nerve Tracing* (1911) First edition - Palmer [red and black cover].

☐ 38. Vol. 7 *Chiropractic Symptomatology* (1914) First edition - Firth [blue cover].

☐ 39. Vol. 7 *Chiropractic Symptomatology supplement to the 1914 first edition* (1919) - Firth.

☐ 40. Vol. 7 *Chiropractic Symptomatology* (1919) Second edition - Firth [soft brown cover].

☐ 41. Vol. 7 *Chiropractic Symptomatology* (1919) Second edition - Firth.

☐ 42. Vol. 7 *Chiropractic Symptomatology* (1920) Second edition - Firth.

☐ 43. Vol. 7 *Chiropractic Symptomatology* (1921) Second edition - Firth.

☐ 44. Vol. 7 *Chiropractic Symptomatology* (1925) Second edition - Firth.

☐ 45. Vol. 7 *A Text Book Chiropractic Diagnosis* (1929) Third edition - Firth.

☐ 46. Vol. 7 *A Text Book Chiropractic Diagnosis* (1937) Fourth edition - Firth.

☐ 47. Vol. 7 *A Text Book Chiropractic Diagnosis* (1948) Fifth edition - Firth [red cover].

☐ 48. Vol. 7 *A Text Book Chiropractic Diagnosis* (1948) Fifth edition - Firth. [blue cover].

☐ 49. Vol. 8 *Chiropractic Physiology* (1916) First edition - Vedder [red cover].

☐ 50. Vol. 8 *Chiropractic Physiology* (1918) Second edition - Vedder [red cover].

☐ 51. Vol. 8 *Chiropractic Physiology* (1918) Third edition - Vedder [1920 on spine].

☐ 52. Vol. 8 *Chiropractic Physiology* (1921) Fourth edition - Vedder.

☐ 53. Vol. 8 *Chiropractic Physiology* (1922) Fifth edition - Vedder.

☐ 54. Vol. 9 *Chiropractic Anatomy* (1918) First edition - M.H. Palmer.

☐ 55. Vol. 9 *Chiropractic Anatomy* (1919) Second edition - M.H. Palmer.

☐ 56. Vol. 9 *Chiropractic Anatomy* (1919) - M.H. Palmer [soft brown cover] *suspected.

☐ 57. Vol. 9 *Chiropractic Anatomy* (1920) Third edition - M.H. Palmer [1919 on spine].

☐ 58. Vol. 9 *Chiropractic Anatomy* (1920) Fourth edition - M.H. Palmer [1920 on spine].

☐ 59. Vol. 9 *Chiropractic Anatomy* (1920) Fourth edition - M.H. Palmer [1922 on spine].

☐ 60. Vol. 9 *Chiropractic Anatomy* (1923) Fifth edition - M.H. Palmer.

☐ 61. Vol. 10 *Chiropractic Spinography* (1918) First edition - Thompson [booklet].

☐ 62. Vol. 10 *Chiropractic Spinography* (1919) Second edition - Thompson.

☐ 63. Vol. 10 *Chiropractic Spinography* (1919) Second edition - Thompson [soft brown cover].

☐ 64. Vol. 10 *Chiropractic Spinography* (1921) Third edition - Thompson.

☐ 65. Vol. 10 *Chiropractic Spinography* (1923) Fourth edition - Thompson.

☐ 66. Vol. 11 *Chiropractic Chemistry* (1919) First edition - Burich.

☐ 67. Vol. 11 *Chiropractic Chemistry* (1919) First edition - Burich [soft brown cover].

☐ 68. Vol. 11 *Chemistry Supplement to the first edition* (June 1925) - Burich [booklet].

☐ 69. Vol. 11 *Chiropractic Chemistry* (1920) Second edition - Burich.

☐ 70. Vol. 11 *Chiropractic Chemistry* (1920) Third edition - Burich [1921 on spine].

☐ 71. Vol. 12 *Chiropractic Gynecology* (1919) First edition - Vedder.

☐ 72. Vol. 12 *Chiropractic Gynecology* (1919) - Vedder [soft brown cover] *suspected.

☐ 73. Vol. 12 *Chiropractic Gynecology* (1920) Second edition - Vedder.

☐ 74. Vol. 12 *Chiropractic Gynecology* (1921) Third edition - Vedder.

☐ 75. Vol. 12 *Chiropractic Gynecology* (1923) Fourth edition - Vedder.

☐ 76. Vol. 12 *Chiropractic Gynecology* (1929) Fifth edition - Vedder [published while leading Lincoln Chiropractic College].

☐ 77. Vol. 13 *A Textbook on the Palmer Technique* (1920) First edition - Palmer.

☐ 78. Vol. 14 *The Spirit of P.S.C.* (1920) First edition - Nixon.

☐ 79. Vol. 14 *Chiropractic Textbook* (1927) First edition - Stephenson [396 pages, 1927 on spine].

☐ 80. Vol. 14 *Chiropractic Textbook* (1940) Second edition - Stephenson [414 pages, 1927 on spine].

☐ 81. Vol. 14 *Chiropractic Textbook* (1946) Third edition - Stephenson [1927 on spine].

☐ 82. Vol. 14 *Chiropractic Textbook* (1948) Fourth edition - Stephenson [1927 on spine].

☐ 83. Vol. 15 *A Textbook on Chiropractic Orthopedy* (1921) First edition - Craven.

☐ 84. Vol. 15 *A Textbook on Chiropractic Orthopedy* (1922) Second edition - Craven [dark green].

☐ 85. Vol. 15 *A Textbook on Chiropractic Orthopedy* (1922) Second edition - Craven [light green].

☐ 86. Vol. 16 *Chiropractic Advertising* (1924) First edition - Vedder.

☐ 87. Vol. 17 *Malpractice as Applied to Chiropractic* (1924) First edition - Holmes.

☐ 88. Vol. 18 *The Subluxation Specific; the Adjustment Specific* (1934) First edition - Palmer.

☐ 89. Vol. 18 *The Subluxation Specific; The Adjustment Specific* (1934) First edition - Palmer [signed and numbered edition].

☐ 90. Vol. 18 *The Subluxation Specific; The Adjustment Specific* (1977) - Palmer [modern reprint].

☐ 91. Vol. 19 *The Known Man* (1936) First edition - Palmer.

☐ 92. Vol. 20 *Precise, Posture-Constant, Spinograph* (1938) First edition - Palmer [oversized gold spiral].

☐ 93. Vol. 21 *Modern X-ray Practice and Chiropractic Spinography* (1938) First edition - Remier.

☐ 94. Vol. 21 *Modern X-ray Practice and Chiropractic Spinography* (1947) Second edition - Remier.

☐ 95. Vol. 21 *Modern X-ray Practice and Chiropractic Spinography* (1957) Third edition - Remier.

☐ 96. Vol. 22 *The Bigness of the Fellow Within* (1949) First edition - Palmer.

☐ 97. Vol. 22 *The Bigness of the Fellow Within* (1978) - Palmer [modern reprint].

☐ 98. Vol. 23 *Up From Below the Bottom* (1950) First edition - Palmer.

☐ 99. Vol. 23 *Up From Below the Bottom* (1979) - Palmer
[modern reprint, Sherman]

☐ 100. Vol. 24 *Fight to Climb* (1950) First edition - Palmer.

☐ 101. Vol. 25 *Chiropractic Clinical Controlled Research* (1951) First edition -
Palmer.

☐ 102. Vol. 26 *Conflicts Clarify* (1951) First edition - Palmer.

☐ 103. Vol. 27 *History Repeats* (1951) First edition - Palmer.

☐ 104. Vol. 28 *Answers* (1952) First edition - Palmer.

☐ 105. Vol. 29 *Upside Down and Right Side Up with B.J.* (1953) First edition
- Palmer.

☐ 106. Vol. 32 *Chiropractic Philosophy, Science and Art* (1955) First edition - Palmer.

☐ 107. Vol. 33 *Fame and Fortune* (1955) First edition - Palmer.

☐ 108. Vol. 34 *Evolution or Revolution* (1957) First edition - Palmer.

☐ 109. Vol. 34 *Chiropractic Orthopedy* (1956) First edition - Pharaoh.

☐ 110. Vol. 35 *History In the Making* (1957) First edition - Palmer.

☐ 111. Vol. 36 *Palmer's Law of Life* (1958) First edition - Palmer.

☐ 112. Vol. 37 *The Glory of Going On* (1961) First edition - Palmer.

☐ 113. Vol. 37 *Healing Hands* (1959) First edition - Maynard.

☐ 114. Vol. 37 *Healing Hands* (1977) Second edition - Maynard.

☐ 115. Vol. 37 *Healing Hands* (1982) Third edition - Maynard.

☐ 116. Vol. 37 *Healing Hands* (1991) Fourth edition - Maynard.

☐ 117. Vol. 38 *The Great Divide* (1966) First edition - Palmer.

☐ 118. Vol. 39 *Our Masterpiece* (1966) First edition - Palmer.

☐ 119. *Correlative Chiropractic Hygiene* (1946) First edition - Pharaoh
[dark green cover].

☐ 120. *Correlative Chiropractic Hygiene* (1946) First edition - Pharaoh
[light green cover].

☐ 121. *Art of Chiropractic* (1927) First edition - Stephenson.

☐ 122. *Art of Chiropractic* (1947) Second edition - Stephenson
[revised by Quigley, green cover].

☐ 123. *Art of Chiropractic* (1947) Second edition - Stephenson
[revised by Quigley copper cover].

Appendix 7
The Science, Art and Philosophy of Chiropractic by D.D. Palmer: Identification and Rarity of Editions in Print with a Survey of Original Copies

Introduction

The Founder's original tome, *The Science, Art and Philosophy of Chiropractic*, is an exceptionally rare book. It was originally copyrighted by Palmer in 1910. Due to its scarcity, a reprint of the book was done in the 1940s and then again in 1966 by the Founder's grandson, Dr. Dave Palmer. An original printing of the book is highly sought after in the world of chiropractic collectibles. Chiropractic historian, Joseph Donahue, stated in 1990 that only seven original copies of D.D. Palmer's book are known to exist. Intrigued by that statement, the authors, who had been collaborating on collecting and documenting Palmer's books for several years, took survey of known original 1910 copies in chiropractic colleges. This article reviews some of the details of D.D. Palmer's publishing and distribution activities in order to understand how many books may have been printed, and it examines the various reprints, with emphasis on how to tell them apart. The remarkable similarities between the original 1910 and reprints makes documenting original 1910 editions difficult.

D.D. Palmer Prints His First Chiropractic Book

While in Portland, the Founder of chiropractic completed and published his 1910 tome. At around 1000 pages, it was a conglomeration of material from his Portland based monthly journal publication, "The Chiropractor Adjuster," various letters and correspondence between health professionals and chiropractors, as well as discussion of many topics relevant to

Republished with permission from the Association for the History of Chiropractic. Cite as: Faulkner, T., Foley, J. (2015). *The Science, Art & Philosophy of Chiropractic by D.D. Palmer*. Chiropractic History, Vol. 35, No. 1, pp. 36-45.

chiropractic. In addition to the book's formal title, *Text-Book of the Science, Art and Philosophy of Chiropractic for Student and Practitioners* (SA&P), D.D. also labeled it *The Chiropractor's Adjuster.* D.D. Palmer considered it his duty to "adjust" or correct the writings of other chiropractors. As the Founder and originator of chiropractic, he felt it was his right and obligation to make these corrections as he was the ultimate authority on anything chiropractic. D.D. Palmer used his monthly publication and then this 1910 book to comment on others in the profession. Naming the 1910 book *The Chiropractor's Adjuster,* the same basic name as his monthly publication, also allowed him to easily use the material he had previously written in the Portland monthly journal.

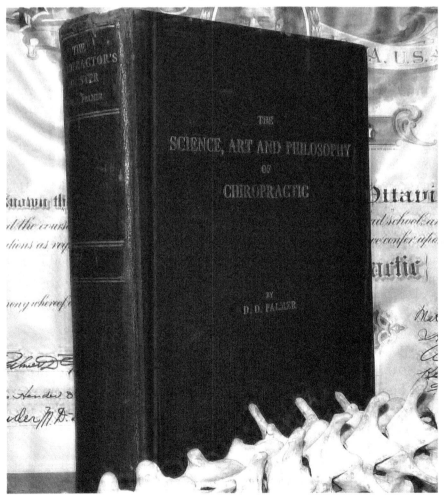

Image 1 – Text-Book of the Science, Art and Philosophy of Chiropractic

D.D. Palmer announced his plans to publish a book in the December 1909 edition of his Portland-based monthly "The Chiropractor Adjuster." In the February 1910 edition of "The Chiropractor Adjuster," he indicated progress and a chosen name of The Science and Art of Chiropractic. Based on material in the book, it appears that he was still gathering material into at least late June of 1910. Limited copies of his monthly "The Chiropractor Adjuster" are known to exist. The February 1910 edition is the last known volume of this publication, and it appears that D.D. Palmer stopped producing this journal well before his book was completed. According to a circa 1911 D.D. Palmer business card, he was still in Portland, and his book was available for purchase from him for $10.

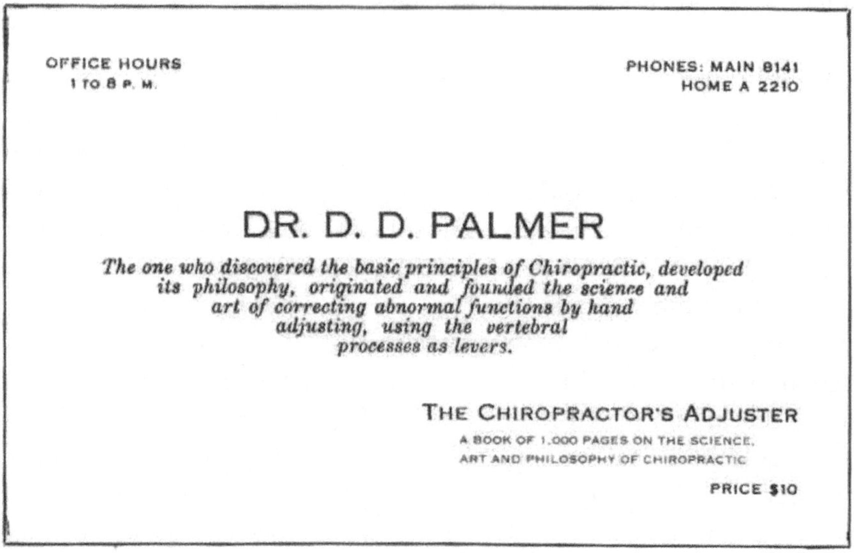

| OFFICE HOURS | PHONES: MAIN 8141 |
| 1 TO 8 P. M. | HOME A 2210 |

DR. D. D. PALMER

The one who discovered the basic principles of Chiropractic, developed its philosophy, originated and founded the science and art of correcting abnormal functions by hand adjusting, using the vertebral processes as levers.

THE CHIROPRACTOR'S ADJUSTER

A BOOK OF 1,000 PAGES ON THE SCIENCE, ART AND PHILOSOPHY OF CHIROPRACTIC

PRICE $10

Image 2 – The phone number used in this business card matches the number used by D.D. Palmer while in Portland in 1911.

Though evidence suggests that Palmer sold his own books, a definitive distribution system of the book has not been documented. One possibility is that chiropractic schools could have distributed them. Potentially the Universal Chiropractic College (UCC) in Davenport may have carried it since Joy Loban, the UCC President, seemed to have a favorable relationship with D.D. Palmer. Evidence of their positive relationship includes a shared strong disdain for B.J Palmer, the fact that Loban served as executor of D.D. Palmer's estate, and that D.D. Palmer taught on several occasions in Davenport at the UCC between 1911–1913. It is very unlikely that other chiropractic schools would carry the

Founder's book for distribution. They would have to enter into a business agreement with D.D. Palmer to sell a book in which he was disparaging or "adjusting" nearly everyone in the profession. D.D. Palmer was at odds with all the other major schools' leaders, so they were not going to help him sell his book.

Another possibility is that a medical book company had the Palmer book listed for sale in its catalogue, but a clear example has yet to be documented. So it is most likely that D.D. Palmer sold his books by mail order using his established mailing lists. Palmer solicited the names and addresses of any known chiropractors so he could send them his promotional material. It is possible that he sold his book in person to his students. Another possibility is that he sold books at various lectures as he traveled and spoke about chiropractic. It would be very difficult for a man in his 60s to have a large number of books readily available as he traveled because they were big, heavy books and walking into a lecture with multiple copies of them would have been difficult. Alternatively, D.D. could have taken orders and collected payment, shipping the book when he returned home. If this was truly the book's distribution system, it would be very difficult to support the rumor that the 1910 book was bought up by those people that D.D. Palmer offended in its pages, in an effort to keep the book from wide circulation in the profession. To do that, his detractors could not just go to the book store and purchase the store's stock; one would have to buy it directly from D.D. Palmer and that would be a challenging activity for those that hated D.D. Palmer. Whatever his distribution system was, book sales were disappointing for D.D. Palmer. In a letter to P.W. Johnson in May 1911, Palmer wrote, "It is STRANGE TO ME WHY EVERY CHIROPRACTOR DOES NOT WANT A COPY OF MY BOOK."

An interesting observation is a signed copy of this book is not known to exist at this time. If Palmer was taking book orders and then sending the books to the buyer himself from his established mailing list, or selling them in person at lectures, it is logical to think he would follow the common practice of signing or inscribing the books with a short note from the author. The low number of original 1910 copies in print supports the concept of a limited distribution system. While Palmer was living in Los Angeles, he had a promotional card made that mentioned *The Chiropractor's Adjuster.*

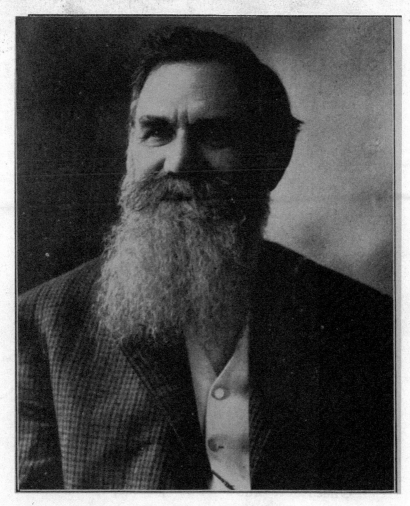

D. D. PALMER

FOUNDER OF CHIROPRACTIC
THE CREATOR OF CHIROPRACTIC SCIENCE
THE ORIGINATOR OF VERTEBRAL ADJUSTING.
THE DEVELOPER OF CHIROPRACTIC PHILOSOPHY.

THE FOUNTAIN HEAD OF THE PRINCIPLES OF CHIRO-
PRACTIC, THEIR SKILLFUL APPLICATION FOR THE USE OF
HUMANITY AND THE REASONS WHY AND HOW THEY GOV-
ERN LIFE IN HEALTH AND DISEASE.

LECTURER AND DEMONSTRATOR ON THE SCIENCE,
ART AND PHILOSOPHY OF CHIROPRACTIC.

HOME ADDRESS, 4339 S. GRAND AVE., LOS ANGELES, CAL.

Image 3A. Front of an advertising card for D.D. Palmer saying
"U need to own Chiropractor's Adjuster"

U N E E D I T .

Uneed Chiropractic.

Uneedit daily.

Uneedit in every case.

Uneedit for improvement.

Uneedit in your practice.

Uneedit as an investment.

Uneedit as a science and an art.

Uneedit because it is progressive.

Uneedit to insure success.

Uneedit to inspire confidence.

Uneedit to increase your business.

Uneedto learn of the founder.

Uneedto adjust for all diseases.

Uneedto take the special course.

Uneedto to know of its philosophy.

Uneedto keep abreast of the times.

Uneedto see Chiropractic demonstrated.

Uneedto own the Chiropractor's Adjuster.

Uneedto embrace the present opportunity.

(OVER)

Image 3B. Back of an advertising card for D.D. Palmer saying
"U need to own Chiropractor's Adjuster"

The Science, Art and Philosophy of Chiropractic has several variations and printings which can be difficult to tell apart. We will attempt to reveal the distinguishing features of the various printings so the books can be properly identified.

Original Green 1910

This book has green cloth boards with gold print, the spine stating "The Chiropractor's Adjuster" by D.D. Palmer, 1910, Portland Printing Company. The inside papers are dark green. This edition will have the thin red on white striped headband or binding threads, as well as the printed script inscription in the front that starts "With my kindest regards…" centered on the page at 2.5 inches from the top of the page to the top of the inscription "With." It has a 29 December 1910 official copyright date registered with the Library of Congress with two copies arriving from Portland on 1911 January 18.

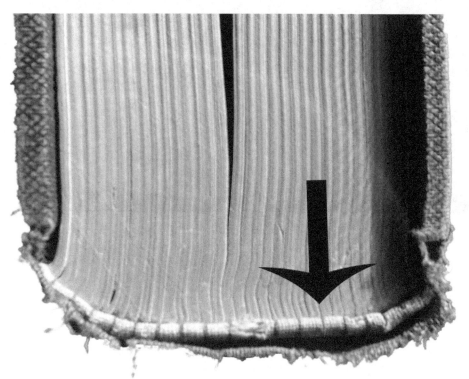

Image 4 – The headband or binding threads can be found along the top and bottom of the spine.

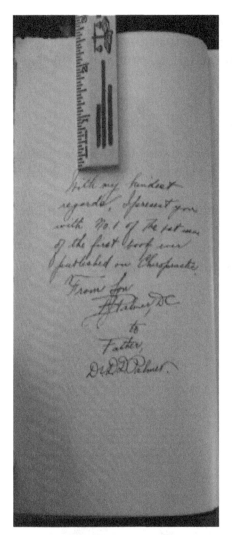 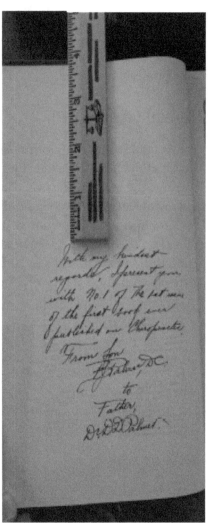

Image 5a (left) & 5b (right) – Comparison of the placement of the printed inscription found in the front of the SA&P. The original 1910 has the inscription centered top to bottom, starting 2.5 inches from the top and in the 1940s it is in the lower half of the page, 3.875 inches from the top of the page.

1940s Reprint

The Chiropractic Research Foundation (CRF) which was the non-profit arm of The National Chiropractic Association (NCA) reprinted the book in the middle to late 1940s. Beginning in 1940, the NCA initiated a plan to reprint the book because of its rarity and to allow the Founder's true chiropractic message to be available to the profession. D.D. Palmer's 1910 book was so rare that at the time of this effort, the profession had never seen or read about chiropractic from the Founder. Some in the profession questioned what was considered true chiropractic and what was not chiropractic, as stated by the Founder. With a new reprint being planned, B.J. Palmer was concerned that his father's writing not be revised or edited by the NCA in an effort to show D.D. Palmer was in line with that association's views or thoughts on chiropractic. C. Sterling Cooley led the NCA push to reprint the book. Dr. Cooley and his father, Edward, had been students of D.D.'s at the Palmer–Gregory Chiropractic School in Oklahoma City. B.J. was reassured by Cooley that an exact photographic reproduction of the original tome would be printed. In 1921, B.J. had published a sanitized version of his father's books as Vol. 4 of the Green Book series. B.J. removed many of his father's negative comments about B.J. and the others D.D. "adjusted" within the text of his 1910 book. This was not a true reprint, as much of the material was changed by B.J.

The NCA ran frequent ads about the book in its monthly journal and solicited orders. They announced that the book would be reprinted when sufficient orders were placed to cover the costs, and only enough books would be printed to satisfy the pre-orders. The cost was $10. Like the 1910 original, it was a small run of books and is also difficult to find by today's collectors. Dr. Cooley, the driving force behind reprinting D.D. Palmer's book, left the NCA in a dispute over the direction of chiropractic in 1945, and the book is not mentioned in NCA publications after he left the organization. It is unclear exactly when the CRF received enough orders and actually had the book printed. One statement implies it was 1949, nine years after the NCA initially advertised the plan to reprint.

This 1940s reprinted book is almost exactly the same as the original. The book's size, cover color, paper thickness and text font is all nearly identical to the original 1910 edition, making it nearly impossible to tell them apart. The 1940s reprint gives no indication within the book text,

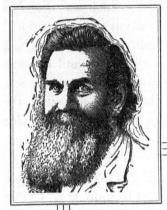
JOURNAL FOR SEPTEMBER, 1940   43

Image 6 - NCA Journal Advertisement (Sep 1940 page 43)

itself, that it is a reprint. The copyright page is identical to the 1910 original book and states a 1910 copyright. There was a small card pasted on the inside of the book indicating that this book was reprinted for historical purposes by the CRF. Over the decades these cards have fallen off and have been discarded, leaving some of the books with only a smudge of glue on the right side of the first page inside. Also of note is in the 1940s reprint, the printed script inscription by B.J. Palmer DC. "From son to father" is in the lower half of a front page, 3.875 inches from the top of the page to top of the W in "With my kindest regards." In the original 1910 it is centered 2.5 inches from the top of the page.

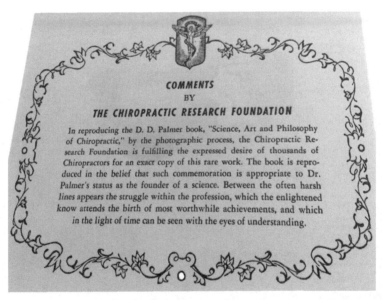

Image 7 – The CRF card that was glued into the 1940s reprint. Most of these have fallen off leaving only a glue smudge.

There is one conclusive way to tell the 1940s reprint apart from the original 1910 book. A close examination of the color of the headband or binding threads can tell the difference between an original 1910 and the 1940s reprint. The original 1910 printing is white with thin red threads and the 1940s printing is thick blue and white threads. There is always an exception. The authors have a 1940s book identified by the placement of the inscription page, however, the binding threads are red and yellow. They are a thicker red then the 1910 and look just like the 1940s blue and white, only they are red and yellow.

The Grandson's 1966 Edition

The 1966 reprint done by Dr. Dave Palmer is what most of the profession has seen. It has the addition of a foreword in the front of the book containing a message from Dr. Dave and a 1966 date at the end of that page. The copyright page still says 1910. This version was the first of the Founder's books made readily available to the profession. The book has been printed numerous times over the 40 plus years since the 1966 printing. The headband in the spine in this book will have yellow and red stripes.

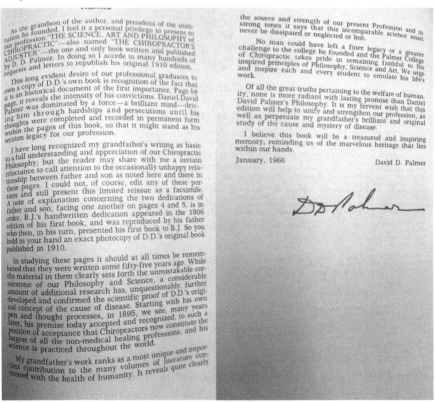

Image 8a & 8b – Dr. Dave Palmer's letter in the front of his 1966 reprint.

1911 Over Stamped

On some of the original books, a small purple inked 1911 is stamped over the printed 1910 on the copyright page of the book. It is unclear why some copies have these distinctive four dots over the printed 1910 and a 1911 next to it. It is possible that D.D. Palmer had the book typeset in 1910, but the actual printing was not done until 1911, so the books were stamped with a 1911, over the printed 1910 copyright, to reflect that they were printed in 1911. However, that would not explain why some of the books do not have the 1911 overstamp. It could be speculated that D.D. Palmer placed the first order for his book in late 1910 and an initial order was filled by the printer. After selling books from that initial order, D.D. Palmer placed a second order with the printer and those were done in early 1911. Rather than changing the printing plates, those books were handstamped 1911. Whether the 1911 overstamp was done by D.D. Palmer or by the printer is unknown. One copy with the 1911 overstamp contains a statement for the original buyer saying they received the book in January of 1911. This seems to support the theory that books purchased in 1911 contained this 1911 overstamp.

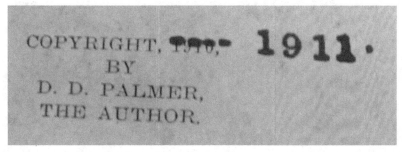

Image 9 - 1911 overstamp of original 1910 copyright

In 1910, realize the demands and risks of D.D. Palmer of theoretically ordering 500 books in an initial order. The printer delivers them and he has 500 very large books in boxes that he has to pay for and deal with logistically. It is a very common practice to order a smaller amount of books in small printing runs. That makes it easier to physically handle the volume of books and gauge sales. If you sell the books on hand, another order is placed for more books. To be clear, a second order is not a second edition or a revised edition, it is just a second printing of the first edition. If this is true, it supports the idea that D.D. Palmer was ordering a small amount of his books from the printer at one time. Based on the known copies revealed in this survey, there appears to be a fairly equal split between the 1910 and the overstamped 1911 copies. The Science, Art and Philosophy copy that the Palmer archives had is the 1911 overstamped edition; a decision had to be made on Dr. Dave Palmer's reproduction in 1966 whether to leave the 1911 overstamp on the copy or not. Numerous 1966 copies were printed, all without the 1911 overstamp, leaving it true to 1910.

1910 and 1911 Red Volume

There are two known red leather copies of the original 1910 Palmer book. It was common for printers to make special "presentation" copies of ordered books. The author would have received a book or two that was bound in leather or with some special aspect of the book to keep as their personal copy or to sell as a special edition. Of these two documented red leather bound books, one is overstamped 1911 and the other is not. Again, this supports the idea that Palmer's book had at least two different printing runs.

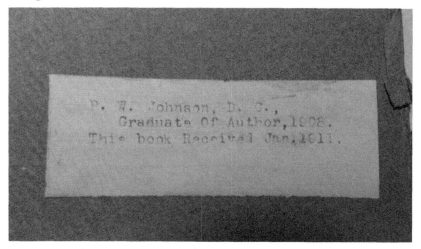

Image 10 – Writing found in P. W. Johnson book 1911

Survey of Chiropractic Colleges Collections

A search on WorldCat.org, an internet based catalog of library holdings, showed 35 copies of the 1910 book worldwide. Seven of the books listed on WorldCat were at chiropractic colleges. Contacting the schools directly revealed all total 28 copies of the 1910 SA&P were listed in the various North American chiropractic colleges. Understanding that both the 1940s and 1966 reprints have the 1910 copyright date listed and the 1940s reprint has no other obvious indications of being a reprint, the authors suspected at least some of the chiropractic college's library holdings were not the original 1910, but were actually the 1940s or 1966 edition.

Identifying Feature	Original 1910	Original 1911	Reprint 1949	Reprint 1966
Headband Thread Colors	Thin Red on a White Base	Thin Red on White Base	Thick Red on a Yellow Base or Thick Blue on White Base	Thick Red on a Yellow Base
BJ to DD Inscription Location	Centered on Page	Centered on Page	Low on Page	Centered on Page
Board Colors	Green Cloth or Red Leather	Green Cloth on Red Leather	Green Cloth	Green Cloth
Dr. Dave Palmer Foreword	No	No	No	Yes
Inside Front Card or Glue Smudge	No	No	Yes but not All	No
1911 Purple Over Stamped	No	Yes	No	No

Table 1. Chart for Identifying Variations of DD Palmer's tome

Chiropractic colleges have their original 1910 D.D. Palmer books in the archives or special collections. The authors contacted the schools to talk to the archives, special collections or library staff in charge of the schools' collections. For this survey, the schools were emailed with follow up phone calls to discuss identification details or the school library was visited in person by the authors. After examining the books in their collections, the libraries emailed their findings to the authors. The schools that listed a 1910 SA&P, without exception, all thought they had an original 1910 book. With the exception of Palmer, they all were not aware of the 1940s reprint, nor did they know how to tell the difference.

The majority of the books could be accurately identified by the color of the headband. We did find a few books that had been recovered, so we had to use the position of the printed script inscription to properly identify the book. The glue smudge where the 1940s card has fallen off is the least accurate method. Some of these old books have many discoloration and stains, and we have seen 1940s editions with the card and no glue smudge.

Only three chiropractic colleges (Palmer, Northwestern and Canadian Memorial) collections held original 1910 Palmer books. The data does not seem to support the idea that the older the school, the more likely it is that they have an original 1910 edition. Besides Palmer, none of the other early schools had an original 1910 edition.

Final Thoughts

A total of four copies of D.D. Palmer's 1910 *The Science, Art and Philosophy of Chiropractic* book were documented in the various North American chiropractic colleges. About 14% of the books listed as 1910 at these chiropractic colleges turned out to actually be original 1910 printings. The others 86% were incorrectly identified and cataloged. WorldCat lists 35 D.D. Palmer 1910 *The Science, Art and Philosophy of Chiropractic* books in libraries worldwide. Given the fact that only about 14% of the books in chiropractic colleges turned out to be original 1910 books, it is likely that an even lower percentage of these books outside of chiropractic schools would turn out to be actual 1910 books. However, further investigation is needed.

Of the four original books documented in the colleges, three have the 1911 overstamp and one does not have it. Ten other original 1910 *The Science, Art and Philosophy of Chiropractic* are currently known by the authors to be in private collections, pushing the known total 1910 original books to fourteen. The total count of known books is six without the 1911 overstamp and eight with the 1911 overstamp.

A total of fourteen copies are known in North American chiropractic school libraries and private collections. Based on the authors' experience in collecting rare and scarce chiropractic books, the availability of the tome over the last twenty years, and the onset of the internet during this period increasing the availability and resultant knowledge of more books in collections, we generously estimate there are fewer than thirty-five of the original 1910 books in existence today, with the bulk being in undocumented private collections. Given the fact that B.J. Palmer ordered his 1906 *The Science of Chiropractic* in print runs of 50 books, the authors speculate that D.D. Palmer printed, at the most, two runs of 50 books each: The first run printed in late December 1910 and the second run in January of 1911. The books printed in 1911 were overstamped with 1911. The Founder's original tome, *The Science, Art and Philosophy of Chiropractic*, is an exceptionally rare book.

Selected References

Bovine, G. (2013). John Atkinson (1854-1904), The English Bonesetter of Park Lane: His Visit to America, Bonesetting Techniques, and the Atkinson Connection to Chiropractic. *Chiro Hist.* 33(1).

Breig, A. (1978). *Adverse mechanical tension in the central nervous system: An analysis of cause and effect.* Stockholm: Almqvist & Wiksell International.

Canguilhem, G., Fawcett, C. R., Cohen, R. S., & Foucault, M. (1989). *The normal and the pathological.* New York: Zone Books.

Capra, F. (1996). *The web of life: A new scientific understanding of living systems.* New York: Anchor Books.

Carver, W. (2010). *History of chiropractic: Online edition.* InstituteChiro. com: National Instititute of Chiropractic Research.

Cooley, C. (1938). Daniel David Palmer was the first true "basic scientist.". *The Chiropractic Journal* (NCA), 7(3), 9-13.

Cooley, C. (1948). Letter to B.J. Palmer. Papers of C. Sterling Cooley: Texas Chiropractic College Library, Nov 29.

Cooley, C. (1949). Why should the kettle call the pot black? *The Record.* Sep, 80.

Crile, G.W. (1926). *The bipolar theory of living processes*: The Macmillan Company.

Davis, A.P. (1909). *Neuropathy: The new science of drugless healing amply illustrated and explained embracing ophthalmology, osteo-pathy, chiropractic science, suggestive therapeutics, magnetics, instructions on diet, deep breathing, bathing etc.* Cincinnati, Ohio: F.L. Rowe.

Del Pino, M. (1955). Questions and comment regarding research of Dr. Hans Selye. *The Chiropractor.* 51(2);12.

Donahue, J. (1990). The man, the book, the lessons: the chiropractor's adjuster, 1910. *Chiro Hist.* 10(2);35-43.

Drain, J. (2014). *Chiropractic thoughts. Second edition.* Asheville, NC: The Institute Chiropractic.

Dye, A. (1939). *The evolution of chiropractic: Its discovery and development.* Philadelphia: A.E. Dye.

Faulkner, T. (2017). T*he Chiropractor's Protégé: The Untold Story of Oakley G. Smith's Journey with D.D. Palmer in Chiropractic's Founding Years.* Rock Island, Ill: Association for the History of Chiropractic.

Faulkner, T., & Foley, J. (2015). The science, art, and philosophy of chiropractic by D.D. Palmer: Identification and rarity of editions in print with a survey of original copies. *Chiropr Hist.* 35(1);36-45.

Firth, J. (1914). *Chiropractic symptomatology* (Vol. 7). Davenport: Palmer College of Chiropractic.

Foley, J. (2016). The chiropractor 1914: Revealed. *Chiropr Hist.* 36(1).

Foley, J. (2018). Dr. Atkinson... Found? *Chiropr Hist.* 38(1).

Fuller, R. (1989). *Alternative medicine and American religious life.* New York: Oxford University Press.

Funk, M. F., Frisina-Deyo, A.J., Mirtz, T.A., & Perle, S.M. (2018). The prevalence of the term subluxation in chiropractic degree program curricula throughout the world. *Chiropractic manual therapies.* 26(1), 24.

Gaucher-Peslherbe, P. (1993). *Chiropractic: Early concepts in their historical setting.* Chicago: National College of Chiropractic.

Gaucher-Peslherbe, P., Wiese, G., & Donahue, J. (1995). Daniel David Palmer's medical library: The founder was "into the literature." *Chiropr Hist.* 15(2);63-69.

Geilow, V. (1981). *Old dad chiro: A biography of D.D. Palmer founder of chiropractic.* La Crosse (WI): Fred Barge.

Gibbons, R. (1995). Universal College: brief history, deep legacy. *Chiro Hist.* 15(1);10-11.

Gliedt, J., Hawk, C., Anderson, M., Ahmad, K., Bunn, D., Cambron, J., Perle, S. (2015). Chiropractic identity, role and future: a survey of North American chiropractic students. *Chiropractic & Manual Therapies.* 23(1);1.

Harper, W. (1964). *Anything can cause anything: A correlation of Dr. Daniel David Palmer's priniciples of chiropractic.* Texas: William D. Harper.

Holmberg, W., & Callender, A. (2003). B.J. of Manistique: The summer of 1901. *Chiropr Hist.* 23(2);49-53.

Keating, J. (1997). *B.J. of Davenport: The early years of chiropractic.* Davenport, Iowa: Association for the History of Chiropractic.

Keating, J., Callender, A., & Cleveland, C. (1998). *A history of chiropractic education in North America.* Davenport, IA: Association for the History of Chiropractic.

Keating, J., Charlton, K., Grod, J., Perle, S., Sikorski, D., & Winterstein, J. (2005). Subluxation: dogma or science. *Chiropractic & Osteopathy.* 13(17).

Keating, J., & Foderaro, F. (1999). C. Sterling Cooley, DC, FICC: politician, innate fundamentalist and Palmer historian. *Chiropr Hist.* 19(1);75-95.

Keating, J., Green, B., & Johnson, C. (1995). "Research" and "Science" in the first half of the chiropractic century. *J Man and Phys Ther.* 18(6);357-378.

Landois, L. (1889). *Textbook of human physiology.* Philadelphia: P. Blakiston, Son & Company.

Langworthy, S. (1902). Letter to D.D. Palmer. April 20. In: Faulkner, T. (2017). *The Chiropractor's Protégé.*

Linniker, C. (1908, November 21). [Letter from Chas Linniker to B.J. Palmer].

Loban, J. (1911). Chiropractic Reasoning. *International Chiropractic Journal.* 1(1).

Lubka, B. (1939). Prof. A.D. Speransky's research and chiropractic. *The Chiropractor.* 35(1);5.

Martin, S. (1994). "The only true scientific method of healing": Chiropractic and American science. *Isis.* 85(2);207-227.

Maslow, A. (1968). *Toward a psychology of being.* New York: D. Van Nostrand Co.

Maturana, H., & Varela, F. (1980). *Autopoiesis and cognition: The realization of the living.* Dordrecth: D. Reidel Pub. CO.

Maynard, J. (1982). *Healing hands: The story of the Palmer family discoverers and developers of chiropractic*. Revised edition. MS: Jonorm Publishers.

McDowall, D., Emmanuel, E., Grace, S., and Chaseling, M. (2017). Tone as a health concept: An analysis. *Complementary therapies in clinical practice*. 29;27-34.

Morat, J.P. (1906). *Physiology of the nervous system*. London: Archibeld Constable.

Morikubo, S. (1907). The Motive of Conspiracy. *The Chiropractor*, 3(11).

Murphy, D., Schneider, M., Seaman, D., Perle, S., & Nelson, C. (2008). How can chiropractic become a respected mainstream profession? The example of podiatry. *Chiropractic & Osteopathy*. 16(10).

Nelson, C., Lawrence, D., Triano, J., Bronfort, G., Perle, S., Metz, R., .LaBrot, T. (2005). Chiropractic as spine care: a model for the profession. *Chiropractic & Manual Therapies*. 13(1);9.

Peters, R. (2014). *An early history of chiropractic: The Palmers and Australia*. Asheville, NC: Integral Altitude, Inc.

Peterson, A., Watkins, R. J., Himes, H., & College, C. M. C. (2013). *Segmental neuropathy: The first evidence of developing pathology*: Online Edition. InstituteChiro.com: CMCC/TIC.

Piaget, J. (1971). *Genetic Epistemology*. New York: W.W. Norton & Company, Inc.

Prigogine, I., & Stengers, I. (1984). *Order Out of Chaos*. In. New York: Bantam Books, Inc.

Quigley, W. (1989). The last days of B.J. Palmer: Revolutionary confronts reality. *Chiropr Hist*. 9(2);11-19.

Richard, S., & Goodwin, B. (2000). *Signs of Life, How Complexity Pervades Biology*. New York: Basic Books.

Schneider, M., Murphy, D., Perle, S., Hyde, T., Vincent, R., & Ierna, G. (2005). 21st century paradigm for chiropractic. *Journal of the American Chiropractic Association*. Jan/Feb;8-15.

Senzon, S. (1999). Causation related to self-organization and health related quality of life expression based on the vertebral subluxation model, the philosophy of chiropractic, and the new biology. *J Vertebral Subluxation Res*. 3(3);104-112.

Senzon, S. (2004). The spiritual writings of B.J. Palmer: The second chiropractor. Asheville, NC: Self published.

Senzon, S. (2010). B.J. Palmer: An integral biography. Journal of Integral Theory and Practice, 5(3), 118-136.

Senzon, S. (2014). *D.D. Palmer's traveling library*. Asheville, N.C.: The Institute Chiropractic.

Senzon, S. (2015). Chiropractic and systems science. *Chiropractic Dialogues*. December 25;9-20.

Senzon, S. (2018). The chiropractic vertebral subluxation part 1: The Need for a Complete Historical Record. *J Chiropr Hum*. 25.

Senzon, S. (2018). The chiropractic vertebral subluxation part 2: The Earliest Subluxation Theories from 1897-1907. *J Chiropr Hum*. 25.

Sheldrake, R. (2012). *The presence of the past: Morphic resonance and the memory of nature*. New York: Simon and Schuster.

Sherrington, C. (1966). *The integrative action of the nervous system*. Cambridge: Cambridge University Press Archive.

Smallie, P. (1963). *The guiding light of Ratledge*. Self-published.

Smallie, P., & Ratledge, T. (2014). *Ratledge philosophy Volume 1*: Second edition. Asheville, NC: The Institute Chiropractic.

Smith, O., Langworthy, S., & Paxson, M. (1906). *A textbook of modernized chiropractic*. Cedar Rapids (IA): American School of Chiropractic.

Sole, R., & Goodwin, B. (2000). *Signs of life: How complexity pervades biology*. New York: Basic Books.

Speransky, A. (1943). *A basis for the theory of medicine*. USA: International Publishers Co, Inc.

Stephenson, R. (1927). *Chiropractic textbook*: Vol. 14. In. Davenport: Palmer School of Chiropractic.

Strauss, J. (1994). *Refined by fire: the evolution of straight chiropractic*. PA: Foundation for the Advancement of Chiropractic Education.

Taylor, E. (1999). *Shadow culture; Psychology and spirituality in America*. Washington, D.C.: Counterpoint.

Terrett, A. (1991). The genius of D.D. Palmer: An exploration of the origin of chiropractic in his time. *Chiropr Hist*. 11(1);36.

Thompson, E. (1918). *Chiropractic Spinography: Vol. 10.* Davenport: Palmer College of Chiropractic.

Troyanovich, S., & Keating, J. (2005). Wisconsin versus chiropractic: the trials at LaCrosse and the bilth of a chiropractic champion. *Chiropr Hist.* 25(1);37-45.

Turner, C. (2006). *The Rise Of Chiropractic. Second edition.* Kessinger Publishing.

Vedder, H. (1916). *Chiropractic Physiology: Vol. 8.* Davenport: Palmer College of Chiropractic.

Walton, S. (2017). *The complete chiropractor: RJ Watkins, DC, PhC, FICC, DACBR.* Asheville, NC: The Institute Chiropractic.

Waters, T. (2013). *Chasing D.D.* Raleigh, NC: Lulu, Inc.

Weiant, C. (1942). Lessons from Speransky: Some specific applications of chiropractic. *Journal of National Chiropractic Journal.*

Wiese, G., & Lykins, M. (1986). A bibliography of the Palmer green books in print, 1906-1985. *Chiropr Hist,* 6;65.

Wikipedia. (2018). *Spiritual but not religious.*

Wilber, K. (1981). The Pre/Trans Fallacy. *J Hum Psych.* 22(2);5-43.

Wilber, K. (2017). *Religion of Tomorrow.* Boston: Shambhala.

Zarbuck, M., & Hayes, M. (1990). Following D.D. Palmer to the west coast: The Pasadena connection, 1902. *Chiropr Hist.* 10(2); 17-19.

*We are very grateful to the Palmer Archives for scanning the images on the following pages: 8, 19, 26, 27, 33, 35, 39, 40, 42, 44, 45, 46, 48, 50, 52-55, 56 58, 61, 63, 65, 66, 76, 82, 101, 102, 104, 106, 107, 108, 112, 115, 116, 118, 119, 121-127, 129, 132, 134, 135, 136, 138, 139, 141, 144, 146, 147, 149, 152, 153, 154, 156, 157, 161, 164, 166, 168, 169, 171, 174, 175, 176, 179, 181, 182, 183, 185-187, 194-196-200, 202, 205, 208, 209, 212, 215, 217, 218, 220, 222, 225, 227, 230, 233, 238, 239, 240, 242, 243, 246, 247, 248, 249, 251, 252, 254, 256, 257-261, 263-273, 275, 276, 278, 282, 283, 290, 291, 296-298, 301-304, 305, 317-319, 323, 324, 325, 333, 335, 340, 342, 344, 345, 348, 352, 353, 354, 358, 361, 362, 369-372, 377, 382, 427, 454 , 470.

Made in the USA
Monee, IL
16 July 2025

21269231R00331